Digital Forensics

Digital Forensics

Edited by André Årnes
Norwegian University of Technology and Science (NTNU), Norway
and Telenor Group, Norway

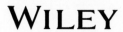

Registered Offices
John Wiley & Sons, Inc., 111 River Street, Hoboken, NJ 07030, USA
John Wiley & Sons Ltd, The Atrium, Southern Gate, Chichester, West Sussex, PO19 8SQ, UK

Editorial Office
The Atrium, Southern Gate, Chichester, West Sussex, PO19 8SQ, UK

For details of our global editorial offices, customer services, and more information about Wiley products visit us at www.wiley.com.

Wiley also publishes its books in a variety of electronic formats and by print-on-demand. Some content that appears in standard print versions of this book may not be available in other formats.

Library of Congress Cataloging-in-Publication Data

Names: Årnes, André, 1976- editor.
Title: Digital forensics / edited by André Årnes.
Description: Hoboken, NJ : John Wiley & Sons Inc., 2018. | Includes
    bibliographical references and index.
Identifiers: LCCN 2017004725 (print) | LCCN 2017003533 (ebook) |
ISBN 9781119262381 (paperback) | ISBN 9781119262404 (Adobe PDF) | ISBN 9781119262411 (ePub)
Subjects: LCSH: Computer crimes–Investigation. | Computer security.
    | Electronic discovery (Law) | Forensic sciences. | BISAC: MEDICAL / Forensic Medicine.
Classification: LCC HV8079.C65 D53 2018 (ebook) | LCC HV8079.C65 (print) | DDC 363.25/968–dc23
LC record available at https://lccn.loc.gov/2017004725

ISBN: 9781119262381

Cover Design: Wiley
Cover Images: (Background) © alengo/Gettyimages;
Figures: Courtesy of Petter Bjelland

Set in 10/12pt WarnockPro-Regular by Thomson Digital, Noida, India

10 9 8 7 6 5 4 3 2 1

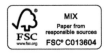

Contents

Preface

You are holding in your hand a copy of the *Digital Forensics* textbook written by faculty, associates, and former students of the Norwegian Information Security Laboratory (NISlab) at the Norwegian University of Science and Technology (NTNU). Some of the authors of this textbook have themselves studied digital forensics at NISlab. The textbook is based on teaching material, academic research, experiences, and student feedback over almost ten years of teaching digital forensics, and it represents our common philosophy of how digital forensics should be learned.

Digital forensics is a unique field of research, in that new information technology and new ways of exploiting information technology are introduced at an astonishing rate. Both researchers and practitioners regularly face new technical challenges, forcing them to continuously develop their inquisitive and creative abilities. While digital forensics requires a strict adherence to process and procedures, it is the creative abilities that will make one excel in this area.

This textbook starts with an introduction of forensic sciences that establishes the foundation for understanding the more specific area of digital forensics (Chapter 1). We introduce the fundamental principles of digital forensics, evidence dynamics, and chain of custody, followed by the digital forensics process, introduced by Anders O. Flaglien in Chapter 2. The introductory chapters introduce the main building blocks of any digital investigation, and these serve as a common thread through all the chapters in this textbook.

With the forensic principles and process in mind, Inger Marie Sunde, a Professor of law, takes us through a deep dive into the legal aspects of cybercrime and digital evidence, supported by a range of international examples and legal provisions. Chapter 3 serves as a comprehensive overview of the areas that will benefit technical, legal, and tactical professionals alike.

Further building upon the digital forensics process and the legal framework, Ausra Dilijonaite introduces us to the area of digital forensic readiness in Chapter 4. While we are often left with the impression that investigations depend on ingenious and heroic efforts after the fact, we intuitively understand that the key to successful investigations is the readiness of people, processes, and tools. Ausra builds the case for planning and preparations as a key success factor for digital forensics.

The three technical chapters in this textbook are written by digital forensics practitioners – Jeff Hamm, Jens-Petter Sandvik, and Petter Christian Bjelland. They discuss in detail how to handle evidence in computer systems (Chapter 5), in embedded and mobile devices (Chapter 6), and on the Internet (Chapter 7). The chapters leverage the forensic process and share a common format. However, the evidence dynamics and the technical expertise required for the three areas are quite different.

Following the technical chapters, we provide an overview of research topics and open research questions within the field of digital forensics, supported by examples from research at NTNU. The purpose of Chapter 8 is to provide inspiration for further research for the readers of the textbook.

In the final chapter (Chapter 9), Stefan Axelsson provides advice and "lessons learned" to the educators and students using this textbook. Stefan is currently teaching digital forensics using an early version of this textbook as the curriculum, and he has played an important role in ensuring that the textbook is suitable for educational use. As inspiration to future studies and research, his chapter provides references to the main conferences, journals, and training programs in the field of digital forensics.

We would like to thank the chapter authors for their dedicated and collaborative efforts over more than one year of writing, proofreading, and editing, as well as the proofreaders Carl Leichter, Tyler Maldonado, Svein Johan Knapskog, and Arlene Marie Pearce for their contributions to this book. The Digital Forensics classes of 2015 and 2016 also provided important feedback and guidance with regard to the scope of the book.

We are grateful for the support from our publisher, John Wiley & Sons, Inc., who chose to believe in our proposal and who has provided valuable support over the course of one year. We are further grateful for the financial support provided by the Norwegian Information Security Laboratory at NTNU, the Centre for Cyber and Information Security (CCIS), the Testimon Forensic Group, the Norwegian Police Directorate, and the Norwegian Research Council toward this work.

Finally, on behalf of the authors, we would like to thank our loved ones, family, and friends for their support and for bearing with us during the preparation of this textbook.

Good luck with learning *Digital Forensics*!

André Årnes and Katrin Franke
Testimon Forensic Group
Norwegian Information Security Laboratory
Norwegian University of Science and Technology
Norway, September 2016

List of Contributors

This textbook has been written as a collaborative project with contributions from academic, law enforcement, and industry experts in the field.

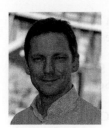

André Årnes, PhD, Siv.ing. (MSc) – Oslo, Norway
Associate Professor, Testimon Forensic Laboratory, Norwegian University of Science and Technology (NTNU); and Senior Vice President and Chief Security Officer, Telenor Group, Oslo, Norway

- Telenor, 2010–*current*: currently Senior Vice President and Chief Security Officer (from 2015)
- National Criminal Investigation Service (Kripos), 2003–2007: Special Investigator within computer crime and digital forensics
- PhD and MSc in information security from NTNU; visiting researcher at University of California, Santa Barbara, USA, and Queens's University, Canada
- GIAC Certified Forensic Analyst (GCFA), IEEE Senior Member, and member of the Europol Cyber Crime Centre (EC3) Advisory Group for communications providers.

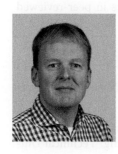

Stefan Axelsson, PhD, MSc – Gothenburg, Sweden
Associate Professor, Norwegian Information Security Laboratory (NISlab), Norwegian University of Science and Technology (NTNU), Gjøvik, Norway

- Blekinge Institute of Technology, 2007–present: Associate Professor
- Research in computer security since 1996
- Worked in telecoms industry seven years with security and forensics
- Research cited more than 2000 times
- Program committee member of DFRWS and IFIP WG 11.9.

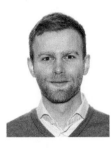

Petter Christian Bjelland, MSc – Oslo, Norway
Manager, Fraud Investigation & Dispute Services, Ernst & Young AS

- Advisor, National Criminal Investigation Service (NCIS Norway/ Kripos), 2015-2016 Norwegian Defense, 2011–2015: Senior Software Engineer
- MSc in Digital Forensics from Gjøvik University College, 2014
- Peer-reviewed paper at DFRWS Europa 2014 and in Elsevier Digital Investigation.

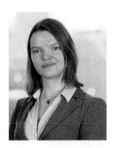

Ausra Dilijonaite, MSc – Oslo, Norway
Manager, Cyber Risk Services, Deloitte AS

- MSc in Digital Forensics from Gjøvik University College, with a thesis on Forensic Readiness in Digital Forensics
- Deloitte AS, Cyber Security Services, 2016–current: roles include Manager and Senior Consultant
- Mnemonic AS, Governance, Risk Management and Compliance, Managed Security Services, 2011–2016: roles include Senior Security Consultant and Consultant-Analyst
- Ernst & Young Baltics UAB, Technology Risk Security Services, IT Risk Advisory, 2007–2010: roles include Senior Consultant and Consultant
- Various professional certifications, including CISA, ISMS (ISO 27001) auditor/lead auditor, and RSA Certified Security Professional.

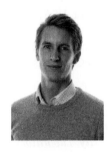

Anders Orsten Flaglien, MSc – Oslo, Norway
Security Architect, Central Bank of Norway

- Central Bank of Norway, 2016–current: Security Architect
- Accenture, 2010–2016: Security Consultant
- Gjøvik University College, 2012–2015: Teaching Coordinator in Digital Forensics
- Best Master Thesis award (2010), and papers in peer-reviewed publications
- CISSP Certified.

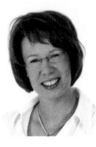

Katrin Franke, PhD, MSc – Gjøvik, Norway
Professor, Head of Testimon Forensics Group, Norwegian University of Science and Technology (NTNU)

- PhD in Artificial Intelligence, University of Groningen, The Netherlands; and MSc in Electrical Engineering, Technical University Dresden, Germany
- Fraunhofer Society, Germany, 1994–2006: Researcher, then Scientific Project Manager
- Joined the Norwegian Information Security Lab in 2007; mission to establish research and education in digital and computational forensics

- 20+ years of experience in basic and applied research, working closely with financial services and law enforcement agencies in Europe, North America, and Asia
- Founding member and first chair of the TC6 on Computational Forensics under the auspice of the International Organization of Pattern Recognition (IAPR)
- IAPR Young Investigator Awardee in the year 2009 for contributions on computational forensics.

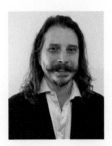

Jeff Hamm, A.S. Criminal Justice – Mainz, Germany
Manager of Consulting Services, Mandiant, a FireEye company

- Mandiant, 2010–current: Manager of Consulting Services in digital forensics and incident response
- NTNU, 2011–current: Adjunct Lecturer in Digital Forensics
- Paradigm Solutions, 2008–2010: Senior Forensic Computer Analyst
- Oakland County Sheriff's Office, Michigan, USA, 1997–2008: Sergeant.
- GCFE (current) and GCFA, and EnCE (expired).

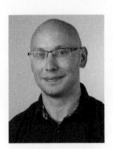

Jens-Petter Sandvik, Cand.scient. – Oslo, Norway
Senior Engineer in Digital Forensics, National Criminal Investigation Service (Kripos)

- NTNU, 2017-current: PhD student in Digital Forensics for IoT
- Norwegian Criminal Investigation Service, 2006–current: Senior Engineer in Digital Forensics
- Malware Detection, Norman ASA, 2001–2005: Software Developer
- Cand.scient., University of Oslo, 2005.

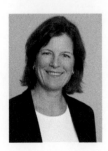

Inger Marie Sunde, PhD, LL.M, Cand.jur. – Oslo, Norway
Professor, Norwegian Police University College

- Norwegian Parliamentary Intelligence Oversight Committee: Member
- Økokrim, 1994–2005: Head of Police Computer Crime Center and Senior Public Prosecutor
- Studied at Harvard, University of Oslo, and Norwegian Defense University College
- Author of several books and academic papers.

List of Figures

List of Tables

List of Examples

List of Definitions

List of Abbreviations

5WH	Who, Where, What, When, Why, and How
ADB	Android Debugging Bridge
ADS	Alternate Data Stream
API	Application Programming Interface
AS	Autonomous System
ATA	Advanced Technology Attachment
AuC	Authentication Center
BCD	Binary Coded Digit
BGA	Ball Grid Array
BSC	Base Station Controller
BSS	Base Station Subsystem
BTS	Base Transceiver Station
CDMA	Code Division Multiple Access
CHS	Cylinder, Head, Sector
CN	Core Network
CPU	Central Processing Unit
DDoS	Distributed Denial of Service
DFRWS	Digital Forensics Research Workshop
DFU	Device Firmware Upgrade Read-Only Memory
DST	Daylight Savings Time
ECHR	European Convention of Human Rights
EDGE	Enhanced Data Rates for GSM Evolution
EFS	Encrypted File System
EIR	Equipment Identity Register
eMMC	Embedded Multimedia Card
EPC	Evolved Packet Core
EPS	Evolved Packet System
ESD	Electrostatic Discharge

E-UTRAN	Evolved Universal Terrestrial Radio Access Network
exFAT	Extended FAT File System
EXT	Extended File System
FAT	File Allocation Table
FTL	Flash Translation Layer
GMSC	Gateway Mobile Services Switching Center
GPRS	General Packet Radio Service
GPS	Global Positioning System
GPT	GUID Partition Table
GSM	Global System for Mobiles
GUID	Globally Unique Identifier
HLR	Home Location Register
HSS	Home Subscription Server
HTTP	Hypertext Transfer Protocol
IC	Integrated Circuit
ICCID	Integrated Circuit Card ID
ICS	Industrial Control System
IDE	Integrated Drive Electronics
IEC	International Electrotechnical Commission
IMEI	International Mobile Equipment Identity
IMSI	International Mobile Subscriber Identity
INDX	Index Record
IoT	Internet of Things
IP	Internet Protocol
IPC	Interprocess Communication
ISO	International Organization for Standardization
JTAG	Joint Test Action Group
LiME	Linux Memory Extractor
LBA	Logical Block Addressing
LTE	Long-Term Evolution
LUN	Logical Unit Number
LVM	Logical Volume Management
MAC	Modified, Accessed, Changed Times
MBR	Master Boot Record
MFT	Master File Table
MME	Mobile Management Entity
MS	Mobile Station

MSC	Mass Storage Device Class
MSC	Mobile Services Switching Center
MSD	Mass Storage Device
MSISDN	Mobile Subscriber ISDN
MTP	Media Transfer Protocol
NAT	Network Address Translation
NSRL	National Software Reference Library
NSS	Network and Switching Subsystem
NTFS	New Technology File System
OBEX	Object Exchange
OMC	Operation and Maintenance Center
ONFI	Open NAND Flash Interface
OOB	Out of Band
OOV	Order of Volatility
OS	Operating System
OSI	Open System Interconnection
OSS	Operation Subsystem
PCB	Printed Circuit Board
PCM	Phase Change Memory
PCRF	Policy Control and Charging Rules Function
PDU	Protocol Data Unit
PE	Portable Executable
PF	Prefetch
PGP	Pretty Good Privacy
PII	Personally Identifiable Information
PIN	Personal Identification Number
PRNG	Pseudo-Random Number Generator
PUK	PIN Unlock Key
RAID	Redundant Array of Independent Disks
RAM	Random Access Memory
RDP	Remote Desktop Protocol
ReFS	Resilient File System
RF	Radiofrequency
RNC	Radio Network System
RPMB	Replay Protected Memory Blocks
RSS	Radio Subsystem
SaaS	Software-as-a-Service

SAE	System Architecture Evolution
SAS	Serial Attached SCSI
SATA	Serial AT Attachment
SCADA	Supervisory Control and Data Acquisition
SCSI	Small Computer System Interface
S-GW	Service Gateway
SID	Security Identifier
SIM	Subscriber Identity/Identification Module
SLA	Service-Level Agreement
SMS	Short Messaging Service
SMSC	Short Messaging Service Center
SoC	System-on-a-Chip
SOP	Standard Operating Procedure
SSD	Solid-State Drive
TAP	Test Access Port
TCP	Transmission Control Protocol
TP	Transport Layer Protocol
TSOP	Thin Small Outline Package
UDH	User Data Header
UE	User Equipment
UFS	Universal Flash Storage
UICC	Universal Integrated Circuit Card
UMTS	Universal Mobile Telecommunication Service
USB	Universal Serial Bus
UTC	Coordinated Universal Time
UTRAN	Universal Terrestrial Radio Access Network
VBR	Volume Boot Record
VCN	Virtual Cluster Number
VLS	Visitor Location Register
VPN	Virtual Private Network
VSS	Volume Shadow Service
YAFFS	Yet Another Flash File System

1

Introduction

André Årnes

Testimon Forensic Laboratory, Norwegian University of Science and Technology (NTNU), Gjøvik, Norway; and Telenor Group, Oslo, Norway

The world is becoming increasingly interconnected. We find connected devices in virtually every home, and computer networks are the nervous systems of corporate and government organizations everywhere. According to Internet Live Stats (2016), there are almost 3.5 billion Internet users in the world as of August 2016, covering close to 50% of the world's population. The Internet is, however, a network of networks consisting of competing and concurrent technologies with users from different organizations and countries. Unfortunately for the investigator, the Internet was designed for robustness and redundancy, rather than security and traceability. This increases the complexity and uncertainty of digital investigations and represents a formidable challenge for digital forensics practitioners.

Digital forensics is becoming increasingly important with the escalation of cybercrime and other network-related serious crimes. Understanding the laws and regulations governing electronic communications, cybercrimes, and data retention requires the continuous acquisition of new knowledge, methods, and tools. Digital evidence is everywhere and plays an important role in virtually any criminal investigation, from petty crimes to cybercrime, organized crime, and terrorism. It is therefore critically important that students of computer science and security acquire a fundamental understanding of digital forensics, in order to take part in the public debate and to act as experts in a legal context.

1.1 Forensic Science

Forensic science is a branch of science that is widely popularized in fiction and in contemporary media, ranging from Sir Arthur Conan Doyle's first Sherlock Holmes novel *A Study in Scarlet* published in 1887 to today's *CSI* and similar crime shows. It is commonly understood that forensic science is both highly inquisitive, requiring a creative mindset, and formalistic, requiring a strict adherence to established processes. An authoritative textbook in the field, *Criminalistics* (Saferstein, 2007), states that "forensic science in its broadest definition is the application of science to law." The terms *criminalistics* and *forensic science* are used interchangeably, although criminalistics has a

Digital Forensics, First Edition. Edited by André Årnes.

stronger flavor of the services of a crime laboratory. For the purpose of this book, we will only use the first term, as defined in Definition 1.1.

Definition 1.1: Forensic Science

The application of scientific methods to establish factual answers to legal problems.

A forensic scientist is responsible for the important task of establishing facts related to questions such as: what has happened, how did it happen, who has been involved, and when did it occur? To solve such problems, a forensic scientist draws on methods and tools from a wide range of theoretical and applied sciences, including biology, medicine, physics, geology, computer science, and electrical engineering. As it is often not possible to answer a problem with full certainty, a forensic scientist is also trained to apply statistics to express the results in terms of probabilities (for a comprehensive discussion, see Aitken & Taroni, 2004).

1.1.1 History of Forensic Science

Forensic science was established as a separate scientific domain during the 1800s and early 1900s. The contributions of this new area of science dramatically changed the effectiveness of law enforcement. A comprehensive overview of the contributions is available in Saferstein (2007), but some notable innovators and milestones are:

- Mathieu Orfila (1787–1853), considered the father of forensic toxicology, published the first scientific text on forensic toxicology in 1814.
- Alphonse Bertillon (1853–1914) developed a method for identification through body measurements and published a system on personal identification in 1879.
- Francis Galton (1822–1911) studied fingerprints as a means of identification and published the book *Finger Prints* in 1892.
- Hans Gross (1847–1915) established the principles for the application of science in investigations in several publications, the first one in 1893.
- Alberts S. Osborn (1858–1946) established scientific principles for document examination and published the book *Questioned Documents* in 1910.
- Leone Lattes (1887–1954) studied characteristics of blood types for identification and created a method for the analysis of blood groups in blood stains in 1915.
- Edmond Locard (1877–1966), recognized worldwide for promoting the scientific method in criminal investigation, established a police laboratory in Lyon in 1910.

1.1.2 Locard's Exchange Principle

Edmond Locard formulated the famous Locard's exchange principle, which has served as an important principle for subsequent research within forensic science. The principle states that "when a person or object comes in contact with another person or object, a cross-transfer of materials occurs" (Saferstein, 2007). In this way, every criminal can be connected to a crime through trace evidence. It should, however, be noted that the principle cannot necessarily be directly applied to digital forensics, as the dynamics of digital evidence is different from that of physical evidence. In this textbook, we will, nonetheless, adopt Definition 1.2.

Definition 1.2: Locard's Exchange Principle

Whenever two objects come into contact with one another, there is an exchange of materials between them.

1.1.3 Crime Reconstruction

Crime reconstruction (or crime scene reconstruction) is the process of determining the most likely hypothesis, or sequence of events, through the application of the scientific method. For the purpose of this textbook, we apply Definition 1.3, based on the book *Crime Reconstruction* by Chisum and Turvey (2008).

Definition 1.3: Crime Reconstruction

Crime reconstruction is the determination of the actions and events surrounding the commission of a crime.

A crime reconstruction can leverage a wide range of forensic methods, for example firearm ballistics tests, statistical simulations, and biological experiments. The objective is to establish a hypothesis about the event or sequence of events and then to test whether the hypothesis is possible or not. If the hypothesis is confirmed, then one possible explanation has been identified. If it is refuted, then the explanation is not possible and other hypotheses will have to be considered.

1.1.4 Investigations

An investigation is a systematic examination, typically with the purpose of identifying or verifying facts. A key objective during investigations is to identify key facts related to a crime or incident, and a common methodology used in this textbook is referred to as *5WH* (Stelfox, 2013; Tilstone *et al.*, 2013), as defined in Definition 1.4.

Definition 1.4: 5WH

5WH defines the objectives of an investigation as *who, where, what, when, why,* and *how.*

The 5WH formula sets the following objectives (Stelfox, 2013):

- *Who*: Persons involved in the investigation, including suspects, witnesses, and victims
- *Where*: The location of the crime and other relevant locations
- *What*: Description of the facts of the crime in question
- *When*: The time of the crime and other related events

- *Why*: The motivation for the crime and why it happened at a given time
- *How*: How the crime was committed.

1.1.5 Evidence Dynamics

Evidence dynamics is defined as "any influence that adds, changes, relocates, obscures, contaminates, or obliterates physical evidence, regardless of intent" (Chisum & Turvey, 2000). The concept is useful in understanding the actual behavior of evidence and plays an important role in crime scene reconstructions. Although the definition is originally intended for physical evidence, it is equally applicable to digital evidence. For example, evidence dynamics can describe the mechanisms for writing to a sector on a hard drive, or the operations for creating, changing, or deleting a file in a file system. For the purpose of this textbook, we will use Definition 1.5, based on Chisum and Turvey (2000).

Definition 1.5: Evidence Dynamics

Evidence dynamics refers to any influence that adds, changes, relocates, obscures, contaminates, or obliterates evidence, regardless of intent.

1.2 Digital Forensics

Digital forensics refers to forensic science applied to digital information, whereas a *digital investigation* refers to investigations in the digital domain. We will use the definition from the first Digital Forensics Research Workshop (Digital Forensics Research Workshop, 2001), as defined in Definition 1.6.

Definition 1.6: Digital Forensics

The use of scientifically derived and proven methods toward the preservation, collection, validation, identification, analysis, interpretation, documentation, and presentation of digital evidence derived from digital sources for the purpose of facilitating or furthering the reconstruction of events found to be criminal, or helping to anticipate unauthorized actions shown to be disruptive to planned operations.

Other terms, such as *network forensics*, *device forensics*, and *Internet forensics*, are often used to label specialized fields within digital forensics. As information technology has become an integral part of all aspects of society, digital forensics is growing in importance. Most legal cases today have an aspect of digital forensics, involving for example mobile phones, credit card transactions, email systems, Internet logs, and GPS systems. As many types of digital evidence can be volatile and easily manipulated, the trusted preservation of evidence through the use of standardized forensic tools and methods has become essential.

You may have previously seen references to digital archaeology and digital geology when discussing digital forensics. This refers to the analogy introduced in Farmer and Venema (2004), where *digital archaeology* refers to digital traces in computer systems created by human behavior, whereas *digital geology* refers to digital traces created by the computer systems themselves as part of their inherent processes. The goal of digital forensics is usually to gather facts about human behavior (i.e., digital archaeology), but it is a prerequisite to understand how the computer systems behave (i.e., digital geology) in order to interpret digital evidence.

As forensic scientists and forensic practitioners, our role in digital forensics is to establish factual answers to legal problems. This responsibility calls for strong standards for the processing of evidence and for the soundness of the analysis and its conclusions. This textbook will provide a comprehensive introduction to this process and its principles.

1.2.1 Crimes and Incidents

An important consideration for digital forensics is that it is commonly applied both in criminal law and in private law. Law enforcement increasingly depends upon digital forensics to process digital evidence in the context of a *crime* under investigation, whereas public and private companies and organizations depend upon digital forensics as a tool for supporting legal action in the case of an *incident* (e.g., contract or policy violations). Digital crimes and incidents consist of a *digital event* or a sequence of events, as defined in Carrier and Spafford (2004a). For simplicity, we refer to the event investigated as an *incident* in this textbook, unless we are specifically referring to criminal law. The location of the incident is referred to as the *scene of the incident*, or in the case of a crime, the *digital crime scene*.

This textbook addresses the field of digital forensics, with an emphasis on after-the-fact forensic analysis (often referred to as *post mortem*). Digital forensics can be initiated by real-time detection of cybersecurity incidents (e.g., intrusion detection) or as part of security incident handling processes. However, the topics of security monitoring and security incident management are not addressed in this textbook, as these are separate fields with different processes, contexts, and objectives.

1.2.2 Digital Devices, Media, and Objects

A central distinction in digital forensics is that between digital devices, digital media, and digital objects. A *digital device* is a physical object, such as a laptop, a smartphone, or a car. A digital device necessarily contains one or more storage media, such as a hard drive or memory, referred to as *digital media*. The digital media contain data, stored in binary format, referred to as *digital data*. Forensic analysts often work with discrete collections of digital data, referred to as *digital objects* in this textbook, based on the original definition in Carrier and Spafford (2004c).

1.2.3 Forensic Soundness and Fundamental Principles

The scientific method refers to the use of "a method or procedure . . . consisting of systematic observation, measurement, and experiment, and the formulation, testing, and modification of hypotheses" (Turvey, 2008). Ideally, this should also be the gold standard for digital forensics, with the implication that any investigation of digital evidence must be entirely reproducible by a third party. However, our ability to capture digital evidence in real life is far from perfect, and forensic soundness has therefore come to mean that the professionally recognized principles and standards of digital forensics are observed. Our definition of *forensically sound* is thus provided in Definition 1.7.

Definition 1.7: Forensically Sound

An investigation is forensically sound if it adheres to established digital forensics principles, standards, and processes.

The two fundamental principles discussed in this textbook are evidence integrity and chain of custody. *Evidence integrity* refers to the preservation of evidence in a complete form without any intentional or unintentional changes, as defined in Definition 1.8.

Definition 1.8: Evidence Integrity

Evidence integrity refers to the preservation of evidence in its original form.

While evidence integrity is an ideal in digital forensics, it is often not achievable, as data inevitably changes in live computer systems and networks during investigations. Due to this, documentation of all steps in the investigation is an important objective. This is referred to as the *chain of custody*, as defined in Definition 1.9.

Definition 1.9: Chain of Custody

Chain of custody refers to the documentation of acquisition, control, analysis, and disposition of physical and electronic evidence.

It should be noted that there are, of course, many other important principles in digital forensics, some of which are extensively discussed in this textbook. We have, nevertheless, chosen to adopt these two principles as fundamental principles that should be observed throughout all phases of the digital forensics process.

1.2.4 Crime Reconstruction in Digital Forensics

Crime reconstruction can help test hypotheses about a possible chain of events. It leverages the five-step process for event-based crime scene reconstruction as proposed by Carrier and Spafford (2004b).

1) *Evidence examination*: Identify and characterize evidence relevant to an incident.
2) *Role classification*: Examine the role of the evidence as a cause or effect of an event.
3) *Event construction and testing*: Identify events and assess whether they are possible.
4) *Event sequencing*: Combine events into event chains.
5) *Hypothesis testing*: The hypothesis is tested using the scientific method.

The method can also be applied in the case of digital forensics through the use of physical or virtual testbeds set up to perform simulated experiments, as discussed in Årnes *et al.* (2007).

1.3 Digital Evidence

Central to any digital investigation is the notion of digital evidence, which is defined in Definition 1.10, based on the definition by Carrier and Spafford (2004a).

> **Definition 1.10: Digital Evidence**
>
> Digital evidence is defined as any digital data that contains reliable information that can support or refute a hypothesis of an incident or crime.

In digital forensics, we aim to process and store digital evidence in a way that is consistent with the principles of evidence integrity and chain of custody. A number of digital evidence storage and exchange formats have been developed to support this (Flaglien *et al.*, 2011), but close attention to a manual process and detailed documentation of the chain of custody are nonetheless required.

1.3.1 Layers of Abstraction

As you will see in the remaining chapters in this book, it is useful to discuss digital evidence in the context of *layers of abstraction*. This refers to the practice, used in all areas of computing, of hiding implementation details of higher layers of abstraction in order to reduce complexity. A forensic analyst has to analyze and reconstruct data at all layers of abstraction to be able to extract and explain relevant digital evidence. For example, a forensic analyst may have to analyze data at the binary level of a disk drive to reconstruct a text file that contains an email with content relevant to the investigated case. A well-known example from computer networks is the Open Systems Interconnection (OSI) reference model, which divides network protocols into seven layers of abstraction (see also Section 7.3).

1.3.2 Metadata

Metadata is a valuable source of evidence in digital forensics that will be thoroughly discussed in this textbook. Metadata, or *data about data*, contains information about data objects. For example, the metadata associated with a digital photograph can contain the time of taking the photo, the geographical location, and the camera used. The analysis of metadata is an important activity throughout the forensic process, as metadata can contain information that is key to solving a case.

1.3.3 Error, Uncertainty, and Loss

Other aspects of digital evidence that have to be understood by a forensic scientist are error, uncertainty, and loss (Casey, 2002). Such uncertainties can impact the interpretation of timestamps, geographical location, and authorship or ownership of data. This must be understood in the context of evidence dynamics in order to accurately interpret and present digital evidence in a legal context. Failure to do so can lead to a weakened or lost case in court, or even the wrongful conviction of an innocent.

1.3.4 Online Bank Fraud – A Real-World Example

To better facilitate learning across the topics covered in this textbook, we will refer to the real-world online bank fraud example of SpyEye. This case is particularly relevant for us, as it is both legally and technically complex, with relevance to all the chapters in this textbook. The case is well documented, as it has been investigated by the US Federal Bureau of Investigation (FBI) and tried in public court with broad media coverage. The hackers behind the malware were recently convicted to a total of 24 years in prison (US Department of Justice, 2016).

1.3.4.1 Modus Operandi

Online bank fraud is a well-known crime pattern in which a large number of computers are compromised and infected with Trojan malware, allowing their computers to be monitored and remote controlled. The computers are part of a network of infected computers – a *botnet* – and typically controlled by one or more command-and-control centers. Once established, the botnet is continuously monitored to gather personal information and credentials, and to establish an overview of the online bank accounts accessed by the victims through the compromised computers.

At some point during a regular online bank session, when a victim is active, the command-and-control center issues an instruction to initiate a transaction of a specific amount of money from a victim's account. The Trojan malware, having circumvented the security of the online banking session, fools the unsuspecting victim to authenticate and authorize the transaction. When such an illegitimate transaction is completed, an amount of money is transferred to a complicit third party – a *money mule* – whose primary task is typically to withdraw the money and transfer it to a (possibly foreign) account in a jurisdiction that is more forgiving to financial fraud and cybercrime.

The crime pattern involves multiple actors and a long-term commitment, requiring a criminal organization with access to highly specialized competencies and tools. Central actors in such schemes are thus the malware programmers, the command-and-control center managers, the mules, as well as the organization that is recruiting the mules and profiting from the operation. Access to the required botnet, consisting of the command-and-control center and a network of compromised computers with active malware, can be purchased as a service on underground forums, as discussed in Namestnikov (2009). The victims are, of course, both the online bank customers and the financial institutions.

1.3.4.2 The SpyEye Case

The SpyEye case closely followed this pattern, infecting 50 million computers worldwide and compromising at least 10,000 bank accounts. The convicted programmers responsible for the malware and botnets, Aleksandr Andreevich Panin ("Gribodemon") of Russia and Hamza Bendelladj ("Bx1") of Algeria, were subsequently sentenced to a total of 24 years in prison for causing losses to financial institutions and individuals of close to a billion US dollars. One of Panin's clients reportedly made $3.2 million in 6 months (US Department of Justice, 2014).

Due to the scale and complexity of the case, law enforcement agencies from several countries were involved in the investigations, supported by cybersecurity experts from the private sector. From a technical perspective, the investigation ranged from the forensic analysis of a large number of infected computers, to online investigations of their distribution and sale in underground forums, and to tracing and identifying the perpetrators and malware where forensics is complicated by obfuscation and anti-forensic countermeasures.

1.4 Further Reading

We recommend that students of this textbook study supplementary literature to gain a broader understanding of digital forensics. For this purpose, here is a list of textbooks that have previously been utilized, in full or for inspiration, in our digital forensics curriculum:

- *Forensic Discovery* by Dan Farmer and Vietse Venema: used as the main textbook from 2007 to 2011 (Addison-Wesley Professional; Farmer & Venema, 2005).
- *Open Source Forensics* by Cory Altheide and Harlan Carvey: used as the main textbook in 2012 and 2013 (Syngress; Altheide & Harlan, 2011).
- *The Basics of Digital Forensics: The Primer of Getting Started in Digital Forensics* by John Sammons: used as the main textbook in 2014 (Syngress; Sammons, 2012).
- *Guide to Computer Forensics and Investigations – Processing Digital Evidence*, 5th ed., Bill Nelson, Amelia Phillips and Christopher Stewart: supplementary literature (Cengage Learning; Nelson *et al.*, 2015).
- *Incident Response and Computer Forensics*, 3rd ed., by Jason Luttgens, Matthew Pepe, and K. Mandia: supplementary literature (McGraw-Hill Osborne Media; Luttgens *et al.*, 2014).
- *Digital Archaeology: The Art and Science of Digital Forensics* by Michael W. Graves: supplementary literature (Addison-Wesley; Graves, 2014).

We have further utilized a wide range of specialized supplementary literature that is worth studying, including:

- *File System Forensic Analysis* by Brian Carrier (Addison-Wesley Professional; Carrier, 2010).
- *Windows Registry Forensics: Advanced Digital Forensic Analysis of the Windows Registry* by Harlan Carvey (Syngress; Carvey, 2016).
- *Network Forensics, Tracking Hackers through Cyberspace* by Sherri Davidoff and Jonathan Ham (Prentice Hall; Davidoff & Ham, 2012).
- *Practical Mobile Forensics* by Satish Bommisetty, Rohit Tamma, and Heather Mahalik (Packt Publishing; Bommisety *et al.*, 2014).
- *Practical Malware Analysis: The Hands-On Guide to Dissecting Malicious Software* by Michael Sikorski and Andrew Honig (No Starch Press; Sikorski & Honig, 2012).

1.5 Chapter Overview

This book is divided as follows:

- *Chapter 2, "The Digital Forensics Process"*: This chapter provides a comprehensive overview of the digital forensics process and its fundamental principles. A thorough understanding of these aspects is a prerequisite for any forensic practitioner.
- *Chapter 3, "Cybercrime Law"*: This chapter provides an introduction to the legal aspects of cybercrime investigations, with an emphasis on the Cybercrime Convention and criminal law with examples.
- *Chapter 4, "Forensic Readiness"*: With the process and legal considerations covered, it is time to look at the processes and capabilities required to perform a forensic investigation, whether in a government or corporate context. This chapter introduces the concept of forensic readiness and its requirements.
- *Chapter 5, "Computer Forensics"*: This chapter describes the most classic scenario in digital forensics – the forensic analysis of a regular computer. From a technical perspective, this chapter provides a fundamental insight into digital evidence, in preparation for the more specialized technical chapters.
- *Chapter 6, "Mobile and Embedded Forensics"*: This chapter covers digital forensics for mobile devices and embedded systems. As the world is becoming increasingly digital, with personal mobile devices and the "Internet of Things" everywhere, the science of digital forensics is facing a wide range of new challenges.
- *Chapter 7, "Internet Forensics"*: This chapter covers digital forensics on the Internet, with tracing, acquisition, and advanced analytics of networked evidence from various sources, such as open sources, personal services (e.g., email), and cloud services.
- *Chapter 8, "Challenges in Digital Forensics"*: This chapter provides an overview of research topics and open research questions within the field of digital forensics, with an emphasis on computational forensics. The purpose of the chapter is to provide inspiration for further research, and it is supported by examples from research at NTNU.
- *Chapter 9, "Educational Guide"*: This chapter provides guidelines and additional material for educators and students in digital forensics. The chapter includes an overview of available training programs, standards, and supporting literature.

1.6 Comments on Citation and Notation

For the benefit of the reader, the following standards have been adopted in the textbook:

- *Citations*: Citations to authoritative textbooks, research papers, and online sources are provided throughout. Students are encouraged to research the primary sources to better understand the subject matter.
- *Definitions, Examples, and Legal Provisions*: These are highlighted in separate gray boxes throughout the book. Examples can be either real-world case examples or illustrative scenarios.

- *Figures*: All photographs and illustrations are made by the chapter authors, unless otherwise specified.
- *Software*: All references to software and hardware tools are included as examples only. They do not represent a recommendation or preference regarding tool choices, and they should not be interpreted as guidelines or instructions on tool usage.

2

The Digital Forensics Process

Anders O. Flaglien

Security Architect at the Central Bank of Norway

Digital evidence may be found in computers, mobile devices, internet infrastructure, industrial systems, and other digital devices. The application of the forensic process and its underlying principles will ensure that an investigation is forensically sound. In this chapter, we present the five phases of the digital forensics investigation process, based on the principles of digital forensics and common law enforcement and industry practices. The process is considered in the context of digital investigations, and we will look into examples and scenarios that address how investigators work, or should work, and the tools they use.

Just as in our daily lives, from work to school to all kinds of social situations, crimes may involve one or more digital devices and services. Fortunately, many well-established principles of physical investigations and forensic science can also be applied to digital forensics. The motivations for crime do not change much simply because new technology is involved. The traditional robbery of a physical grocery store in pre-digital societies can easily parallel the hacking of web-shops to steal credit card information. Physical criminal activity (e.g., murder) cannot generally be committed with the use of digital services alone, but these services may facilitate the planning or communication for the execution of a crime.

2.1 Introduction

Over the last decade, cybercrime has evolved and will continue to do so. Technically savvy attackers, more advanced technology, and stronger incentives are factors that support this trend. Cybercriminals today conduct sophisticated attacks that exploit vast digital networks and multiple endpoints at the same time, resulting in data breaches and disclosure of data. The existence of cybercrime that results in such data breaches serves to emphasize the importance of well-defined forensic investigation processes. These processes require the availability of appropriate tools for the investigation of the causes and effects of such incidents. Forensic principles targeting specific types of investigations have been established over time, such as for cybercrime investigations (Ciardhuáin, 2004). These are principles that can be applied to computer forensics, Internet

Digital Forensics, First Edition. Edited by André Årnes.

investigations, and mobile device forensics. The tools used can be supported by computational methods and they will have to comply with legal requirements.

How can we trust the information acquired and evidence found during a digital forensics investigation? The uncertainties associated with potential evidence, both physical and logical, accidental and deliberate, must be addressed in any forensic investigation (Casey, 2002).

Example 2.1: Email from Whom?

Imagine investigating a case where a person has received an email with potentially important evidence of a crime. The email was sent over the Internet. Because of this, the origin of the email must be considered uncertain, as must the timestamps, since they could have been tampered with while en route. If the email was in fact sent from a given system, how may one know that it was created by the system's owner and not by some intruder intentionally placing it there? What if the email was sent by a Trojan horse or other malware? This argument can be used as part of a legal defense, often referred to as the *Trojan horse defense* (Brenner *et al.*, 2004).

The digital landscape changes rapidly and so too must digital forensics practices. The adaptation of new technology and new ways of online communication challenges the effectiveness and efficiency of digital forensics investigations. Even though the challenges are increasing, the digital forensic process remains the same. The complexity and resource demands of each phase will, however, vary. Technology continues to change and provide new tools for old crimes.

The Nigerian bank fraud scam is a digital version of the Spanish Prisoner scam from the 1600s, where the victim was, believing there were great rewards to be gained, fooled into raising money for a supposedly wealthy prisoner in Spain. Today, technology (typically e-mail) is used to lure innocent people to transfer money to help a friend in need or to pay a lawyer to release the funds of a dead great-great-grandfather abroad. For the investigator, the complexity of the crime has become much more sophisticated, but so have the tools at the investigator's disposal.

2.1.1 Why Do We Need a Process?

The forensic process defines a structured investigation of digital evidence from any device capable of storing or processing data in a digital form. As noted in Section 2.1, there are many similarities to physical investigation processes. Yet there is one obvious and significant difference that needs to be accounted for: the evidence of interest is *digital*. Because of this, traditional forensics processes are challenged by *how* to gather *what* evidence to support a hypothesis of a crime or incident. The process needs to ensure that whatever digital evidence is identified, it must be managed properly for it to prove a case.

The process is universal in that it can be used for investigations of any kind of crime or incident involving digital devices, such as computer forensics, mobile forensics, Internet forensics, as well as future digital technologies. Accused murderers, robbers, and other criminals may have their electronic devices analyzed in an investigation to identify evidence about a crime. Such evidence can provide answers to the 5WH questions of investigations (see Section 1.1.4): *who* committed the crime, *where* the collaborators of a crime were at the time a suspect called or sent a text message, *what* the facts of the crime were, *when* the crime was committed, *why* the crime was committed (i.e., motives for the crime), and *how* it was committed.

Evidence may be found in diverse places like in a chat session, communication log, or any other digital traces. In the case of corporate investigations, loss or misuse of corporate confidential information is typically discovered by employees, customers, partners, or incident management analysts using security solutions and tools. The digital forensics process can thus be used in criminal investigations, corporate investigations, or even private investigations. The process can be adapted to most, if not all, types of digital investigations.

This chapter presents the process phases typically required to conduct an investigation of a crime or incident. As few crime cases involve electronic devices exclusively, the process needs to interact with traditional physical investigation practices in order to support an end-to-end criminal investigation. As we shall see, there are many pitfalls and risks involved in not following a defined process.

2.1.2 Principles of a Forensics Process

As introduced in Section 1.2.3, a process or method can be considered forensically sound if it adheres to established digital forensics principles, standards, and processes. The investigation should aim to find the strongest evidence with the resources available and also produce appropriate documentation of the investigation's processes, key assumptions, and uncertainties.

As we see in this textbook, many tools exist for data collection, examination, analysis, and presentation of digital evidence. These tools are developed by commercial actors, the digital forensics community, and academic researchers. The trustworthiness of the software should be evaluated by reviewing the tool's code. The National Institute of Standards and Technology (NIST) has established a project to create a set of criteria for evaluating forensics tools.[1]

In the following sections of this chapter, we will review the most common and well-established forensic principles (see Section 1.2.3). The first principle is *evidence integrity*, which refers to the preservation of evidence in its original form. This is a requirement that is equally valid both for the original evidence when it is collected, as well as for the copy of the evidence that is used for analysis and then referred to when evidence is presented to a court. The second principle is *chain of custody*, or the ability to document all actions done to the evidence in order to prove its authenticity and integrity.

2.1.3 Finding the Digital Evidence

We use Definition 1.10, based on Carrier and Spafford (2004a, 2004c), and define *digital evidence* as "any digital data that contain reliable information that supports or refutes a hypothesis about an incident or crime." A closely related term is *electronic evidence*,

---

1 Computer Forensics Tool Testing (CFTT) Project, www.cftt.nist.gov.

which can be defined as "electronically stored information that is admitted as evidence at a trial or hearing" (Johnson, 2013).

In the search for digital evidence, forensic analysts process digital objects as introduced in Section 1.2.2. If a digital object is determined to be relevant to the investigation, then it is considered digital evidence. This principle is emphasized in the ISO 27042 standard in that the digital evidence has been determined, through the process of analysis, to be relevant to the investigation (see ISO/IEC 27042:2015; ISO/IEC, 2015b). Until this time, the digital object can only be considered potential evidence.

Digital evidence can be relevant in two ways. The first is the ontological way, as something we can observe and describe. The second is evidence in the way of recognition, which means what it can tell us about a case.

2.1.4 Introducing the Digital Forensics Process

The digital forensic process presented in this textbook is a normative approach of conducting digital forensics investigations. It is primarily grounded on a traditional physical forensics investigation process and includes all required phases. These phases include the original notification, through the reporting to the final presentation of the findings. As described earlier in this chapter, it is important to act according to a defined process in order to identify digital objects reflecting the facts of interest in criminal or civil courts of law. It is also important for corporate and private investigations to verify the impact of an incident, in order to know whether there were serious breaches, such as loss of confidential data. In this way, the process can be considered as a part of a quality assurance system for digital forensics.

The process is split into five consecutive, but also iterative phases, which we will focus on in this section. The first phase is the *identification* of potential evidence sources from digital devices. Then, we *collect* digital raw data by copying the source in a forensically sound manner. Next, we *examine* the raw data, giving it structure so it is easier to process and understand. Then we conduct the *analysis*, where we seek to gain a better under-standing and to identify digital objects that would ideally be the evidence that is, finally, *presented* to a court of law or the entity of interest. The process is described as a step-by-step process from start to end, but there can and will be multiple iterations of several phases. The process is illustrated in Figure 2.1.

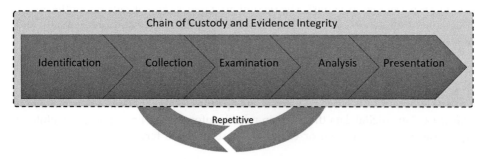

Figure 2.1 The digital forensics process.

Typically, the digital forensics process begins with an observation, alert, or notification of an event or an incident related to a crime. Based on this, a hypothesis about the event or incident is made and the investigation process is initiated.

Research into developing a standard for the digital forensics investigation process has been ongoing since the 1980s. The most well-known processes have been analyzed in order to identify their common characteristics and phases. In this book, we have chosen to focus on the most common five phases and describe the essence of each phase. Typical characteristics of a digital forensics investigation process have been discussed in various research (Yusoff *et al.* (2011), and Carrier and Spafford (2003)) and summarized her for reference:

- Adhere to the leading practice and theory from traditional forensic investigations.
- Be easily adaptable and practically oriented, and support traditional investigation steps.
- Remain independent of technology, product, and procedure.
- Applicable to law enforcement, corporate, and incident investigations.
- Support forensic reconstructions.
- Improve proper and efficient identification of facts.
- Limit unnecessary generation of new artifacts.
- Use and support forensic science and technology, and the results must be usable in a court of law.
- Must be capable of being scrutinized by the judiciary if the case is presented in court.

To illustrate the iterative aspect of the process, let us consider a case where we have identified multiple potential evidence sources. For example: we have seized a computer with multiple hard drives from one suspect of a crime, a mobile handset owned by another suspect, an online file share account, and the victim's mp3 player. In this case, one would have to reiterate the process phases for each potential evidence source. Each source will be collected and examined. The analysis for each potential evidence source may be conducted one at a time, but often the data is analyzed simultaneously from several of the collected sources. This occurs since there may be correlating events on the multiple devices that together form the final evidence to be presented in court.

2.2 The Identification Phase

Incidents can be identified based on complaints, alerts, or other indications. The identification phase as described in Definition 2.1 (see Figure 2.2) forms the basis for

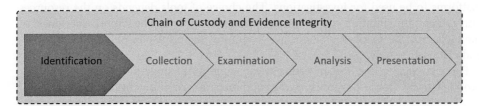

Figure 2.2 The digital forensics process: identification.

all the following phases or activities during the digital investigation. For example, it can be used to identify which evidence or objects to look for during the investigation. The identification of an incident or a crime leads to the formation of a hypothesis about what might have happened.

An investigation can focus on identifying supporting information to prove a case, identifying information that refutes a case, or verifying the validity of any given information. The questions defined by the 5WH model should always be raised during the identification phase. They help us to establish a hypothesis based on the information triggering the investigation.

As investigators, we operate with a preliminary hypothesis about a digital device or system that may contain potential digital evidence. In the case of computer and file system analysis, the identification step includes making a determination about which files on a volume are available, active, or deleted.

Definition 2.1: The Identification Phase

The task of detecting, recognizing, and determining the incident or crime to investigate (Reith *et al.*, 2002).

2.2.1 Preparations and Deployment of Tools and Resources

Proper planning helps prevent poor performance or substandard results in an investigation, and it is a precondition for an efficient and effective investigation. This is applicable for investigations of all types of incidents, including digital crimes. In this section, we will refer to the event-based digital investigation process developed by Carrier and Spafford (2004a) as a well-established reference in the field.

Law enforcement agencies, digital forensic units, and corporate investigators all need to be well prepared before a crime or incident even occurs. A trained team of investigators is crucial for determining what occurred, based on the digital objects at hand. The ability to have access to such a team depends, of course, on the resources available. Since no two cases are the same, it can be difficult to make decisions on investigative resource allocation. As discussed in Chapter 4, a readily available investigative infrastructure, such as a lab and available tools, is an advantage when making such decisions.

Guidelines and principles for building a forensics laboratory are presented in Watson and Johnson (2013). The book assesses the common ISO standards (such as ISO 17020, 17025, 27001, and 27041) and what is required to establish the ideal environment. Many commercial vendors and open source communities provide toolkits and digital forensics platforms to be used for investigations. The choice of tools depends on the resources available and the ambition and objective of the agency or unit. The forensic soundness of the tools must be assessed, as they have to support the principles of evidence integrity and chain of custody.

For a physical crime scene, readiness can range from fingerprint analysis to DNA profiling to any special-purpose imaging equipment for recording the layout of a physical scene. For cases involving electronic devices, it may include tasks such as the setup and configuration of digital forensics software and hardware. All preparations done before the investigation are part of the preparation phase.

In the research of Carrier and Spafford (2004a), a digital crime scene has been classified as a *sub-environment* of a physical crime scene. In an example, a computer located beside a dead body may play a part in an investigation. A digital crime scene requires investigation of the hardware, software, and data that may hold digital evidence. It is an iterative activity, as multiple physical devices may be found and investigated sequentially. An important component of the digital crime scene investigation phase is an understanding of the forensic and core processes for sound investigations. We can generalize the physical and digital crime scene concept to be applicable also for those scenes of incidents that produce corporate investigations, where a policy has been breached.

When an incident is recognized, a confirmation is generally required to authorize and initiate a forensic investigation. For example, if the investigation includes critical IT systems or services, then a corporation may have to authorize the investigator's access to the potential evidence sources. Additionally, if these systems are operational, then special care must be taken and the investigation activities must be coordinated with the system owner.

In criminal cases, seizure of physical items with digital data is performed by law enforcement personnel with appropriate search warrants. It is generally recommended that they are trained in the seizure of digital evidence, or that they consult with digital forensics experts in order to ensure none of the seized evidence is compromised. What can be seized in respect to legal and ethical perspectives must be considered at the scene of the event. Legal considerations and perspectives are further discussed in Chapter 3.

2.2.2 The First Responder

The first responder in a criminal case is typically a police officer, arriving at a physical scene of an event, such as at a crime scene. The first responders are the ones responsible for handling potential evidence, including digital devices. Imagine that you arrive at a crime scene as the first responder, and there is a hypothesis that someone has committed a crime. Evidence of how it happened, when it happened, and who did what might be found in the smartphone laying on the counter, on the compact camera on the shelf, or on the laptop playing music. Perhaps there is even additional evidence at an unknown physical location in a cloud service?

All scenes are different, and so are the digital devices that might be relevant to the case in question. The digital objects found on *one* device might not be the sole source of evidence, or it might not be enough to bring a case to court or convict anyone of a crime. Other evidence sources thus need to be accounted for, reinforcing the need to have a complete perspective of the scene of the event you are investigating. As an aid to the first responder, standard operating procedures (SOPs) should be in place to provide structured evidence identification activities, including documentation, to maintain evidence integrity.

Example 2.2: First Responder Mistake

In a murder trial in the United States, a detective at the crime scene allegedly tried to unlock the mobile phone of the suspect. While doing so, he repeatedly entered incorrect PIN and PUK codes to unlock the SIM card. This led to data relevant to the case being erased. The defense team argued that the police investigation destroyed critical evidence that would have been relevant to the case.[2]

A digital forensics investigation is a response to an observed incident and the first responder must act accordingly. The principles that apply for criminal investigations can be significantly different from those for civil investigations. In any case, a hypothesis must address the goal of the investigation. For example, if a hypothesis states that a hacker used a set of tools to attack a vulnerable service or resource and export data, this could lead to an investigation of a possible confidentiality breach. The goal of the investigation may be to reveal evidence of the incident, to determine the extent and confidential value of the data compromised, and then to estimate the consequences of the attack. The attack might not have violated criminal law, or it might not be economically feasible to investigate it as a crime.

Example 2.3: SpyEye Bank Account Fraud

To illustrate the different definitions and terms in this chapter, let us look at a realistic scenario of bank account fraud (as introduced in Section 1.3.4). The SpyEye incident was a challenge for computer forensics investigators back in 2009. Imagine an incident in which a customer's computer is misused to commit fraud and then reported to you, as a forensic analyst. You investigate the case in order to identify digital objects that can be used as evidence to prove the existence of a criminal fraud.

You identify multiple events while investigating the case, for example the legitimate use of a computer and suspicious traces of emails sent from that computer to numerous email addresses. One or more emails can be represented as one digital object, as SpyEye was shown to be distributed in mass email campaigns. This tells you what you need to know in order to identify who sent emails with suspicious content. The content reflects what the intention of the digital object (email) was: to get the user to access a phishing website exemplified in Figure 2.3 or to execute the attached file containing the SpyEye code. This email is then potential evidence that, together with other evidence from the case, can support the hypothesis of the criminal fraud.

The principle of evidence integrity comes into play when we identify and want to preserve evidence. Imagine that you found a computer that is going to be seized for investigation. Will you touch the machine, unplug it from any cables, or remove any physical hardware from it, affecting the integrity in any way? If so, all precautions must be taken to ensure that you only perform necessary actions that can be justified in hindsight and that do not breach the integrity of the evidence.

---

2 www.justiceforbrad.com.

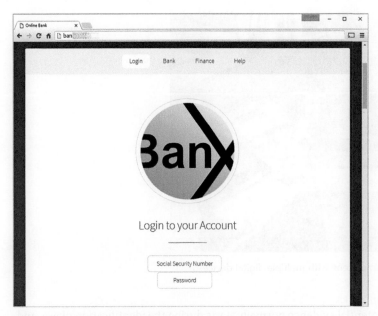

Figure 2.3 Example website directed to from a fraudulent email.

2.2.3 At the Scene of the Incident

A *scene of an incident* is simply the location (or set of locations) where an incident took place or evidence is found. With respect to a digital scene in an incident, it is important to understand typical characteristics of a traditional physical scene or the origin of where we believe it (being a crime, incident, or event) all started.

A great deal of digital evidence can be found in a private home, as illustrated in Figure 2.4. Many of these devices communicate using wireless networks, which in turn connect to other devices outside the physical premises of the residence. Furthermore, adversaries may also access the network, especially where there is a lack of adequate network access control. In addition, extended digital evidence sources such as cloud storage and common email services may be present and linked to individuals with access to the residence.

In a small corporation, digital devices are usually managed and accounted for to some degree. Because businesses operate with individual computers, smartphones, and assigned application, network, and service access, it should be possible to identify and seize additional potential evidence sources. Compared to small businesses, large businesses generally practice stricter control of digital devices and equipment, and they often have separate IT departments. Because of compliance requirements and the computer security threats aimed at today's businesses, they may also have security systems, services, and dedicated security professionals that can support the investigator's identification of potential digital evidence sources. Log analysis has become a fundamental IT operations capability that can also facilitate forensic readiness, as discussed in Chapter 5, 6 and 7. Caution should, however, be taken to closely supervise all actions, as the employees of a business under investigation naturally have loyalties to their employer.

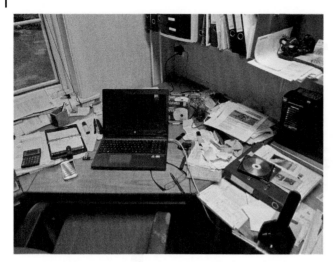

Figure 2.4 Example crime scene with multiple digital devices.

2.2.3.1 Preservation Tasks

The processing of potential evidence normally starts during the identification phase, and it is crucial to preserve the chain of custody and evidence integrity from the very start. This includes activities to isolate, secure, and document the physical and digital devices at hand. Evidence preservation may require the assessment of technologies for subsequent copying of the original media, establishing time synchronization, and any other tasks that facilitate additional forensic activities.

The documentation activities begin from the moment the investigator starts handling the digital devices that will be "touched" during the investigation phases. The documentation enables reproducibility of results and traceability from the physical object's origin to the final evidence presentation. This calls for thorough documentation throughout the digital forensic process.

2.2.4 Dealing with Live and Dead Systems

Physical equipment that holds potential digital evidence is identified either as live (turned on) or dead (turned off, with no power):

- By *live systems*, we mean systems that are running and are at the time of identification potentially holding evidence that may be lost or hard to acquire if the system is shut down.
- By *dead systems*, we mean systems not running. Any data in temporary storage areas such as cache, main memory, running processes, or active application dialogues on a computer will normally be lost when the system is powered down.

Definition 2.2: Post Mortem
Post mortem analysis is, in the context of digital forensics, associated with analysis of a "dead" (not running) computer or electronic device.

Special caution must be taken before any action, regardless of whether the system is live or dead at the time of identification. Critical data may not be retrievable if a system is turned off. Imagine yourself using your computer, not for criminal purposes of course, but for typical tasks such as browsing the web or playing games online. What would happen if the machine was suddenly shut down? Would you be able to recover and continue playing from the level you just reached or continue reading that forum post where you connected through a virtual private network (VPN)? Although this is a rather hypothetical example, it illustrates the considerations that are necessary before you touch or shut down a digital device in practice. Important evidence can easily be lost.

Contrary to the example given here, turning on a system that was initially turned off might also lead to evidence loss. At boot time, a PC, mobile phone, or media player executes boot activities that can overwrite previously cached data.

Cell phones, media players, laptops, or any devices that can communicate over any network can potentially be altered while being seized or even after they have been seized. This can be caused by either deliberate tampering or unintentional changes (e.g., due to humidity or electricity). Because of this, one should consider the use of containers that can shield the device from external radiofrequency (RF) sources, such as a Faraday bag.

2.2.5 Chain of Custody

Let us say we have identified a removable storage media, which we believe has something to do with a crime. As we will further discuss in Section 2.3, we must ensure that we first copy (or "clone") the raw data from the device before we can start searching for evidence of the crime in question. To ensure that we do not alter or change the data stored on the device during the copying process, we can use read-only mode when accessing the data. In turn, this can be enforced through software or hardware that is typically known as *write-blocking technology*. This ensures that the copy represents the exact same data as was stored on the media. Only then can we be sure that what we find while analyzing the copy will match what can be found on the original. The documentation of these tasks is crucial to preserving the chain of custody.

After copying, we generate a *digital signature* of the storage media by using a cryptographic hash function, as described in Section 2.3.5 (see Definition 2.4). By computing a digital signature both for the original storage media and for the copy, we can compare them to verify that the content is identical. This is important information that supports the chain of custody and evidence integrity. It means that we can continue the investigation on a copy, but still confidently refer back to the original source. All changes, such as copying, case information, and information about how it was collected and who was involved, must be documented. Multiple tools can be used to collect the data and to generate a hash to avoid any uncertainties in the tools used (referred to as *dual-tool verification*). Examples of practical implications for different media, such as computers, mobile devices, and online data, are given in the technical chapters of this textbook (Chapters 5, 6, and 7).

Most digital forensics tools have reporting capabilities. These reports are often incorporated into or appended to case reports. Digital forensics software and tools can also provide automated reports, which typically reflect changes made by an investigator while using the tool. Most tools also support forms that the investigator must fill out, related to the case and the investigated physical or digital object in question.

At a minimum, the documented information should cover the following (based on Laliberte & Gupta, 2004):

- the person handling the evidence;
- processes and procedures performed;
- the time and date of evidence acquisition;
- original location of the evidence collected;
- method of collection, examination, and analysis; and
- the reason for collecting the evidence.

Intentional (tampering) or unintentional (accidental) changes to digital evidence, as for physical evidence, is a risk in any digital investigation. In order to maintain the integrity of the evidence, precautions should be taken to ensure that the tools used for acquisition, examination, and analysis of data will not modify it in any unexpected way. To ensure the chain of custody, the use of integrity checks and timestamps of forensic activities should be applied. Various kinds of supporting data and documents may be used for supporting the chain of custody, for example:

- photographs,
- reports,
- laboratory information management systems,
- notebooks,
- checklists,
- log files, and
- videos and screen captures.

The chain of custody is a critical element of the digital forensics process, as we shall see in later sections of this chapter. In some jurisdictions, evidence could be excluded from a case (deemed not admissible) if the vital elements of the chain of custody listed here are not documented.

2.3   The Collection Phase

In a digital forensics investigation, the collection phase (see Figure 2.5) refers to the acquisition or copying of the data. This is when a forensic investigator gains access to the electronic device(s) containing raw data that has been identified as relevant for the specific case. The collection phase of the digital forensics process is common to most literature and scientific research in digital forensics. The majority of literature that discusses the forensics process uses the term *collection*, whereas more technically oriented literature refers to an

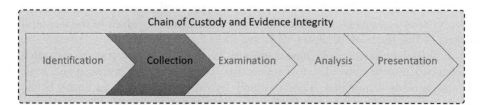

Figure 2.5 The digital forensics process: collection phase.

acquisition and/or *extraction*. Chapters 5, 6, and 7 discuss how the collection method chosen may impact the result of an investigation from a technical perspective.

As discussed in Section 2.2.5, the data being investigated should always be copied[3] to a separate media, and the forensic examination and analysis should always work on a copy. This ensures that there are no accidental data changes to the original during the forensic process. In addition, a write blocker (either in hardware or in software) is typically employed to guarantee that no data is written to the original storage media. Finally, a digital signature (a cryptographic hash) is calculated both for the original media and for the copy, as described later in this chapter.

To support a forensically sound collection, the Digital Forensics Workshop 2001 jointly stated the importance of collecting relevant data using approved methods (Palmer, 2001). On the basis of the concepts and tasks addressed, this book uses the term *collection* as defined in Definition 2.3.

Definition 2.3: The Collection Phase

Collection of data from digital devices to make a digital copy using forensically sound methods and techniques.

Metadata about a case should be tied to the potential evidence, whether it be a physical device or a data file. Such metadata can include the case name, case number, examiner (the digital forensics investigator or investigators), timestamps, case and seizure location, and time zone.

Example 2.4: SpyEye Online Banking Fraud

Online banking fraud cases typically involve multiple parties and sources of evidence. What to search for and how depend on the case in question, the context, and the environment where potential evidence may be found. In the case of SpyEye, many parties, networks, and systems were involved. Results from the investigation revealed that the SpyEye toolkit developer was a central actor who was selling a malware kit to fraudsters via online forums (e.g., darkode). Central command servers were investigated as part of the central management of all SpyEye bots.

Examples of potential evidence sources that could be collected are:

- traces of transactions from the victim's computer,
- bank transaction records from the bank's backend systems,
- malware evidence on victim hosts and the botnet,
- server-side logs at the bank,
- communication with a mule (email, messaging services and phone),
- transactions made by a mule, and
- network monitoring logs from the bank infrastructure, and internet forums.

---

3 The terms *duplication, cloning, bit-stream image, working copy, bit-by-bit copy*, and *raw data copy* are all used interchangeably in the digital forensics literature to emphasize the importance of leaving the original data source alone, while pursuing the investigation with its copy.

Whether data is easy to acquire or not depends in part on whether systems or services have already been prepared for the logging of events and storing or preserving data that will be used in a forensic investigation. If this is the case, potential digital evidence can be quickly made ready for use in a forensic investigation. This kind of preparedness is known as *forensic readiness* and is addressed in Chapter 4.

As mentioned in Chapter 1 (Section 1.3.3), errors, uncertainty, and data loss are common challenges in digital investigations. The data collected will form the basis of information used for the later process phases. Because of this, carefully documenting all the factors that may introduce uncertainty, such as the origin of the collected data, the context of the case, or the location or context in which the digital device was found, can help support further understanding the data collected (Casey, 2002).

2.3.1   Sources of Digital Evidence

As introduced earlier in this chapter, digital evidence includes any digital data that contains reliable information that supports or refutes a hypothesis about an incident. In today's society, digital evidence can be found almost everywhere, and one could write a lengthy separate chapter with a taxonomy of all possible digital evidence sources. We choose to focus on the most well-known sources of digital evidence, to serve as a reference and an inspiration for where one may find digital evidence.

The most common source of evidence has traditionally been hard drives or other computer long-term storage media. An example of a hard disk (as shown in Figure 2.6), and flash storage drives, main memory, GPU (graphics processing unit) memory, or a CPU with a cache (as illustrated in Figure 2.7), are all examples of this. Additional examples are external devices that can be connected to a computer, such as removable media, memory sticks, web cameras, and CDs, DVDs, and Blu-rays.

Embedded devices can have removable and integrated storage media with proprietary connectors and physical interfaces. Imagine a memory chip from a remote-controlled central garage opener, often used in apartment buildings with many

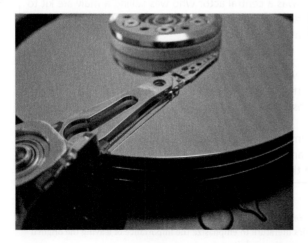

Figure 2.6 A disc from an opened broken hard drive.

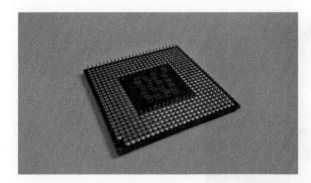

Figure 2.7 CPU with potential cached data.

residents. Such a device can hold information about which remote control keys were in use (if any) to open a gate at the time that a criminal broke into a car. Data from the garage-opening system and toll roads can provide relevant information about the travel path of a car. If this data is combined with data from the vehicle used (if found), along with the driver's log from an autonomous car, then a more complete picture of an incident can be created.

Smartphones and tablets have become almost as widespread as traditional computing devices, such as workstations. These devices are personal and portable, and they will frequently hold a trove of information relevant to a forensic investigation. For example, they may contain evidence of geographical movement and mobile network communications. In Figure 2.8, we can see a smartphone that has been disassembled to gain access to the physical storage device within. Chapter 6 covers more details on the best practices for digital forensics with mobile devices.

Computer networks can hold vast amounts of digital evidence. Network forensics is often related to the monitoring and analysis of volatile and dynamic network traffic. Network data can be wiretapped, as illustrated in Figure 2.9. Internet forensics covers both the traffic and the connected systems in digital forensics investigations. This can involve network components (such as switches and routers connecting the devices), the

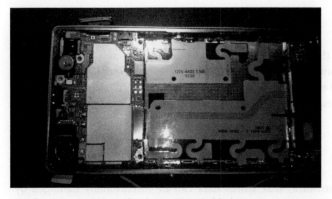

Figure 2.8 A smartphone has been disassembled to gain access to memory chips with digital evidence.

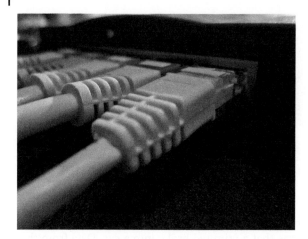

Figure 2.9 Computers and systems are connected to the Internet.

devices themselves (such as web servers and consumer devices), along with the Internet services accessed.

The Internet, the services and applications it offers, along with all users and company-generated data (blogs, online shops, forums, and chat services) provide additional sources of evidence. More information about Internet forensics can be found in Chapter 7.

2.3.2 Systems Physically Tied to a Location

In many cases, it is not possible to move, or remove, a system or digital device from its physical location. In such cases, the data needs to be copied at the physical location itself. A typical crime or incident could involve emails from a central corporate email server. The email server will, in most cases, not be removed from its physical location just because of one single email. It is up to the case investigators to determine if it is necessary to physically remove the digital device, in this case the email server.

2.3.3 Multiple Evidence Sources

In an investigation, it is rare that all potential digital evidence is present in a single digital storage device, such as a computer hard disk or a memory card. Figure 2.10 illustrates some typical personal digital evidence sources. Relative to the case investigated, potential digital evidence can be present in multiple devices in one physical location or in several locations across the world.

2.3.4 Reconstruction

The collected media (or hardware) that stores data can be intentionally damaged by suspects trying to destroy evidence, or unintentionally, for example in a fire or accident. We will not go into the details of how to prepare or recover data from broken media in

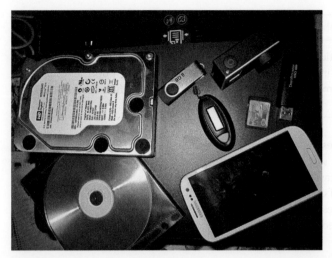

Figure 2.10 An example of seized electronic storage and computing devices to be examined and analyzed.

this chapter, as this is covered in Chapters 5, 6, and 7. However, it is important to be aware of the fact that one cannot always expect to start copying data right away.

2.3.5 Evidence Integrity and Cryptographic Hashes

Evidence integrity is at the core of every forensic investigation, as discussed in Section 1.2.3. This is a requirement that is applied equally to both the original evidence as well as the copy used for analysis. In order to preserve evidence integrity, multiple factors must be considered, such as the integrity of individuals and the processes followed, both physically and logically (Hosmer, 2002).

There are multiple measures to ensure evidence integrity in digital forensics. The intent is to ensure that evidence is neither accidentally nor intentionally changed when collecting digital data from an original source. Evidence integrity can be facilitated by using hardware or software write blockers, which protect the data source from anything but read access. There are software-based write blockers that typically restrict access rights in software to read-only. For example, in UNIX, read-only can be set for each file or a partition in order to preserve evidence integrity.

In order to verify that integrity is preserved, a concept known as *digital fingerprinting* is applied, as introduced in Section 2.2.5. This involves the use of cryptographic (or one-way) hash functions. The input to a hash function is a bit stream, which can come from a file, a disk, or a partition, and the output is the unique hash or signature of that input stream. By comparing the hashes of an original with those of its respective copy, one can verify that a copy is the exact same as the original.

Examples of cryptographic hash algorithms include MD5, SHA1, and SHA256. It should be noted that cryptographic algorithms become outdated over time, due to vulnerabilities in the algorithms, advances in cryptanalysis, and ever-increasing processing power. Both the MD5 and SHA1 functions have been found to be vulnerable to certain attacks (Schneier, 2004), but they are still in widespread use in forensic tools.

Definition 2.4: Cryptographic Hash

A cryptographic hash function is a nonreversible mathematical function that takes an arbitrary amount of data as input and returns a fixed-size string as output. The result is a hash value, and it is mathematically infeasible to find two different files that create the same hash.

Be aware that in some cases, data inevitably changes during acquisition. An example is the case of a live computer system with multiple evidence sources that have different levels of volatility. In some cases, memory may have to be accessed in order to acquire a password, for the purpose of opening an encrypted archive file. The evidence integrity of the memory will not be preserved, and the activities required to access the memory, along with the chosen procedure and why, must be documented as part of the chain of custody.

2.3.6 Order of Volatility

Investigations rarely involve just one single digital device. Evidence may be present across multiple devices, such as a workstation, memory stick, and Internet email service. By analogy, if we apply the Heisenberg Principle of uncertainty to digital forensics (as was done in Farmer & Venema, 2004), it is not just difficult but impossible to gather all the information from a computer system without changing its state. For example, data acquisition from one data source in a live computer may impact the data in another. Because of this, the term *order of volatility* (OOV) has become a central term in digital forensics.

Definition 2.5: Order of Volatility

Prioritization of the potential evidence source to be collected according to the volatility of the data.

Based on Definition 2.5, we understand that the order of volatility deals with data lifetimes. It is the concept of gathering the most volatile data first, as it will most likely be changed or destroyed first. Any operation will, however, affect data. This means that one has to carefully consider the context and goal of what to extract first to avoid damaging potentially crucial evidence.

Data stored on disk is less volatile than data stored in memory. In cases where only data on a disk is to be extracted in a postmortem investigation, extraction of data from this media will be prioritized. Table 2.1, based on the analysis by Farmer and Venema (2004), lists typical storage devices and media and their expected data longevity (the life expectancy of the data stored) in a running system. All lifetimes depend upon the influence of external factors, such as the use of the media, the SLA (service-level agreement) for cloud storage, or magnetic-field influences on tape media.

In practice, it is difficult to determine what source is likely to be the most valuable. If time is critical, one may choose to pay less attention to the volatility perspective based on

Table 2.1 Examples of order of volatility.

Type of storage media and data	Typical storage lifespan and longevity (dependent on usage)
System registers, peripheral memory, and caches	Nanoseconds
RAM	Ten nanoseconds
Network state	Milliseconds
Running system processes	Seconds
Data on disk (cache)	Minutes
Cloud storage	Months to years
HDD data storage	Years
Floppies and other magnetic tape–based media	Years to decades
CD-ROMs, DVDs, print-outs,	Decades
Read-only memory; flash and SSD data storage	Decades to centuries

the situation, the crime in question, and the hypothesis of where relevant evidence can be found. Imagine that you are investigating a crime where you are presented with a live computer that may hold vital evidence for the crime in question. You do not know where the evidence can be found or what data you need. For example, the evidence you need might not be stored locally on the machine, but in encrypted cloud storage with encryption keys stored in a computer's RAM. Shutting down the machine will destroy the keys.

As we have seen, in order to access the most relevant data, we need to consider different factors before starting the collection process. Some methods have a given probability of succeeding for a given type of information. As shown in Table 2.2, we can

Table 2.2 Some factors that affect information availability.

Factor	Description
Order of volatility	The most volatile data should be acquired before less volatile data.
Access restrictions and encryption	Restricted or encrypted information should be acquired early if we cannot ensure access later.
Powered on	Keeping a device on can make the data available at a later time, but running processes might overwrite data.
Shutdown	Powering off a device might overwrite data. Pulling the battery (or power) will delete data from RAM that is not written to nonvolatile memory.
Physical interface	Different data can often be acquired from different interfaces.
Communication protocol	Different data can often be acquired using different communication protocols.
Lab resources	Availability of lab resources will often be a limiting factor when selecting acquisition method. Time is also a resource.
Interpretation	The data can be just gibberish if we are not able to interpret it correctly.

look at this as a matrix of information availability, where each factor affects the availability of the acquired information.

2.3.7 Dual-Tool Verification

Digital forensics is conducted using software applications and tools, often made by third parties. This is because data is preferably analyzed at higher layers of abstraction to make it easier to understand for the investigator. An investigator must trust the technology to present the information with a high level of data integrity.

Dual-tool verification can be applied as a means to detect errors from one tool by using another tool to confirm the results. For example, during a forensic investigation, an investigator is extracting evidence from a broken memory stick. Through the use of an imaging tool to acquire a copy of the memory stick's data storage, only 70% of the original storage space is collected. In order to check if a human or software error was the cause of this, another imaging tool could be used and the results compared. If there is a deviation between the results, further analysis will be needed to understand the root cause.

In cases where dual-tool verification is conducted, tools from different vendors or organizations should be used to avoid any common vendor weaknesses or interference between the tools' capabilities. Dual-tool verification can be valuable in all phases of the digital forensics process, not just in the collection phase.

2.3.8 Remote Acquisition

Physical collection is not always feasible as it often requires traveling to a location to identify and collect devices of interest, such as the hard drives of a set of computers. Remote forensic acquisition can increase the speed of the investigation and reduce expenses. Furthermore, the more time it takes to arrive on-site and begin the collection, the more data may be lost. In case of data stored in cloud services, it may not be practically feasible or even possible for an investigator to enter a data center. There are several important considerations that are worth noting, including:

- To enable remote acquisition, software will have to be installed on devices or systems to support remote acquisition.
- Data must be transmitted over a network, which can breach confidentiality, integrity, and availability.
- Trust is reduced as we are not in possession of the physical device and a complete collection of data may be infeasible.
- It is dependent upon the hardware of the device as tools are running on the IT.

Many forensic software vendors include remote forensics capabilities in their tools, such as Guidance Software (EnCase), Accessdata (FTK), and FireEye. An investigator can also collect data by secure shell access (SSH) or Powershell. These tools along with an incident response capability in an IT security department of a company provide quicker response times to initiate forensic analysis of devices in remote locations.

Remote acquisition can also be applicable in cases where you have physical possession of the device of interest. Remote forensics laboratory tools can transmit binary copies of collected data from one device to another. Netcat is one tool that is often used for this purpose. Data should be hashed before it is sent over a network, to verify the evidence integrity when it is received and to support the chain of custody.

Most people who use the web today use cloud services. These can be common email services, file storage services, social media (such as Facebook and Twitter), and corporate services hosted online in locations far removed from the users. The legal aspects of cloud services investigations are complex and can restrict access to potential evidence. Service providers may provide their services from foreign physical locations that are subject to laws of countries other than the one where the actual crime is believed to originate from. Chapter 7 discusses more of these concerns as well as how to go about investigating across physical and legal borders.

2.3.9 External Competency and Forensics Cooperation

In global or multinational criminal cases, the involvement of forensics units in other countries can be necessary to solve a case. The Internet poses a unique challenge for digital forensics investigations. Cybercrime is one type of crime that can rarely be solved by police investigators from only one country, as the origin of the attack can be in one country, but the crime has an effect in another country. Arenas for global cooperation include Interpol, Europol, Eurojust, the G8 Subgroup on High Tech Crime, as well as bilateral and multilateral relations.

Example 2.5: Sony's Collaboration with the FBI

In 2008, Sony Computer Entertainment America suffered from extensive distributed denial of service (DDOS) attacks against their online gaming servers. At its height, this attack affected 60,000–80,000 users. In the investigation of the attacks, Sony and their security incident response team collaborated with and helped the FBI in their forensic investigation of the cyberattacks, leading to the prosecution of the attackers. The data collected from these particular attacks also provided the FBI with valuable information for other ongoing investigations at that time (Proctor, 2014).

In the case of SpyEye, many national law enforcement agencies were involved from all around the world. In addition, commercial security companies were part of the investigation of the malware and evidence identified on compromised machines and servers.

2.4 The Examination Phase

All data collected must be examined and prepared for later analysis as part of the examination phase (see Figure 2.11). As with all phases in the digital forensics process, it is important to document your actions and handling of the data to support the chain of custody. The examination often requires restructuring, parsing, and preprocessing of raw data to make it understandable for a forensic investigator in the upcoming analysis. To facilitate this phase, an analyst typically uses forensic tools and techniques appropriate for extracting relevant information. As stated in ISO/IEC 27041:2015

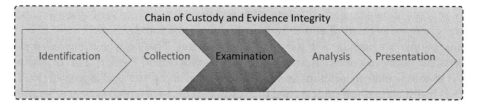

Figure 2.11 The digital forensics process: examination.

(ISO/IEC, 2015a), we are attempting to "retrieve relevant potential digital evidence from one or more sources." We define the examination phase in Definition 2.6, based on National Forensic Science Technology Center (NFSTC) (2009) and Carrier and Spafford (2004a).

Definition 2.6: The Examination Phase

Preparation and extraction of potential digital evidence from collected data sources.

2.4.1 Initial Data Source Examination and Preprocessing

A copy of the data source can be considered a "black box" of unstructured, binary data. The objective of the initial, basic examination of the data is to make it more structured and readable. Digital forensics tools automate much of these preliminary examination and preprocessing tasks. This reduces the manual task load for the investigator, and reduces the likelihood of mistakes, such as overlooking essential evidence or damaging it. However, the value of manual examination should not be underestimated, as algorithms cannot necessarily substitute for the intuition of an experienced forensic investigator.

As the data loads increase exponentially with Moore's law, *triage* has become an increasingly important part of digital forensics. The analogy relates to the triage of patients, where treatment is prioritized based on the severity of the patient's condition. With respect to digital forensics, triage is the process that aims to identify the most relevant data as quickly as possible. The purpose is to manage situations where one has a finite amount of time and resources to carry out an investigation (Roussev *et al.*, 2013). Digital forensic tools support this need, for example by extracting the most recently changed files from a computer.[4]

Another technique that can be useful for the initial examination is to use known case information to identify data of interest, such as malicious executable files or contraband image files. There are typical web and Internet activity characteristics that can prove fruitful for an investigation, such as email for communication, cached websites, bookmarks, and cookie files for web activity. In general, the more the examination phase can structure and organize the data for the investigators, the better the overview will be for later analysis of the actual content of the data objects.

File hashes can be used to identify files that you are searching for, such as known images (e.g., contraband images) or known documents (e.g., manuals that describe how

---

4 Autopsy User Documentation, version 3.1, http://sleuthkit.org/autopsy/docs/user-docs/3.1/.

to perform a crime). A similar example for targeted examination is to use a known keyword database to search for suspicious activity in general or for the specific case in question.

Forensic tools generally add metadata to each digital object, including references to databases with known hashes and key words. The added metadata is stored in common forensic file formats and can be used during further examination of the evidence.

2.4.2 Forensic File Formats and Structures

Many digital forensics toolkits and software suites come with their own file formats or databases to store information that has been collected in a structured manner. The forensic format used can have an impact on the effectiveness of the forensic analysis. It is important that the formatting of the copied data clearly reflects the evidence tied to the incident investigated and provides as much additional information as possible.

There are many different digital forensics formats, and the information storage capabilities of these formats have different impacts on the investigation results. First and foremost is the raw data format, which is used to copy the data source "as is." The more extensive storage formats are EnCase, SMART, AFF, and Prodiscover, as discussed in Flaglien *et al.* (2011). The latter formats add more information and flexibility to the extracted and examined data; this serves to improve subsequent analysis. Examples of such additional information include metadata extractions, integrity checks, archive decompressions, and file decryptions.

In cases where huge volumes of data are being copied for the investigation, examination can be difficult, and it is sometimes impossible to analyze the data in one single image file. Because of this limitation, some forensic file formats support splitting of image files, so that they can more easily be shared. If such file formats are used, one needs to ensure that image splitting doesn't affect the integrity of the data.

Forensic file formats typically support the most common data sources, such as block devices, hard disk images, and computer memory. However, not all formats support all file systems.

2.4.3 Data Recovery

Most computer systems, digital devices, and file systems are typically designed to treat information in the most efficient way to enhance performance and the user experience. As a result, they are not designed to securely wipe or destroy data upon request. In most modern file systems, only the pointer to the file is marked "available" or "unallocated." This results in the space being available, and a new file can overwrite the previous file. Data can thus be recovered from the storage area even after deletion of a file, as long as the data area was not overwritten.

For example, if an image were deleted years prior to an investigation, parts of the image might still be extracted. The image data can be rebuilt in a viewer, and it will represent the original material and its content, even though other details or portions of the data are missing. An example of this is shown in Figure 2.12.

In cases of deleted files, it is essential to carefully document traceability to the original data source, since methods used for examination may change the state of data. These actions need to be documented to maintain evidence integrity.

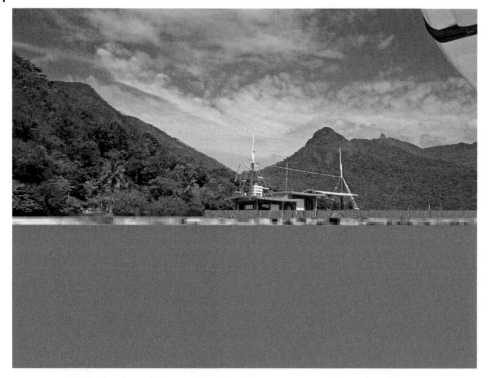

Figure 2.12 Illustration of a partially broken image file.

2.4.4 Data Reduction and Filtering

Large amounts of data present a challenge for effective digital forensics investigations. A single digital device may hold terabytes of data from billions of files. All methods for safely reducing the data volume should be considered. Filtering is an example of a method that can be used during examination.

A well-known filtering or hash lookup technique is based on databases with cryptographic hash values from *known files*. Many files in a computer belong to the operating system, software, and other applications. These files usually do not contain any useful evidence, and they can safely be ignored in the examination/analysis. The use of known file databases, in combination with digital forensic tools, makes it possible to improve the understanding of files that are known to be good or simply to filter them out if considered useless.

There are two categories of known files: known bad files and known good files. *Known bad* hash databases can also be used to identify suspicious files like malware and rootkits as well as images known to be associated with criminal activities. The National Software Reference Library[5] is an example of a library that provides datasets of *known good* files that can be used to filter out operating system files, application files, and more, leaving only files of interest for further analysis. Figure 2.13 shows how known good files might be removed to reduce the total amount of data.

---

5 National Software Reference Library, www.nsrl.nist.gov.

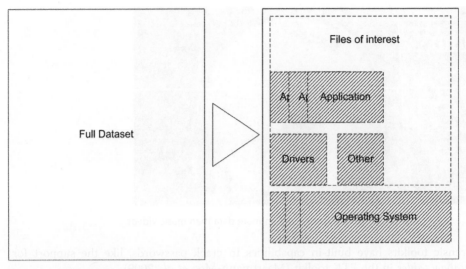

Figure 2.13 Illustration of filtering using known good file datasets.

2.4.5 Timestamps

A systems internal clock should always be noted, as should any deviations in time zones or suspicions of incorrect system clocks. The recording of correct timestamps in an investigation can help identify correlations across multiple data objects. In addition, adjustments have to be made if the clock of one digital device is off and not synchronized relative to accurate time sources. The investigator also needs to know whether the forensic tool being used will display and support different time zone settings, and how these relate to local machine times and UTC (coordinated universal time).

2.4.6 Compression, Encryption and Obfuscation

During the examination phase, compressed files should be uncompressed, and encrypted files should be decrypted if possible. Compressed files are not necessarily difficult to handle as long as one knows the compression algorithm and has tools to decompress the file. If proprietary compression algorithms are in use, it can be more difficult and time-consuming to uncompress the data. It can also be that obscurity techniques have been applied to complicate the identification of potential evidence. If pictures or executable files are renamed and their extensions are changed to appear as text documents, they need to be preprocessed before the upcoming analysis. Many tools support file type extension matching to detect if a file is what its extension claims it to be.

Encryption can be used by corporations to secure their assets, by individuals for privacy protection, and by criminals for anti-forensics. The encryption algorithm, key format, and length used may make the examination of encrypted data simple, complex, or even impossible to accomplish within a reasonable period of time and scope of resources. The increasing use of encryption and obfuscation techniques is starting to become a serious challenge in digital forensics. To help the forensic investigator, some

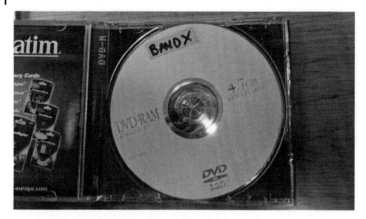

Figure 2.14 A music DVD, which may contain more data than music videos.

forensic toolkits have built-in capabilities to crack passwords, like the support for *rainbow tables* in the FTK toolkit (Maartmann-Moe *et al.*, 2009).

Steganography is a method for concealing a hidden message, image, or other information in another file, message, image, or video. For example, in digital pictures it is possible to store textual information in "hidden layers" not visible to the eye or to typical photo applications such as MS Paint. Special tools exist to make this possible, such as DeepSound,[6] which is a tool to conceal information in audio or music files (exemplified in Figure 2.14). The benefit of using steganography over encryption is that it does not attract attention. This introduces an additional complexity for digital forensics.

2.4.7 Data and File Carving

When data is collected from a data source, a forensic investigator may find it unstructured and difficult to interpret. One might view files, such as photos and documents, with a computer browser, but a collected data image can contain broken files, deleted files, scattered data elements, and objects that stem from many years of using a computer or handheld digital device. In order not to overlook potential evidence, there are tools and techniques available for parsing or carving unstructured and sometimes raw binary data, as illustrated in Figure 2.15, based on a similar presentation in Richard and Roussev (2005).

Media file parsers use techniques to identify patterns or signatures associated with particular file formats and types. Most file types contain headers and footers that make them readable to the applications handling them; these applications render the file as intended for use by the user. The use of carving tools allows forensic examiners to select a set of file types to recover from a piece of media. Media carving can be quite useful in order to acquire deleted files such as previously deleted images.

Other parsers are useful for examining one of the most common electronic communication protocols: email. Email parsers can crawl through the raw data copied from a digital device and render individual emails in a manner that makes it easier to analyze them in later phases of an investigation.

---

6 DeepSound overview, http://jpinsoft.net/DeepSound/.

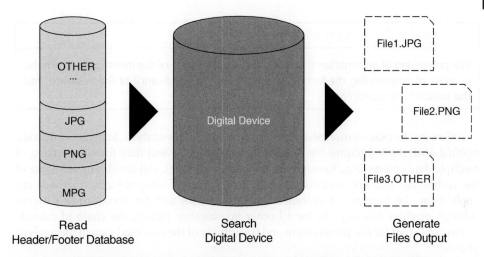

Figure 2.15 File carving with database read and search in a digital device for relevant files.

The parsing of standard, well-known file types is one thing; the parsing of proprietary files and objects is a different matter. More manual work is required to examine the information contained within the files and to ensure that they can be presented in a format that is as readable as possible for a forensic analyst.

2.4.8 Automation

Automation is an objective in itself during the examination phase, for reasons of both forensic soundness and efficiency. Most of the tasks in the examination phase can be automated using scripts or programs. File parsing, string searches, and extraction of compressed files will significantly reduce the manual task load on an investigator, in particular when working with large datasets. The most common digital forensic tools, such as EnCase, offer special-purpose scripting languages to help automate tasks.[7]

2.5 The Analysis Phase

In the analysis phase (see Figure 2.16), forensic investigators determine the digital objects to be used as digital evidence to support or refute a hypothesis of a crime, incident, or event, as defined in Definition 2.7, based on Yusoff *et al.* (2011).

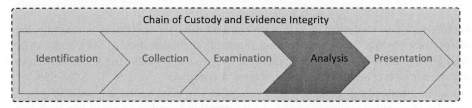

Figure 2.16 The digital forensics process: analysis.

---

7 https://www.guidancesoftware.com/encase-forensic.

> **Definition 2.7: The Analysis Phase**
>
> The processing of information that addresses the objective of the investigation with the purpose of determining the facts about an event, the significance of the evidence, and the person(s) responsible.

Following the examination phase, the data is prepared for analysis. Statistical methods, manual analysis, techniques for understanding protocols and data formats, linking of multiple data objects (e.g., through the use of data mining), and timelining are some of the techniques that are used for analysis. In Chapter 8, computational methods are applied for the purpose of automating analysis tasks and for recognizing patterns through machine learning. As for all other investigative phases, the chain of custody is also important for the preservation and traceability of the collected data in the analysis phase.

The analysis phase is an iterative process in itself. We often operate with preliminary hypotheses about data that may potentially contain evidence, but during the analysis one forms new hypotheses about the case that may require collection of additional data objects. Investigations proceed in this manner until the results can be considered sufficient for the purpose of the investigation, though in many cases this might be practically infeasible.

2.5.1 Layers of Abstraction

What you see is not always what you get. One has to recognize this as a fact when analyzing digital media, regardless of the storage media chosen. In the case of file system forensics, data seen by an application is not the same as what is seen by an operating system and, again, not the same as what is actually stored in bits and bytes on the storage device. A deleted file, for example, can be fragmented over multiple sectors of a hard drive, and new files might overwrite some of the sectors fully or partially. However, this does not mean that one cannot get access to those sectors or even parts of sectors that have not yet been overwritten. Figure 2.17 illustrates different layers as they can be interpreted by end-user applications, file systems, and hardware (based on a similar example from Farmer & Venema, 2004).

2.5.2 Evidence Types

Any case will have its own evidence, depending on the type of crime. For example, the evidence of a physical crime, where clues regarding the motivation of the crime can be found in a digital device owned by the suspect or the victim, will be much different from the evidence of a cybercrime conducted from a computer.

Imagine investigating a case where a computer has been seized for you to analyze. Examples of potential evidence can be the information found in an email file, such as a message that was sent from a specific email address. The address can then be linked to one person and sent to another person's email. Another example can be a malicious

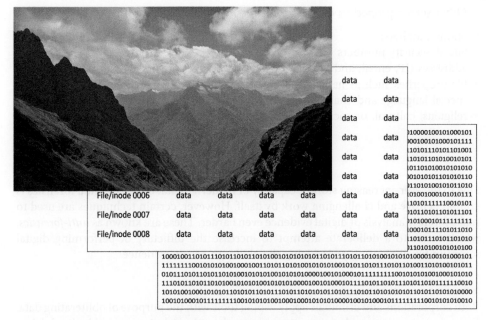

Figure 2.17 Image as seen by users, by the operating system, and in hardware.

application that was found installed on a system unbeknownst to the person owning that system. The Trojan horse defense (Brenner *et al.*, 2004) is a well-known concept intended to complicate digital forensics investigations. To prove or disprove the validity of a Trojan horse defense requires thorough analysis.

2.5.3 String and Keyword Searches

String and keyword searches may simplify the analysis. This is a targeted analysis technique that can be used if one knows what to look for. Imagine an illegal drug case where the investigation was triggered based on a reported crime with specific information about a person and a certain drug or its code name. The name of the person or the drug can be used as a keyword to search through the potential evidence media sources. Keyword searches can be automated or scripted with the use of forensic tools.

Pattern matching is a similar method that can be applied. Depending on the scope and the task of an investigation, some patterns can be more interesting than others. For example, Social Security numbers can be relevant for identity theft cases, and account numbers or credit card numbers for fraud cases. Regular expressions are used to automate the search for all strings with the pattern that you are searching for. Consider an electronic fraud case where one has information about bank accounts, credit card numbers, IP addresses, and URLs. These parameters can be searched for by using regular expressions. If some of the identifiers are known, then the values can be directly searched for to identify whether any of these values were present in the system or device analyzed.

Other search properties or regular expressions of interest can be:

- phone numbers;
- Social Security numbers (SSNs);
- addresses (IP, email, and physical home or work, along with website URLs);
- file properties such as name, type, size, date of creation, and when accessed;
- special language and characters; and
- religious, cultural, or social relations and characteristics.

2.5.4 Anti-Forensics

Due to the ever-increasing storage capacity of modern digital devices, digital forensics is comprehensive and challenging work by itself. However, certain techniques are used to make forensic analysis of digital evidence even harder. These are known as *anti-forensics*, which refers to a deliberate attempt to increase the difficulty of performing digital forensics by eliminating or reducing the ability to access evidence.

2.5.4.1 Computer Media Wiping

Both corporations and criminals apply wiping tools with the purpose of obliterating data. For companies, these techniques are used to reduce the risk represented by hard drives and other media containing sensitive corporate information when outside their control. Another typical example of wiping, used by both corporations and personal users, is remote wiping of lost or stolen devices. The degree of how much data may be permanently removed varies among the techniques and tools used. These tools can be both software and hardware based, functioning on different levels of the target: file level, device level, or component level.

2.5.4.2 Analysis of Encrypted and Obfuscated Data

Malware developers have for a long time utilized anti-forensics mechanisms and techniques. This makes forensic analysis of both the functionality and origin of malicious software difficult. Encryption of configuration files is a typical technique, especially for botnet malware where the botnet masters want to avoid breaches of the command-and-control mechanisms used to control the bots.

As forensic analysts, we should separate the use of encryption for anti-forensics purposes from the use of encryption to secure data. Corporations may encrypt digital devices to avoid a data breach when a device is stolen. In this case, there are typically recovery keys centrally stored to recover the files if necessary. These keys may be accessed by forensic analysts, provided that authorization is provided. In contrast, where criminals have used encryption, the investigator may not be able to acquire or recover the keys without obtaining the passwords from the owner of the digital device.

As introduced in the examination phase (Section 2.4), steganography is another technique that can be used to complicate forensic analysis. This can be done by a range of data-hiding or steganography applications by storing files in nontraditional storage locations, changing file formats, or including a hidden message in photographs to avoid suspicion.

2.5.5   Automated Analysis

Large data volumes, obfuscated malware, and techniques to remove their traces make it time-consuming, costly, and difficult for forensic personnel to identify and analyze relevant evidence. This is especially difficult when evidence is present over a large collection of computers, as discussed in Flaglien *et al.* (2011). Computational forensics, as discussed in Chapter 8, discusses methods for analyzing large amounts of data or highly unstructured datasets that are otherwise difficult to analyze manually. Data mining, especially link-mining techniques, can be applied to the large and complex datasets collected during investigations.

Manual analysis is time-consuming, and analysts often develop scripts and program code to automate their tasks, such as when they search for relevant forensic artifacts. Digital forensic tools are being introduced with more forensic analytics capabilities to reduce the manual efforts of analyzing large data volumes.

2.5.6   Timelining of Events

Timelining is a powerful tool for forensic analysis and contextual awareness. Many forensic tools can automatically structure files and data based on the time they were accessed, last changed, or deleted. Figure 2.18 shows an example of a file timeline using Autopsy,[8] based on when each file was last modified. Whether timestamps can be linked to a digital object depends on the metadata tied to the object. In file system forensics, timestamp metadata is generally available.

A timeline of a chain of events can include physical events, as well as digital events. Imagine a case where a murder has been committed and you investigate the cell phone of the victim. The activity revealed on the cell phone, such as call logs, can provide relevant evidence related to the timeline of the crime.

Analyzing system and application logs can provide a structured chain of events in time. Logs are useful when trying to trace recent or past activities and system behavior related to system users or abnormal users. The content of such logs may vary and depends on the log's primary purpose. For example, for critical systems that require a high level of protection, firewall, or intrusion detection, system logs may reveal the potential origin of a cyberattack. Legal and commercial requirements often exist to ensure that corporations are able to quickly ascertain the chain of events when an incident or crime occurs.

2.5.7   Graphs and Visual Representations

The relationships between data objects, individuals, files, and network interactions are all easier to grasp when presented graphically. Many applications and tools exist to present data in a visual manner that is based on a set of common attributes, such as email addresses found across a set of digital devices related to a crime or an incident. Visualizing the sending and receiving entities of those emails may reveal that one entity

---

8 Image courtesy Brian Carrier; for additional information, see http://www.sleuthkit.org/autopsy.

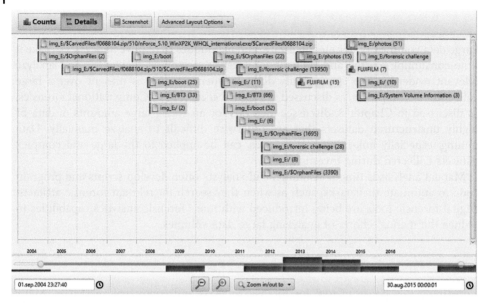

Figure 2.18 Example timeline from file system forensics in Autopsy.

was more involved than others, or is even the hub of all communication with all other entities.

2.5.8 Link Analysis

Link analysis is a powerful and emerging discipline in digital forensics. The goal of link analysis is to produce a structured presentation of interconnected and linked objects. One can gain a better understanding of the relationships and associations among them when links are visualized in graphs, for example where nodes in the graph represent entities and objects. Link analysis is a valuable tool for digital forensics, law enforcement, and intelligence, as illustrated in Figure 2.19 using the tool Maltego.[9] It is also frequently applied in the field of social networks, the World Wide Web (e.g., interconnected by hyperlinks), medical domains, and financial and bibliographic domains.

Example 2.6: Linking Entities in a Drug-Trafficking Case

A case study was conducted that dealt with a drug-trafficking case, as described in Mena (2002). The responsible police department had huge amounts of information available about the crime, but did not have an adequate method for analyzing the links associated with the crime. The solution to this limitation was a web-based application for querying and searching for links within the large amounts of data stored in the database. This gave the investigators a better view of the crime.

---

9 Image courtesy Paterva; for additional information, see https://www.paterva.com/web6/products/maltego
.php.

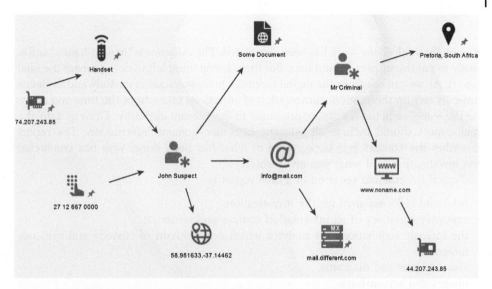

Figure 2.19 Graphical representation of connected entities in digital evidence with Maltego.

2.6 The Presentation Phase

Following the analysis phase, theories have been developed and hypotheses tested. The presentation phase (see Definition 2.8 and Figure 2.20) involves the final documentation and presentation of the results of the investigation to a court of law or other applicable audiences, such as a corporation's top management or crisis management team. The presentation is based on objective findings with a sufficient level of certainty, based on the analysis of digital evidence.

It is important that the findings are summarized and that all actions performed during the investigation are accounted for and described in a fashion understandable by the audience.

Definition 2.8: The Presentation Phase

The process by which the examiner shares results from the analysis phase in the form of reports to the interested party or parties.

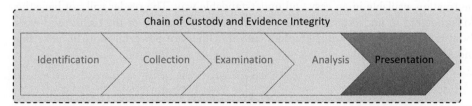

Figure 2.20 The digital forensics process: presentation.

2.6.1   The Final Reports

You might think all the work has been completed. The evidence is "in your hands" and is ready to put the suspect behind bars. But there is one thing left to do – prepare the final report. As we can see from the digital forensics process, chain of custody and evidence integrity rely on thorough documentation of all actions taken from the time you arrive "at the scene" until the results are presented to the relevant authority. To wrap it up, the final report should include all relevant case management information. The report describes the context and background of what has been done, who has conducted the investigation, and what was investigated.

Typical information required in a final report is:

- roles and tasks assigned for the investigation;
- executive summary of all information sources and evidence;
- the forensic acquisition and analysis, which reflect chain of custody and evidence integrity;
- visualizations and diagrams;
- images and screenshots;
- information that supports repeatability or reproducibility of the analysis;
- tools used; and
- findings.

Many digital forensics tools have reporting functionality that documents and summarizes all the interactions that have been carried out. This alone is not enough, especially since you may have used a variety of tools, manual tasks, and analyses during the process. This means that the investigator must be able to prepare this information so that it is understandable to a third party. Ultimately, this is the purpose of the investigation: to present the findings in a clear and understandable manner. It is also important for the report to sufficiently document reproducibility. Given your report of the methods used and the same evidence, a skilled third party should, in principle, be able to reproduce the findings. An example report generated by the digital forensic analysis tool Autopsy is shown in Figure 2.21.[10] The preparation of the final report can be time-consuming, especially for large and long-lasting investigation.

2.6.2   Presentation of Evidence and Work Conducted

A wall of text is no good for anyone. As we saw from the analysis phase of the digital forensics process, visualization techniques are valuable in order to identify patterns and information that are not immediately obvious. Presenting the final report professionally and in a format that is rich with visual aids will make the complex and unstructured information available in an easy and understandable way. The reader will not have the skills required to understand all the technical tasks conducted or the technical details about the evidence. Diagrams, graphics, and timelines are powerful tools to make the findings more accessible.

---

10 Image courtesy of Brian Carrier; for additional information, see www.sleuthkit.org/autopsy.

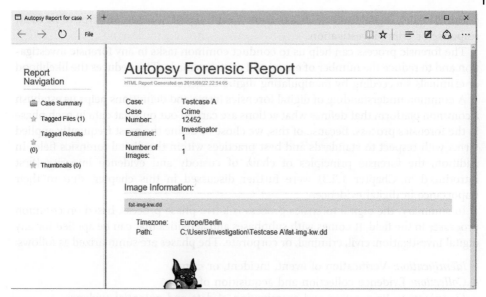

Figure 2.21 Example report generated by Autopsy.

2.6.3 The Chain of Custody Circle Closes

The documented chain of custody is the glue that holds the forensics process together and supports the final evidence integrity so that it can be presented as trustworthy evidence in court. If you have not documented all activities, a court could claim that a critical task did not occur. No matter how carefully the work has been completed, an inability to document the chain of custody for all phases could compromise the trust in the authenticity and integrity of the evidence in court.

The documentation made throughout the digital forensics investigation, together with recommendations and expert testimony, will form the final presentation. The evidence and methods used to find it are presented to a court of law or to a corporate audience (depending on the context of the investigation).

2.7 Summary

In this chapter, we have described the phases, principles applied, and techniques used in the digital forensics investigation process. Understanding the digital scene of the incident, as well as the physical scene, has shown to be crucial for the digital forensics process. The people applying the processes, and the technology supporting them are also fundamental aspects of forensically sound investigations. Examples and scenarios have been presented to emphasize the relevance and importance of having a process to structure the work conducted and the results presented.

Cybercrime has over the last decade evolved and continues to do so. As digitalization is all-encompassing and the Internet is available to both law-abiding actors as well as criminal actors, digital forensics has become a central part of nearly any type of incident response or crime investigation.

The forensic process can help us to conduct common tasks in any forensic investigation and to reduce the number of errors and mistakes made. This reduces the likelihood of criminals succeeding by manipulating digital evidence.

A common understanding of digital forensics terms and definitions helps us establish a common platform that defines what actions are carried out on what data in each phase in the forensics process. Because of this, we chose to define the most frequently applied terms with respect to standards and best practices within the digital forensics field. In addition, the forensic principles of chain of custody and evidence integrity (first introduced in Chapter 1.2.3) were further discussed in this chapter, due to their importance in digital evidence.

In summary, the digital forensics process is a five-phase process, based on common processes in the field. It comes with subphases and activities that can be applied for any digital investigation: civil, criminal, or corporate. The phases are summarized as follows:

- *Identification:* Verification of event, incident, or crime.
- *Collection:* Evidence collection and acquisition of data.
- *Examination:* Preparation and examination of data and potential evidence.
- *Analysis:* Use of scientific methods to determine the facts about an incident or crime (if any) and the significance of the evidence.
- *Presentation:* Documentation and reporting of evidence found.

We would like to note that there are multiple challenges to the forensics process and principles presented. These need to be accounted for through the utilization of tools, processes, and digital forensics research. Adaptation of new technology, ways to communicate online, use of the Internet, shared services, cloud services, the Internet of Things, and big data, together with all the heterogeneous devices, platforms, and technology available, make digital forensics a highly complex undertaking.

Immense amounts of data will challenge the effectiveness of forensic analysis. To complicate matters further, we have seen that Internet crime and cybercrime can rarely be solved by investigators from one country alone. When encryption, obfuscation techniques, and other means are used to complicate analysis, investigators have to be prepared and account for the order of volatility for any given case where data objects are present in multiple digital devices. Finally, errors, uncertainties, and losses associated with evidence recovery give us a more complete picture of the issues that investigators have to deal with.

Even though there are many challenges, they are not insurmountable, and we hope you feel more confident about how an investigation of a digital crime or incident works after reading this chapter.

2.8 Exercises

This section contains a few exercises that touch upon the topics in this chapter. They can be used for reviewing the chapter or as a basis for discussion. The questions do not necessarily have one single correct answer, as the answer might vary with the assumptions made. As an extra challenge to all the questions, one might find it interesting to identify these assumptions and to assess how changing the assumptions might influence the answer.

1   There are five phases in the digital forensics process. List them, and explain what their key activities are.

2   Sometimes it is required to do a dual-tool verification. What does this mean?

3   Provide examples of how errors, uncertainties, and doubt can impact the evidence integrity and forensic soundness.

4   In selected cases, anti-forensics techniques may have been used and lead to a resource-intensive investigation. In what digital forensics process phase would you have to deal with this, and how?

5   Name at least five challenges of digital forensics.

6   A murder has occurred. The victim is identified to be the national chief of defense. Not long afterwards, a security breach in the IT systems of the department of defense is detected. The suspected perpetrator appears to be an outside hacker. What would be your hypothesis, and how would you investigate the case?

7   As part of a drug cartel case, you have been asked to seize all digital devices from one of the potential drug dealers' homes. The "dealer" was caught sitting in the living room, and he was brought to custody. What devices would you look for, and what would you have to consider in order to obtain all evidence relevant to the drug cartel case?

8   What are some of the benefits of investigating incidents in corporate environments, compared to civil cases, where only personal digital devices and services have been used?

9   You are involved in the analysis phase of an investigation of a cyberattack. All potentially relevant data objects have been collected and examined. In order to proceed, what do you need to ensure with regard to the evidence integrity? How will you do this, and why?

10   A bank has registered an incident, and it has been reported to a national financial crime agency in which you are working. Imagine that you, as a digital forensics investigator, are engaged to investigate the online banking fraud case. Describe how you would go about solving the case, finally presenting the evidence to a court of law and to the bank executives.

3

Cybercrime Law

Inger Marie Sunde

Professor, Norwegian Police University College, Oslo, Norway

This chapter explains the fundamentals of cybercrime law. The general starting points are the universal principles of human rights, the rule of law, and the Cybercrime Convention. The chapter explains how the international legal framework links into national legal systems. It does not, however, have *any particular* national legal system in mind. *Specific cases* must always be solved according to the law of the relevant national jurisdiction. This requires familiarity with legal textbooks and primary sources of that jurisdiction. Such information is not provided here.

3.1 Introduction

The expression *cybercrime law* is applied to signify the "legal regulation of digital crime and digital evidence." Crime and evidence are different phenomena governed by different sets of legal rules. Whereas provisions of *substantive criminal law* describe the criminal offenses, rules concerning the collection and use of evidence in criminal investigation and prosecution are laid down in *rules of procedural (criminal) law*.[1] There is a close factual relation between criminal offenses and evidence. The law defines criminal offenses by description of the conditions that the perpetrator must fulfill. Conviction of a crime requires proof beyond any reasonable doubt. The prosecutor has the burden of proof and must prove each condition of the crime(s) included in the criminal charge. Proof is a product of evidence. Importantly, a criminal investigation must keep focus on *legally relevant* conditions, and ensure that the evidence collected *covers them all*. This is, of course, generally important to any digital investigation, in the sense that one should seek for evidence that covers all aspects of the hypothesis that motivates the investigation (see Chapter 1).

The *principle of legality* requires that criminal offenses are laid down (described) in formal legislation on a national level. The legal provision must be in force at the

---

1 Some jurisdictions have a single procedural code that governs both civil and criminal cases, whereas others apply a procedural code for civil cases and a criminal procedural code for criminal cases. For example, the USA, Sweden, and Denmark use single codes, whereas Norway and Germany use different codes.

Digital Forensics, First Edition. Edited by André Årnes.
© 2018 John Wiley & Sons Ltd. Published 2018 by John Wiley & Sons Ltd.

time when the crime was committed. Thus, a criminal offense can be defined as in Definition 3.1.

Definition 3.1: Criminal Offense

A criminal offense is defined by the conditions set out by a provision laid down in formal legislation of the national legal system. The provision must be in force when the crime was committed.

Provisions of substantive criminal law are usually gathered in the criminal code of the national jurisdiction, such as the German Strafgesetzbuch (StGB), the 18 US Code Part I – Crimes (USC), the Norwegian and the Danish Civil Criminal Codes.[2]

Legal competence to investigate, prosecute, and adjudicate is limited to the territory of the nation state.[3] It means that the scope of procedural criminal law is territorially limited. However, the substantive criminal law of a nation state may extend to encompass crimes committed abroad.[4] A nation state always applies its own substantive criminal law provisions, and a wide range of offenses are criminalized regardless of where they are perpetrated. This means that the perpetrator can be prosecuted when she shows up on the territory, (unless there is basis for extradition). As nation states do not extradite their own nationals, the possibility to prosecute crimes committed abroad secures that criminal liability is not evaded by going abroad.

The term *nation state* is formal, often used in relation to matters of sovereignty, such as when entering into an international convention (e.g., the Cybercrime Convention). Usually one can use *state*, *nation*, or *country* instead.

Now, having established some basic legal notions relevant to cybercrime, the chapter continues like this:

- Section 3.2, "The International Legal Framework of Cybercrime Law"
  Main principles of human rights and the rule of law in relation to criminal investigation and prosecution are covered, along with the international legal instruments that specifically address online crime and digital evidence. The principles covered apply to both common law and civil law systems. Importantly, as emphasized in Chapters 1 and 2, skills and knowledge regarding computer forensics and digital investigation are relevant to investigating criminal cases in general, not only "cybercrimes."

---

2 Germany and the USA are federal nations, with formal legislation on both federal and state levels. Legal issues that follow from the interrelation of legislation on different levels are not dealt with here.

3 With respect to legal rules, the old device "no rule without exception" is adequate, and the law of jurisdiction is of course no exception to the rule. Given that this cybercrime chapter is aimed at international students of computer forensics, the main rules are in focus. After all, lawyers spend years to acquire knowledge about the exceptions.

4 The national criminal code (or some other body of formal law) may lay down provisions that determine the scope of substantive criminal law of the national jurisdiction. The Cybercrime Convention addresses the issue in article 22.

Space does not permit a comprehensive description of every international instrument of relevance. The description of the fundamental human rights and the rule of law rests primarily on the European Convention of Human Rights of 4 November 1950 (ECHR).The principles and values are widely recognized, often enshrined in national constitutions regardless of whether the state is party to the convention or not; see for example the US Bill of Rights.[5] Moreover, the convention is unique in that *it has its own court* (the European Court of Human Rights, or ECtHR), which produces extensive case law. The ECHR is thus a dynamic instrument able to take account of the impact of new technology on fundamental rights. In the context of cybercrime law, this point is of particular significance to investigation methods relating to digital evidence.

The ECHR was adopted by the Council of Europe (CoE), "the European continent's leading human rights organization," founded in 1949 (Council of Europe, 2016).[6] The CoE includes 47 member states, all of which are party to the ECHR. The Coe and teh EU should not be confused woth each other. The EU developed as a political union in postwar Europe and currently includes 28 member states.[7] All members of the EU are members of the CoE as well. The EU produces legislation applicable to its member states, and its court, the European Court of Justice (ECJ), interprets EU law, including the Charter of Fundamental Rights of the European Union (the European Charter, 2000/C, 364/01). The ECHR/ECtHR and the European Charter/ECJ form part of distinct legal systems.

As regards the special framework of cybercrime law, the Cybercrime Convention from 2001 remains the most widely recognized international instrument, notwithstanding the technical development over the last decades. The convention was drawn up by the CoE in 2001 (CETS 185) and supplied with an Additional Protocol concerning racist and xenophobic speech in 2003 (CETS 189). Its Explanatory Report provides background information to the provisions, and T-CY Guidance Notes [Cybercrime Convention Committee (T-CY), 2014] explain their application to new forms of digital crime.[8] The convention is open also to accession by nonmember states of the CoE. As per 2016, 49 nation states have ratified, including nonmember states such as Japan, the USA, Australia, and Canada.[9]

---

5 "The first 10 amendments to the [US] Constitution make up the Bill of Rights" (The Bill of Rights Institute, 2016). See https://www.billofrightsinstitute.org/founding-documents/bill-of-rights/k. The information provided above should not be understood to imply that the Bill of Rights has been inspired by the ECHR. To the contrary, the Bill of Rights, adopted in 1791, has strongly influenced human rights law in other parts of the world. This is also the case for the ECHR, which dates from 1950.

6 http://www.coe.int/en/web/about-us/who-we-are.

7 https://europa.eu/european-union/about-eu/eu-in-brief_en.

8 The guidance notes include a preamble that states that they "represent the common understanding of the Parties . . . regarding the use of the Convention." The legal sources mentioned in this section are available on the website of the Treaty Office of the Council of Europe, and related sites that are linked to it. Of particular interest is the *Cybercrime website*, which provides updates about recent initiatives, upcoming conferences, reports by the Cybercrime Convention Committee (T-CY), etc.: http://www.coe.int/en/web/cybercrime/home.

9 The number soared to 49 in 2016, when Israel and Lichtenstein ratified. Six other nations have signed but not yet ratified (Andorra, Greece, Ireland, Monaco, Sweden, and South Africa).

- Section 3.3, "Digital Crime – Substantive Criminal Law"
  The Cybercrime Convention contains a catalog of cybercrime concepts. The number of criminal offenses is limited, only nine in total.[10] One may take the view, though, that the offenses are even more important today, given that digital devices are increasingly widespread and society is increasingly interconnected. Identity infringement (or *ID theft*) emerged as a significant problem after adoption of the convention. Frequently the offense is an integral part of online fraud, and it is described here. The convention permits its parties (states) to rely on their traditional legal concepts, provided certain minimum conditions are fulfilled.
- Section 3.4, "Investigation Methods for Collecting Digital Evidence"
  The Cybercrime Convention describes methods for collecting digital evidence in the course of a criminal investigation. These methods are also applicable to the investigation of crime in general, that is, they are not reserved solely for cybercrimes. Moreover, they are *coercive* and *can be applied in secret*. The methods must fulfill conditions that are compatible with fundamental rights, in order to be lawful. By authorizing lawful application of the methods, states improve the legal framework for international cooperation in criminal investigation of transborder crime. The convention does not regulate the treatment of evidence *after* it has been collected. Treatment of evidence *ex post* is regulated by national procedural rules in light of the *right to fair trial* pursuant to ECHR article 6 (see Sections 3.2.3.8 and 3.2.3.9). The digital forensic process described in Chapter 2 is a *de facto standard* that must be fitted into the legal framework.
- Section 3.5, "International Cooperation in Order to Collect Digital Evidence"
  Due to the territorial limitation of jurisdiction when investigating and prosecuting crime, procedures for international cooperation have been developed. These procedures operate on legal and practical levels, as described in Section 3.5.

3.2 The International Legal Framework of Cybercrime Law

The rules flowing from the international legal framework belong to general and special parts of the law. The general framework concerns the fundamental human rights and the rule of law. The special framework concerns digital crime and digital evidence, and the Cybercrime Convention is the main legal instrument of this framework.

3.2.1 The Individuals Involved in Criminal Activity and in Crime-Preventing Initiatives

The legal framework is relevant both to the individuals involved in criminal activity, and to those engaged in crime prevention initiatives. Crime is committed by individuals, often somewhat vaguely referred to as *criminals*. In procedural terms, such an individual may be a *suspect*; be *charged*; be a *perpetrator, criminal offender, accused,* or *defendant*; or, as the case may be, a *convict*.

---

10 The criminal offenses are set out in articles 2 through 10. Criminalization of racist and xenophobic speech as addressed in the Additional Protocol has not reached the same degree of international consensus, because of differences between national safeguards concerning the freedom of speech.

Professionals conducting criminal investigation, prosecution, and adjudication hold a formal position, such as *criminal investigator, computer forensic expert, public prosecutor,* or *judge.* Except for the judge, they are representatives of *law enforcement agencies.* At the stage of the criminal trial, the roles of the *judge* and the *jury* (laymen) are crucial, in addition to the roles of the public prosecutor and the *defense lawyer.* A third party may become involved by happenstance, for instance a *witness* who noticed the presence of the suspect at an Internet café, or an Internet service provider (ISP) whose service has been used by the suspect. However, a third party may also be engaged pursuant to a formal mandate issued by the aforementioned professionals. One example is an *expert witness* who completes a report pursuant to a formal mandate regarding the analysis of digital evidence, and subsequently testifies in court.

The officials of the police and the public prosecutors form part of the executive branch of the state. The organization and division of powers between the police and the prosecution are particular to each national legal system. This chapter applies the term *law enforcement* in order to encompass both the police and the prosecutors.

The society at large, as well as individual citizens, need protection against crime. There is a tension between the need for protection and the right to be free from injustice and arbitrary interference. The fundamental human rights and the rule of law seek to strike a balance between these competing interests. The legal implications for an individual are quite different, however, depending upon whether she is engaged in criminal activity or performs tasks on behalf of law enforcement or the judiciary. In the former capacity, she is treated as a private individual, whereas in the latter, as a representative of the state. While crime is a *personal responsibility*, criminal investigation, prosecution, and adjudication are *state responsibilities.*

The state must act through *public officials* (servants of the state) and assumes responsibility for their acts. This responsibility also extends to encompass professional private sector forensic experts, insofar as they serve pursuant to a formal mandate by the court or law enforcement. For instance, a digital forensic expert from a global auditing corporation, who undertakes a formal assignment as expert witness in a criminal proceeding, acts on behalf of the state.[11]

3.2.2 The National Legal System versus the International Legal Framework

A national legal system *in its pure form* is an entity separate from rules on the international level. Individuals are subject to the rules of the legal system of the nation where they reside. The rules emanate from a parliament (i.e., the *legislative body*, or *lawmaker*, in democratic societies). A nation state's authority to create binding rules on its citizens is associated with sovereignty. Basically, the state may decide "the law of the land" without taking external considerations.

---

11 National legal systems may permit expert testimony without a formal mandate by the judge or the public prosecutor, for instance adduced by the defense lawyer. Legal responsibility may in this case be different from that described in this section. The present outline concerns *main rules and principles*, so one always has to check the legal regulation of the relevant national jurisdiction.

In practice, national legal systems in pure form do not exist, as mutual interests give rise to international rules that facilitate international order and conduct. This explains why nation states enter into agreements with each other (via *conventions* and *treaties*). The nation state becomes a "party" to a convention or treaty.[12] Agreements between nation states are binding on the state as such, without any direct applicability to individuals. The Cybercrime Convention is an example in point.

Example 3.1: The Binding Effect of the Cybercrime Convention

The Cybercrime Convention is an agreement between states. The parties to the convention must criminalize certain cybercrimes in their national substantive criminal law. Individuals are not parties and cannot be punished for committing the crimes included in the convention, only because the nation state has entered into the convention. For the individual to be criminally liable, the provisions of the convention must first be implemented as criminal offenses in the substantive criminal law of the national legal system where that individual resides.

There is also the option *not* to become party to a convention. The nation state may prefer to adopt legislation similar to the contents of a convention, while retaining the freedom to omit parts it finds unsuitable. It follows that a nation state is free to adopt legislation concerning cybercrime and digital evidence, without having to become party to the Cybercrime Convention. It may, for instance, adopt a criminal provision concerning computer intrusion or a procedural provision concerning computer searches. Indeed, one must assume this is not unusual, given that nation states in all parts of the world have passed cybercrime legislation, but only 49 of them have ratified the Cybercrime Convention.

3.2.3 Fundamental Rights Relating to Cybercrime Law – The ECHR

Every individual is entitled to enjoy the fundamental human rights and protections conferred by the rule of law. Contrary to conventions that are binding on nation states, these rules *give rights to the individual regardless of whether they have been formally implemented in the national legal system or not.* It is widely held that fundamental rights and the rule of law flow from natural law. According to this view, conventions are not necessary in order to *create* such rights, because those rights exist independently of any written legal framework or convention. Still, if nothing else, international legal instruments are at least helpful in *describing* the rights.

The general starting point is the Universal Declaration of Human Rights of 10 December 1947, according to which all human beings are born free and equal in dignity and rights (article 1), and are entitled to fundamental rights and freedoms (article 2). The fundamental rights are *universal* because they apply to every person regardless of age, gender, race, nationality, or domicile. Consequently, also *criminals* have fundamental rights.

---

12 They can be referred to as a *member state, High Contracting State,* and so forth, but *party* suffices.

The United Nations (UN) followed up with two "International Covenants" dated December 16, 1966 (Economic, Social and Cultural Rights; and Civil and Political Rights). Moreover, numerous international instruments have been created, often (1) limited in scope to focus on special topics (e.g., the UN Convention on the Rights of the Child of 1989) or (2) geographically limited to a region [e.g., the African Charter on Human and Peoples' Rights of June 27, 1981, aka the Banjul Charter; the Arab Charter on Human Rights of September 15, 1994; the ASEAN Charter of November 20, 2007, article 1(7), article 2(2)(h)–(j), and article 14; and the European Charter of 2000].

The ECHR stands out as particularly important. Its court, the ECtHR, is of crucial importance for the fundamental rights to be effective in practice. It is also instrumental to the dynamic development of the human rights. The latter point is addressed first.

3.2.3.1 The ECtHR as a Driving Force for Development of Human Rights

The ECtHR constantly produces new case law. Thus, it is a driving force in the development of fundamental rights, including assessing the impact of new technology on those rights (see, e.g., European Court of Human Rights Research Division, 2015).[13] The dynamics carry over to other international instruments, since they often refer to the ECHR.

An example in point is the Cybercrime Convention, which is mindful of "the need to ensure a proper balance between the interests of the law enforcement and respect for fundamental rights as enshrined in the [ECHR]" (preamble, seventh paragraph). According to article 15, which concerns coercive investigation methods for collecting digital evidence, a party has an obligation to "provide for the adequate protection of human rights and liberties, including rights arising pursuant to obligations it has undertaken under the [ECHR]."

The EU has formally recognized ECtHR case law. The European Charter states that its fundamental rights shall be interpreted in light of the ECHR and its case law (preamble, fifth paragraph). For instance, in 2014 the ECJ declared void the so-called *Data Retention Directive* (2006/24/EC), for the reason that its interference with the right to private life was not sufficiently justified. The ECJ reached the result partly by referring to ECHR article 8 and ECtHR case law.[14] However, legal influence goes both ways, as the ECtHR in its interpretative method regularly gives weight to so-called *common positions* among the European states when reaching its decisions, including the positions of the ECJ.

3.2.3.2 The Right to Bring a Case before the ECtHR

First and foremost, the ECtHR provides a means of redress for individuals whose fundamental rights have been violated. A party to the ECHR must abstain from violating fundamental human rights. Moreover, a party has an obligation to secure the fundamental rights for "everyone within [its] jurisdiction" (ECHR article 1). This means that its obligation encompasses all individuals on its territory. In the event that a party allegedly

---

13 Available in English, French, and Russian. http://www.echr.coe.int/Documents/Research_report_Internet_ENG.pdf (English version).
14 Judgment by the ECJ, Grand Chamber of 8 April 2014, paragraphs 35, 47, 54 and 55.

has violated a right covered by the ECHR, the individual may lodge a complaint against the party (nation state) before the ECtHR.[15]

Most European states have been convicted at one time or another for violation of the ECHR. It should not lead one to infer that European national legal systems, in general, largely ignore fundamental human rights. Normally, only a change in law or practice is required to make amends.

An individual cannot bring a complaint before the ECtHR regarding an alleged violation perpetrated by a state that is not a party to the ECHR. For instance, the ECtHR may not assume jurisdiction of a complaint by a US national who claims to have been subject to unlawful search or seizure by the Federal Bureau of Investigation (FBI). She must avail herself of the judicial remedies provided for in the USA, regarding alleged violations of the Fourth Amendment of the Bill of Rights (unreasonable search and seizure).

3.2.3.3 A Special Note on Transborder Search and Surveillance

Global integration in terms of digital networks and services exposes individuals to invasive online investigation methods *by law enforcement agencies of other states.* Assuming that a law enforcement agency of a European country is carrying out a transborder investigation and targets *an individual residing outside Europe*, then the question is whether that individual may bring a complaint before the ECtHR invoking ECHR article 8 (the right to private life).

Absent valid permission from the state in which the individual resides, transborder investigation amounts to a violation of sovereignty. A violation of sovereignty may give rise to a claim by the aggrieved nation state, but not by the individual, and the ECtHR does not hold any jurisdiction in such matters.[16] The individual is also barred from availing herself of the courts in her jurisdiction, because the interference was not caused by anyone working for law enforcement authorities in the state in which she resides. Hence, in order for the right to private life to become effective, the individual certainly has a legitimate need to bring a complaint before the ECtHR. Her access to the court, however, is contingent *that the ECtHR may assume jurisdiction over the case.* The main rule is that the complainant must be residing in Europe in order to have access to the ECtHR. The issue, however, has been assessed by the European Court of Human Rights Research Division (2015), which reasons as follows: The obligation to secure the fundamental rights "within their jurisdiction" (ECHR article 1) cannot be interpreted so as *to authorize* a party to the ECHR to perpetrate violations of the convention in another state. As the right to private life is protected by the ECHR, it is not "*a priori*, out of the question that an act committed in the territory of another State should fall within the '*jurisdiction*' of a [party to the convention] as an 'extraterritorial act.'"

In other words, it is not out of the question that an individual residing in a state that is nonparty to the ECHR, has access to the ECtHR, in the event that she has been targeted by an invasive transborder investigation method that originates from a party to the ECHR.

---

15 The national remedies must have been exhausted by the individual. For instance, that a complaint has been dealt with by the national Supreme Court with negative outcome.

16 Disputes concerning violation of sovereignty are a matter between nation states, which can be brought before the International Court in The Hague. http://www.haguejusticeportal.net/index.php?id=305.

The case *Weber and Saravia v. Germany* deals with the admissibility of a complaint filed by two individuals living in Uruguay, one a German, the other a national of Uruguay.[17] The complaint concerned alleged violation of article 8, due to strategic surveillance (signal intelligence) carried out by Germany. Germany asserted the complaint inadmissible because the complainants were residing outside the jurisdiction (territory) of the ECHR.[18] The complainants asserted that they were entitled to avail themselves of the ECtHR, due to the universality of the fundamental rights, and because one of them was a German national. The ECtHR declared the complaint inadmissible, as "manifestly ill-founded," but not – notably – because of lack of jurisdiction. The reason was that its case law had already settled that Germany's strategic surveillance was lawful. However, the court readily spent 156 paragraphs over 37 pages on two residents of Uruguay, in order to reach a conclusion *that was held to be crystal clear*. If it had been easier to throw the case out of court due to lack of jurisdiction, the solution would probably have been preferred. Thus, the decision may be interpreted so as to leave scope for assuming jurisdiction for extraterritorial acts. The interpretation is supported by the legitimate need for such a remedy, strongly reinforced by the technological development since 2006 when the decision was made.

Internationally the issue, so briefly dealt with here, is highly contested. There are tensions between the need for reasonably effective crime prevention and prosecution, respect for sovereignty, and the need to control the law enforcement in order to prevent abuse of secret investigation methods to the detriment of privacy.

However, the basic – and traditional – main rules are not suited to deal with new matters: (1) a "cyberspace" without borders (problem with territorial jurisdiction). (2) Computer data in the "cloud" as objects of seizure (because they are not precisely "located" in the manner that we are used to for physical objects). (3) Subscribers (suspects) to cloud services offered by foreign corporations may be residents of the state of the law enforcement in charge of the investigation, and so "virtually" be considered to be under its jurisdiction. For example, a UK resident with a Facebook profile is under investigation by UK law enforcement. UK law enforcement may not feel compelled to ask abroad for permission to search the user account of a UK suspect *regardless of who offers the service*. (4) Direct online accessibility to computers worldwide makes traditional procedures for international cooperation impracticable as compared with the freedom enjoyed by criminals to make use of services anywhere. Arguably, the situation features a certain lack of fairness.

Time-consuming cooperation procedures may result in unsuccessful investigations, because evidence (data) located abroad may not be collected within the relevant time frame *or* the data (evidence) was deleted in the meantime. As described in Section 7.5, one may for instance have to trace identity data in several steps in order to identify an online perpetrator. Data loss in one of the links is sufficient to break the chain, resulting in a "cold case." However, many different kinds of interests come into play, and lack of fairness is but one of them. It is also important to take problems of maintaining control with online investigation into account. Ultimately, the rule of law is at stake.

---

17 *Weber and Saravia v. Germany*, decision June 29, 2006, ECtHR (third section).
18 *Ibid.*, paragraph 66.

3.2.3.4 The Connection between Fundamental Rights and the Rule of Law

As a check against the arbitrary exercise of sovereign power, *the law* features prominently in the system of fundamental rights. Fundamental rights cannot arbitrarily be put aside by a power apparatus. Any interference with fundamental rights must be authorized by law. The legislative procedure ensures democratic control of invasive investigation methods. In a democracy, the majority vote shall prevail. Unchecked majority rule, however, can put the minority at risk. In order to prevent abuse, national legislation must live up to certain standards and conditions. Importantly, any interference with the fundamental rights must have a legitimate aim and be necessary in a democratic society. Thus, the fundamental rights and the rule of law go hand in hand. The law is binding on every citizen, including government officials, members of Parliament, members of law enforcement, and judges.

3.2.3.5 The Principle of Legality in the Context of Crime

According to the *principle of legality*, conduct is not criminal unless it is defined as a criminal offense pursuant to legal provisions in the national legal system. The criminal provision must also have entered into force (ECHR article 7).[19]

Legal Provision 3.1: No Punishment without Law

"No one shall be held guilty of any criminal offence on account of any act or omission which did not constitute a criminal offence under national . . . law at the time when it was committed."

ECHR, article 7 (excerpt)

Crime and criminal policy attract media attention. With respect to criminal liability in the case of an incident, the distinction between the *law in force* as opposed to the *law as it ought to be* is crucial. Often the focal point of public debate is *legal policy*, for instance illustrated by the proposition that "cybercrime is a byproduct of new technology." If it refers to conduct that *ought to be punishable*, then the issue concerns the need for *new criminal provisions* in order to punish new phenomena enabled by new technology. If the issue instead concerns *conduct that is criminal*, then it is simply implied – or taken for granted – that the *law in force* makes cybercrime illegal and punishable.[20]

The law in force shall be clear, stable, and accessible. The notion of crime rests on the concepts of morality and choice, which presuppose that the individual is able to foresee and comprehend the limits of the law. The rationale entails that provisions of criminal

---

19 The principle is also laid down in the UN Declaration article 11; the International Covenant on Civil and Political Rights article 15; and the European Charter article 49.

20 The distinction between future and existing law is marked by the terms *de lege ferenda* (future law) and *de lege lata* (existing law).

One should be aware that "old" provisions may be applicable to online crime. A phenomenon that is new due to new technology is not per definition new in a legal sense. The applicability depends on interpretation of the national criminal provisions (see Section 3.2.5.2).

law must be of such good quality that the citizens, in the due course of normal life, do not easily run the risk of overstepping the legal limits. However, questions regarding interpretation of substantive criminal law invariably arise; see Example 3.2.

Example 3.2: The Blog Case

A Norwegian male was arrested for having urged the murder of two police officers in a blogpost. Utterance "in public" of such content is criminal pursuant to the Norwegian criminal code, and the police petitioned the local court for permission to keep him detained. Dispute arose regarding the interpretation of "in public." The Supreme Court concluded that a blogpost could not be regarded as made in public within the meaning of the criminal code (dissent 2–1). The interpretation required *simultaneous exposure* of the blogpost to a large number of people, while Internet technology only provides for *individual* connection. Hence, he had to be let go. Had the court concluded in the opposite (which arguably was an option, given the dissent), the act would have been criminal and the blogger detained. The blogger was probably just as surprised by the outcome as many others. He had in fact succeeded in his efforts to reach out to a large number of people as thousands had visited the blog. The law was amended shortly afterward in order to comprise blogposts and other modes of speech in public on the Internet.

HR-2012-1554-U

Due to the legislator's efforts to provide for clear legal provisions, paired with the importance of foreseeability, the *exact wording of the criminal provisions* weighs heavily as a legal source of interpretation (see Section 3.2.5.1). This is one of the reasons why the text of many laws is quite complex; it is an attempt to *precisely* specify what is criminal behavior.

3.2.3.6 The Principle of Legality in the Context of a Criminal Investigation

Methods for securing digital evidence during a criminal investigation frequently interfere with the *right to private life* (ECHR article 8(1)). The coercive investigation methods mentioned in the Cybercrime Convention are cases in point. An investigation method is regarded as *coercive* if it interferes with the right to private life, liberty, or property rights, *and* can be applied without the consent or cooperation of the individual who is subject to it.[21] Thus, it can be defined as in Definition 3.2.

Definition 3.2: Coercive Investigation Method

An investigation method is coercive when it lawfully can be applied against an individual without her consent or cooperation, despite that her right to personal liberty, property, or private life is interfered with.

---

21 Protection of liberty is laid down in by ECHR article 5. Protection of property rights is laid down in article 1 of the Protocol from 1952 to the ECHR.

The coercive investigation methods mentioned in the Cybercrime Convention are search and seizure of computer systems (online and physical), interception of electronic transmissions, real-time collection of traffic data, and production orders regarding traffic data (e.g., an ISP that is ordered to expose a person's usage of electronic communication services). The convention does not mention computer surveillance, which nevertheless belongs in the same category.

Given that the ECJ declared void the Data Retention Directive (Section 3.2.3.1) and data protection falls within the scope of article 8, then a *preservation order* concerning *personal data* must be deemed to constitute an interference with article 8 (see Harris *et al.*, 2009, p. 412). The Cybercrime Convention, however, does not limit a preservation order to personal data (article 16), and insofar as an order concerns other data, an interference with article 8 is not clear. Rather, it may interfere with *property rights* protected by article 1 of the 1952 Protocol to the ECHR. Still, legal basis is necessary.

Essentially, a criminal investigation is all about collecting information that can shed light on a suspect's identity, whereabouts, and motive (remember 5WH in Definition 1.4); hence, privacy is always at stake. However, the right to private life is not interfered with, when personal information is given out freely and voluntarily. For instance, a celebrity who blogs about her personal life does not have her privacy interfered with because a police investigator follows the blog. Having said that, one should note that *data protection rules* are always applicable to *storage and use* of personal data by a law enforcement agency, regardless of whether the data is collected from publicly accessible websites or from other sources. Data protection rules are not addressed here.

The scope for carrying out coercive investigation methods *pursuant to consent* is very limited. A valid consent must be free and voluntary. The pressure, sense of surprise, and powerlessness that a criminal investigation may bring about give reason to doubt that consent was actually voluntary, particularly when obtained from the suspect.

Generally, for the above-mentioned methods to be lawfully applied, conditions concerning *legitimate aim*, *legal basis*, and *proportionality* must be fulfilled (ECHR article 8(2)).

Legal Provision 3.2: The Right to Respect for Private life

1) "Everyone has the right to respect for his private and family life, his home and his correspondence.
2) There shall be no interference by a public authority with the exercise of this right except such as is in accordance with the law and is necessary in a democratic society in the interest of . . . the prevention or disorder of . . . crime . . . , or for the protection of the rights and freedoms of others."

The ECHR article 8 (excerpt)

Crime prevention, investigation, and prosecution are *legitimate aims*, so the aim is not an issue. The condition "in accordance with the law" concerns the legal basis for the application of a coercive method. It requires that the method is adequately described and authorized in national legislation. This is the *procedural aspect of the principle of legality, in casu* protecting the individual from arbitrary interference with the right to respect for private life.

Example 3.3: Computer Search "in Accordance with the Law"

The Cybercrime Convention article 19 confers an obligation on the nation state to authorize computer search as an investigation method. In order to comply with the principle of legality, the national legal system must authorize the method in its procedural law in concordance with its formal legislative procedure. The mere act of entering into the convention does not fulfill the legality requirement (unless it follows from national legislation that the text of the convention operates directly as part of the body of national legislation, as per ratification).

The condition "necessary in a democratic society" concerns necessity and proportionality, and it is closely linked to the aforementioned conditions. The legislator, law enforcement agencies, and courts must demonstrate necessity and proportionality. The *legislator* must show that the *method is necessary*, taking into account the suitability (or shortcomings) of other methods available in the legal system. Moreover, legal conditions and safeguards must secure against the risk that legally authorized methods are applied when necessity and proportionality are not present. For instance, invasive secret methods such as computer surveillance and interception of communication must be restricted to serious crime. When petitioning for permission to use the methods in the investigation of a crime, law enforcement must also show that other less intrusive methods are not suitable, and that the interference is not disproportionate in relation to the aim sought to achieve. For example, in light of the circumstances, granting permission to intercept 10 cellphone numbers for 4 weeks may be deemed disproportionate, but interception of 7 numbers for 2 weeks may be acceptable.

Finally, the case law of the ECtHR has established that inherent in article 8(2) are conditions relating to the rule of law. Thus, legal guarantees and safeguards that prevent arbitrary or massive indiscriminate use must be in place.[22] Independent judicial review *ex ante* is crucial. In addition, independent *ex post* control is required for methods that are *used in secret*. For this purpose, national oversight or control committees may be established.

3.2.3.7 The Positive Obligation of the Nation State

As fundamental rights, including the rule of law, are placed on top of the hierarchy of norms, they cannot be suppressed, declared invalid or otherwise be made ineffective by provisions in national law. Moreover, the nation state has *a positive obligation* to "secure" the fundamental rights "to everyone within their jurisdiction" (ECHR article 1). It is not sufficient for national law merely to *recognize* fundamental rights, nor is it sufficient that the state merely *abstains* from unlawful interference. A party to the ECHR

---

22 In a judgement against Bulgaria, the ECtHR commented that "the system of secret surveillance in Bulgaria is, to say the least, overused, which may in part be due to the inadequate safeguards which the law provides." *Association for European Integration and Human Rights and Ekimdzhiev v. Bulgaria*, June 28, 2007 (paragraph 92).

must also – within reasonable limits – *actively make an effort* to ensure that the rights become effective in practice.[23] This positive obligation requires the nation state to initiate effective protective measures, in both the legal and practical sense.

Example 3.4: The Positive Obligation to Provide Subscriber Information

A complaint against Finland was brought before the ECtHR, for alleged breach of the obligation to secure the right to private life of a 12-year-old boy (the complainant). An unknown person had posted an email on a website in the complainant's name, also providing his home address and telephone number. The email indicated that the boy was interested in engaging in sexual activities with adults. The unlawful publication interfered with the boy's right to private life. Pursuant to Finnish law, the act was a "misdemeanor," and not of a sufficiently serious nature to lift the duty of confidentiality with respect to electronic communications in order to inform the police of the subscriber's identity. Legal priority was thus given to the subscriber's right to privacy, at the expense of the victim's need for protection and redress. The ECtHR found that the crime was *serious* despite that national criminal law defined it as a misdemeanor. Finnish law did not adequately protect the boy's right to respect for private life, on account of the absolute character of the confidentiality rule. The ECtHR held that Finland had violated the positive obligation to *actively* protect a victim's right to private life. Finland consequently had to amend its confidentiality rules.[24]

K.U. v. Finland, **judgment 2 December 2008**

3.2.3.8 The Right to Fair Trial

The *right to fair trial* is a bundle of rights enshrined in article 6 of the ECHR. The Due Process Clause in the Fifth Amendment of the US Bill of Rights is a conceptual counterpart.

Legal Provision 3.3: The Right to Fair Trial

1) "In the determination of . . . any criminal charge against him, everyone is entitled to a fair and public hearing within a reasonable time by an independent and impartial tribunal established by law. . . .
2) Everyone charged with a criminal offence shall be presumed innocent until proved guilty according to law.
3) Everyone charged with a criminal offence has the following minimum rights:
   a) [Prompt information] of the nature and cause of the accusation against him;

---

23 The positive obligation does not go so far as to constitute "an impossible or disproportionate burden'" *Osman v. U.K.*, judgment October 28, 1998 (paragraph 116).

24 See also the case of *Söderman v. Sweden*, judgment (Grand Chamber) November 12, 2013, regarding secret video recording of a 14-year-old stepdaughter in the shower, where Sweden's criminal law was regarded as too weak to provide for effective punishment and thus lacked the protective effect required by article 8(1); and *M.C. v. Bulgaria*, judgment December 4, 2003, concerning the "date rape" of a minor. The law enforcement had not fulfilled the positive obligation to conduct an effective investigation, partly due to lack of understanding of the seriousness of this kind of crime.

b) To have adequate time and facilities for the preparation of his defense;
c) To defend himself in person or through legal assistance of his own choosing . . . ;
d) [Right to examine witnesses];
e) [Right to interpretation]."

ECHR article 6 (excerpt)

A procedural guarantee: Fair trial is a procedural guarantee. The ECtHR does not review the merits of a specific case (its substance), but there is no rule without exception. The court has also found against the state because the national judgment, according to the merits of the case, was "arbitrary or manifestly unreasonable" or "grossly arbitrary" (Harris *et al.*, 2009, p. 202). The crucial point is whether the procedural guarantees and safeguards enshrined in article 6 *have been made available* to the defendant. For instance, should a defendant choose not to appoint a defense lawyer, it is her risk, not a matter for article 6(3)(c).

The procedural system as a whole: Article 6 permits the state a wide scope – a wide *margin of appreciation* – to decide the manner in which its courts shall operate. Thus, both common law and civil law systems are compatible with article 6. Differences between national legal systems, for instance regarding evidence rules (addressed below), are not *per se* relevant to article 6. Another example is the differences in the distribution of procedural powers between the professionals involved in criminal investigation and prosecution. Whereas some procedural systems apply a strict division between the criminal investigators and the public prosecutors, others provide for more integrated work models. Some systems confer powers on the magistrate court to order a criminal investigation and to issue criminal charges, while other systems leave this to the public prosecutor and, to some extent, the police. Such differences do not imply that one system is "better" than the others in relation to article 6. Fair trial is concerned with the *system as a whole*. The assessment of an alleged violation of the right to fair trial takes into consideration the guarantees and safeguards provided by the national procedural system, and determines whether the procedural safeguards stemming from article 6 have been complied with, all things considered.

The criminal charge: The right to fair trial is activated once the individual is subject to a criminal *charge* [article 6(2)]. An individual is *charged* when this is formally declared to her; when she is subjected to a criminal investigation *directed at her as a suspect* [even if this has not (yet) been formally declared to her]; and, also when *coercive measures* are applied against her.

A right to trial within reasonable time: The criminal proceedings (trial) must be performed within *reasonable time* from the time that the charge originated [article 6(1)]. Law enforcement agencies are prevented from gaining extra investigation time by deliberately delaying the formal charge, as "charged" is an *autonomous concept* under article 6. It means that the ECtHR determines the charge's point in time, as per the guidelines of case law. This determination is not bound by the formal date that has been set by the national system in question (see Harris *et al.*, 2009, p. 208).

However, the circumstances of the case are relevant to the legal assessment as well. For instance, it matters whether the amount of evidence is large and/or must be obtained from abroad, or is more readily available. In the former instance, a longer time span is accepted as "reasonable" than in the latter. This point is *highly relevant to digital evidence*, as the amount of potential evidence can be massive ("big data"), and the evidence frequently must be obtained by international cooperation (see Section 3.5). The legal assessment, however, must also consider whether the investigation was sufficiently focused and reasonably delimited in light of the seriousness of the crime. Thus, an effort to limit the volume of the data secured in the collection phase of the digital forensic process, is important, in addition to having a plan for the treatment in the subsequent phases of examination and analysis (the phases are dealt with in Sections 2.4 and 2.5). Finally, *time not accounted for* is always a liability in a criminal investigation. If a case has been left unattended without any external cause for the delay, then the limits for reasonable time are easily overstepped. The suspect shall not be burdened by the law enforcement agency's lack of efficiency or problems with prioritization of resources. Ultimately, it is the responsibility of a government to ensure that its law enforcement agencies are suitably organized and equipped in order to carry out the duties against crime in a modern society.

The presumption of innocence and the burden of proof. An individual "charged with a criminal offence" has a right to be presumed innocent *until proved guilty according to law* [article 6(2)]. At trial, the presumption of innocence is safeguarded by placing *the burden of proof* on the public prosecutor. The burden of proof is only fulfilled if guilt has been proved *beyond any reasonable doubt*. Proof beyond any reasonable doubt is a condition regarding the *strength* of the evidence, and is assessed according to its reliability, robustness, and plausibility. Methods for assessing evidence by application of specific criteria for reliability, robustness, and plausibility comprise a distinct research field. The international student may take *Fischer's Techniques of Crime Scene Investigation*, 1st intl. ed. (Tilstone *et al.*, 2013, chapters 1 and 2), as an introduction to the topic. In a Scandinavian context, the works of the professors Christian Diesen (Stockholm University, Sweden) and Eivind Kolflaath (Bergen University, Norway) have contributed to methods for assessing evidence in criminal cases. Specifically, as regards digital evidence and the risk of errors, Ekfeldt (2016) is a recent contribution ("Om informationstekniskt bevis").

Each condition of the criminal provision(s) included in the criminal charge must be proved beyond any reasonable doubt; see Example 3.5, which should be read with the 5WHs in mind (see Definition 1.4).

Example 3.5: Conditions to Be Proved in Relation to Computer Intrusion

A Danish criminal court is going to try a criminal charge concerning illegal access to a computer system. The criminal charge is issued pursuant to the Danish Criminal Code § 263(2).[25] The following conditions must be proved beyond any reasonable doubt:

- That access to "information or programs designated for use in an information system" was obtained.

---

25 Section 263(2) of the Danish criminal code is cited in Example 3.6.

- That the access was unlawful ("unlawfully obtains").
- That the defendant did it. If the access is traced back to the defendant's computer, it must also be proved that the defendant actually used the computer at the critical moment for the criminal purpose. Depending on the circumstances, proof may be established by ruling out all other possibilities (remember that doubt must be "reasonable"). This can also rebut a claim that somebody else used the defendant's computer as intermediary in order to conceal the traces (the Trojan defense; see Brenner *et al.*, 2004).[26]
- That the defendant at the time when access was gained *realized* that she accessed information or programs as mentioned, and that the access was unlawful to her.

In the course of a criminal investigation, people who turn out to be innocent may have been charged. Moreover, third parties not suspected of a crime may endure search and seizure or other measures necessary to secure evidence (they have *witness* status). The presumption of innocence does not prevent such incidents in an investigation. However, a faulty charge may incur liability to pay damages. In addition, those in charge of the investigation have an obligation to limit any interference with the situation of third parties as much as possible. This point is further developed in the context of the Cybercrime Convention, article 15 (Section 3.4.3.4).

The principle of objectivity: An investigation performed in a prejudiced, biased, or otherwise faulty manner entails a risk of wrongful conviction (miscarriage of justice). Requirements as to the impartiality of the court are expressed in article 6(1), with no mention of the investigation. However, safeguards concerning *contradiction* and *equality of arms* operate, at least indirectly, to secure objectivity and quality regarding the investigation (article 6(3)(c)(d) and (e)). This is supported by the right to be presumed innocent, which is activated once the suspect is criminally charged. Thus, *the investigation must be conducted in an impartial and unbiased manner that ensures sufficient quality in the investigative steps*. Routinely, there is a need to proceed with several working hypotheses at the same time, before narrowing down the scope of the investigation to a single hypothesis and, finally, concluding by issuing formal criminal charges (or dropping the case).[27]

It is essential that all steps that have been performed in the course of the investigation *must be documented in the case file*. The need for *detailed documentation produced close in time* with the actual investigative step is also emphasized in relation to the digital forensic process. Thus, by adhering to the process, fundamental principles of procedural criminal law are actively supported. The defendant and the defense lawyer are entitled to examine the documents, a right that is indispensable to a proper defense. Evidence that is not disclosed in the file may normally not be adduced at trial, as the defense cannot be properly prepared. Material omissions of this kind may also call into doubt the overall quality of the investigation, and whether the objectivity standard has been fulfilled. This

---

26 The defendant claims that she mistakenly has been criminally charged, and that the real perpetrator is an unknown third party who, by hacking the computer, brought the defendant in the fry. It is a variant of the SODDI defense ("Some Other Dude Did It").

27 Again, have a look at the 5WH in Chapter 1.

in turn may lead to the conclusion that proof beyond any reasonable doubt is not established. Hence, the defendant is acquitted.

However, people are not perfect, nor are criminal forensic investigators or experts. The law takes a realistic approach to this fact. In the event of a mistake, for instance an unintended deviation from a standard forensic procedure, the significant point is to *disclose the exact treatment of the evidence in reports included in the case documents.* Either that, or omit the evidence. Then it is for the defense lawyer and the court to assess the significance of the mistake. If it does not materially affect the reliability of the evidence, then the mistake may not be legally significant.

Unlawful conduct in relation to methods for securing digital evidence raises the question whether the evidence must be excluded from trial. Exclusion can be justified for preventive and restorative reasons; first, as a disincentive to unlawful conduct, and, second, in order to discontinue the violation of the individual's rights. Whether exclusion will be the final outcome depends upon the circumstances in light of national procedural rules and the case law of the ECtHR. Again, disclosure of the digital investigation steps, including any mistakes made, is important to the outcome. If the evidence is reliable, perhaps supported by other evidence, it may generally be adduced according to the fair trial doctrine. The ECtHR has also accepted unlawfully obtained evidence, which stood alone, on the ground that it was reliable and there was no reason to doubt its authenticity.[28] Conversely, the doctrine of "the fruits of the poisonous tree," developed in relation to the Fourth Amendment of the US Bill of Rights, may regularly declare evidence obtained by unreasonable search and seizure inadmissible, that is, provided the evidence is adduced against a defendant who was victim of such unlawful conduct (Hubbart, 2005, s. 341 et seq.).

3.2.3.9 A Special Note on Evidence Rules in Different Legal Systems

Common law systems adhere to the *admissibility principle* regarding evidence, which means that the *right to adduce the evidence* must be justified. Conversely, in the civil law system, *exclusion of the evidence* must be justified. Despite the difference, both systems are acceptable to the ECHR article 6. What matters is whether the procedural guarantees laid down in article 6 are complied with, not *how* this is achieved.

Some procedures have established themselves as *de facto standards* within the international community of digital forensic investigators and experts (see Chapters 2 and 4). Generally, they must be considered as *guidelines* (*soft law*), the relevance of which is determined according to national procedural law. A variety of situations can be imagined: (1) that the guideline is found to be relevant in order to illuminate a contested procedural issue that is open for interpretation; (2) that the guideline is superfluous because the procedures are already laid down, wholly or partly, in national procedural rules; and (3) that the guideline is dismissed as wholly irrelevant to national law. However, the material issue is, first and foremost, whether the steps of the forensic procedure *exactly as they were actually carried out* have been documented in the case file and disclosed to the defendant and the defense lawyer.

This point is also valid in relation to the *Daubert standard* (or *principle*) regarding expert testimony. The *Daubert standard* in US procedural doctrine is, of course, relevant to criminal trials that take place in the USA. Other jurisdictions, however, apply their

---

28 *Khan v. U.K.*, judgment May 12, 2000.

own national rules regarding expert witnesses. Assuming the *Daubert standard* has established itself as a *de facto standard* within the international forensic community, its legal relevance is the same as for the guidelines mentioned above.

3.2.3.10 Possible Outcomes of a Violation of Fundamental Rights

The nation state is responsible for violations of the fundamental rights. The ECtHR as last resort has competence to declare that the nation state has violated the ECHR. The result may be that a judgment of the national court, for instance a conviction of a crime, is voided. The nation state can also be liable to pay damages (compensation) to the individual and have to implement more effective legal and practical measures for the preservation of the rights that were found to have been violated. The individual who acts in the capacity of a state official is of course responsible for her conduct, but she is not responsible for flaws in national law. Hence, if she has acted in accordance with national law, and the law is flawed, the nation state is responsible. Should she act unlawfully as judged by national law, then a whole range of legal outcomes may be possible, such as criminal liability for deliberate material misconduct, forfeiture of professional position, payment of damages, rebuke, or a mild warning.

3.2.4 Special Legal Framework: The Cybercrime Convention

The Cybercrime Convention is divided in three main parts: (1) a catalog of cybercrimes; (2) a catalog of methods for collecting digital evidence; and (3) international cooperation with respect to collection and exchange of digital evidence.[29]

The convention sets minimum obligations for its parties. Each party must take steps to ensure that their national legal provisions actually criminalize the offenses described in the convention, and that the methods for securing digital evidence are duly authorized. The part concerning international cooperation supports mechanisms and procedures that primarily have developed through other international instruments (see Section 3.5).

Initiatives to counteract cybercrime have also been taken on the EU level, notably by the adoption of the (1) Directive on attacks against information systems (2013/40/EU), and (2) Directive on combating the sexual abuse and sexual exploitation of children and child pornography (2011/92/EU).[30]

Moreover, the UN Convention on the Rights of the Child (1989) is relevant to the issue of online child sexual abuse, especially its Optional Protocol on the sale of children, child prostitution, and child pornography (2000). The Optional Protocol is particularly concerned with Internet-facilitated sexual violence against children (preamble, sixth paragraph). The European Convention from 2007 on the protection of children against sexual exploitation and sexual abuse (CETS 201) should also be mentioned in this context. As previously noted, the contemporary era of globalization and interdependence makes it rational for nation states to enter into such conventions. The backdrop of the Cybercrime Convention is that an individual nation state is incapable of unilaterally protecting its citizens against hazards that originate from abroad through the Internet. Furthermore, states do not extradite their own nationals. Consequently, a "victim state" (State A) needs assurance that the attack will be investigated and

---

29 Formal details about the convention are provided in the introduction of this chapter.
30 The directives replace the Council Framework Decision 2005/222/JHA and 2004/68/JHA.

prosecuted by the "origin state" (State B). The victim state can only reasonably expect aid if it offers reciprocity. Essentially, State A has to *express its sincere willingness to prosecute criminals* who victimize citizens of State B, in order to provide an incentive for State B to prosecute the criminals who have harmed citizens in State A.

Moreover, law enforcement agencies of a nation state may need to collect evidence located outside its borders. The situation also applies to investigations where the law enforcement agencies of the state that will try the case have succeeded in catching the criminal. To understand the necessity of such an arrangement, one only needs to consider the crucial significance of information held by big social media providers (Facebook, Google, etc.). According to principles of international law, the authority of a law enforcement agency to carry out an investigation is limited to the territory of that agency's state. Therefore, law enforcement agencies must cooperate internationally in order to secure and exchange evidence. International cooperation procedures are created by entering into conventions such as the Cybercrime Convention. The Cybercrime Convention seeks to harmonize the contents of cybercrime law on a national level. The catalog of cybercrimes and coercive investigation methods included in the convention serves this purpose. The harmonizing effect should not be overestimated, however. Every national legal system has its traditions and peculiarities. The precise content of an individual nation's criminal laws would still differ, even if all parties made an effort to implement the convention in a literal manner. Nevertheless, implementation of cybercrime law clearly reduces the number of "safe havens" for criminals. Example 3.6 shows some examples of national implementation of the Cybercrime Convention article 2.

Example 3.6: National Implementation of the Cybercrime Convention, Article 2

The Cybercrime Convention article 2: Illegal Access: "Access to the whole or any part of a computer system without right." Optional conditions: "that the offence be committed"

- "by infringing security measures;
- "with the intent of obtaining computer data or other dishonest intent"; or
- "in relation to a computer system that is connected to another computer system."

The USC 1030 18 § 1030 (a)(2)(c): "Whoever intentionally accesses a computer without authorization or exceeds authorized access, and thereby obtains information from a protected computer."

The German criminal code, StGB § 202a(1) Ausspähen von Daten: "Wer unbefugt sich oder einem anderen Zugang zu Daten, die nicht für ihn bestimmt und die gegen unberechtigten Zugang besonders gesichert sind, unter Überwindung der Zugangssicherung verschafft, wird mit Freiheitsstrafe bis zu drei Jahren oder mit Geldstrafe bestraft."

The Norwegian criminal code § 204: Computer intrusion: "Anyone who gains access to a computer system or part of it, by infringing security measures or by other method without right, shall be liable to punishment with a fine or imprisonment for a term up to 2 years."[31]

---

31 Author's translation from Norwegian.

> *The Danish criminal code § 263(2)*: "Any person who unlawfully obtains access to another person's information or programmes designated for use in an information system shall be liable to a fine or to imprisonment for any term not exceeding one year and six months" (cited from Gudmundsdottir, 2015).

Today most crimes involve digital technology. Traditional crime has gone online and developed into "crime-as-a-service." Internet fraud is widespread. Online marketplaces for illegal trade in drugs and weapons, the sale of stolen information or goods (fencing), and the use of online casinos for money laundering are well documented in Chapter 3 in Europol (2014, 2015). Moreover, sexual violations are frequently video recorded on smartphones and distributed, if not committed on demand in front of a web camera. Thus, Europol emphatically claims that "all crime is cybercrime," pointing out the need for being "in the mind frame of thinking 'digital' first." It further notices that "given the continued [technical] development . . . it will be increasingly difficult for digital trace evidence to be entirely removed from the crime scene" (Europol, 2014, p. 84).

The current slogan "Internet is everything" is an eye-opener for the fact that also physical crime may be committed by digital means. It is conceivable that a homicide might be committed by tampering with the Internet connection of a pacemaker. Moreover, organized criminals may prepare burglary by hacking the computer system of a remote door-lock service provider (or the computer system of the host of the door-lock service provider), and disable the entrance locks of a neighborhood (for more elaboration on this point, see Sunde, 2016).

Regardless of whether the crime is considered as "technical" or "physical," digital evidence is regularly available. Email communications and traffic and geolocation data may, for instance, prove that a murder was planned and not – as asserted by the defendant – an act of self-defense. Such evidence may be pivotal, determining whether the outcome be an acquittal or levying the maximum penalty (see Example 3.7).

Example 3.7: Planned Murder or Assisted Suicide?

In a Norwegian case from 2015, the court found a husband guilty of homicide and rape of his wife. The couple had two small children. He admitted to having killed her, but claimed that, as she had not wanted to live anymore, he had assisted her pursuant to her request. Assisted suicide is a crime considered leniently, whereas planned homicide may entail incarceration for 21 years. The investigation uncovered email, Internet logs, and traffic and geolocation data. The digital evidence showed that she had wanted to leave her husband and start over again with a man in Germany. Steps had been taken to rent an apartment for this purpose. Evidently, she had not had any wish to die. Moreover, contrary to the husband's explanation, the digital evidence showed that the murder was planned over time and that he had prepared for it by buying several items needed in order to wrap, strap, and get rid of the corpse. There was no evidence to support that the wife had been aware of, consented to, or participated in the preparations. Her plastic-wrapped body was finally located on the seabed of a fjord. The court sentenced the husband to maximum penalty.

LG-2015-1010

The general importance of digital evidence to criminal investigation and prosecution has been noted in the convention's article 14(2)(c) and article 23. The procedural part of the convention is therefore generally relevant to the investigation of crime.

The UN *Comprehensive Study of Cybercrime* (UNODC, 2013) makes a corresponding observation. The study provides a global overview of common measures and solutions for the purpose of examining options "to strengthen existing and to propose new national and international legal or other responses to cybercrime."

The introduction of the study includes the following statement: "While the Study is, by title, a study on 'cybercrime', it has unique relevance for *all* crimes. As the world moves into a hyper-connected society with universal Internet access, it is hard to imagine a 'computer crime', and perhaps any crime, that will not involve electronic evidence linked with Internet connectivity. Such developments may well require fundamental changes in law enforcement approach, evidence gathering, and mechanisms of international cooperation in criminal matters."[32]

3.2.5 Interpretation of Cybercrime Law

An individual may be criminally liable provided there is sufficient basis for such a finding in substantive criminal law. The judge's application of the law requires interpretation. Interpretation begins with an effort to discern the meaning of the words of the criminal provision. Other legal sources may be relevant as supplements; for instance, preparatory works, the case law of the national jurisdiction, the legal provision's purpose, and the interest in reaching a result that is reasonable and coheres with other provisions of the code.

3.2.5.1 Interpretation of Substantive Criminal Law

The *words* of criminal provisions weigh heavily as source of interpretation. Words can be vague and have several meanings (ambiguity). *Vagueness* implies that a word lacks a definite meaning. The word *object* has caused problems in this respect. While it clearly comprises physical objects, objections have been raised against its applicability to computer data. The question is relevant to interpretation of provisions regarding theft, embezzlement, vandalism, and unlawful use, which often include the word *object* or synonyms such as *thing*.[33] Implementation of article 4 of the Cybercrime Convention (data interference) eliminates the problem as regards the act of vandalism, but not for other offenses. The question is also relevant to confiscation of computer files and filtering of illegal digital content (Sunde, 2010). The legal solution, however, is contingent on the rules of national law.

In *digital forensics*, treating computer data as an "object" seems uncontroversial. As discussed in Section 1.2.2, the conceptual distinction between a *digital device, digital media,* and *digital data* entails that digital data stored on a given medium is a *discrete collection* that is treated as a *digital object* (Carrier flatly says, "Digital evidence is a digital object," in Carrier, 2010, p. 4). This is no different from the manner in which we think of

---

32 At the time of writing, the UN has requested feedback and proposals for initiatives to improve the study in order to publish a final version at a later point in time.

33 Translations in German: *Gegenstand/Ding*; Norwegian: *Objekt/Gjenstand/Ting*; and Swedish: *Sak/Föremål/Ting*.

physical objects. We do not talk of atoms in general, but of objects (made of atoms) that have been identified and specified. Similarly, when we mean data as an object, we do not mean data in general, but data stored on a specified digital medium. Through the relation with the medium, the data is individualized and amounts in aggregate to a specific digital object. Interestingly, and as a final observation, the approach taken in *procedural criminal law* is pragmatic, thus merely adapting the traditional concepts of search and seizure to computer data (Section 3.4.4). It means that, procedurally, a discrete collection of digital data is an object.

Perception of the phenomenon is at least as important to the application of a rule as *interpretation* in light of legal sources. *Description and explanation* form perception. It makes a difference whether computer data is described as "invisible" and "ephemeral" or as follows: "In YAFFS, everything in the file system is an object. An object can, for example, be a file, a directory, a link (both hard and soft), a pipe, or a device. Each object has its own unique Object ID" (see Section 6.3.6). In contrast to the former, the latter description prepares the ground for a perception of computer data as an object with evidentiary significance. Thus, one cannot entirely rule out the possibility that the problem in substantive criminal law is caused by inadequate *description of fact* rather than difficulties with *legal interpretation*.

Another example of vagueness concerns the concept of a "computer system." The definition set out in the Cybercrime Convention article 1(a), does not solve the following problem: how to distinguish a computer system from a network? Earlier, a computer system was a "box" with a clearly delimited perimeter. Today, the computer system of a corporation with a large number of employees may be accessible over a VPN from anywhere, no different from access gained from work stations on its premises. The distributed character of computer systems makes the distinction between a network and a computer system hard to determine. "The Internet is everything" adds to the problem. Thus, it may be difficult to determine the scope of the criminal provision for *illegal access* and for *illegal interception*, respectively. The recurring point is that national law provides the answer. In relation to the Cybercrime Convention, what matters is that both access and interception, without a legal right to do so, are criminal offenses. National legal provisions may clarify the distinction between computer systems and electronic networks in more detail, or, as the case may be, make the distinction irrelevant by including both offenses in a single provision.[34]

An example of *ambiguity* is the expression *electronically stored information*. Legally, the difference between *instructions to machines* on the one hand, and *meaning (information) to humans* on the other may be relevant. The interpretative issue is whether the expression means *computer data*, *humanly perceptible content*, or both. This point is highly relevant in relation to criminal liability for certain forms of speech, robotics, and artificial intelligence (Sunde, 2016).

The *prohibition against analogy* is a general restriction for the application of criminal provisions. Analogy is different from extensive interpretation, which may be permissible.[35] *Analogy* means that a provision is applied to a real-life phenomenon, albeit the

---

34 This is an option according to the convention article 3.
35 Extensive, or broad, interpretation is that the word is understood in a sufficiently broad meaning to cover the phenomenon. A classic example is that 30 pine trees may be regarded as a *forest*; in the digitized society, a smartphone is encompassed by the term *computer system*.

phenomenon is *clearly not covered* by the words of the provision. Analogy is opted for when it is supported by strong reasons, in fact reasons so strong that it seems unreasonable not to apply the provision. Animals once enjoyed better protection against abuse and violence than did children. Animal welfare provisions were then applied, by analogy, in order to provide the same level of protection to children. Today, the application of the word *spouse* to a nonmarried partner would be an analogy. Criminal law has become very detailed in modern society, so analogy, at least to the detriment of the suspect, is not permitted (see Legal Provision 3.4).

Legal Provision 3.4: The Prohibition against Analogy

A court cannot convict a person of a criminal offense if the act falls outside the scope of the words of the criminal provision. The prohibition against analogy flows from the principle of legality.

ECHR article 7 (paraphrased)

It is not always clear whether a problem concerns analogy or extensive interpretation, and the preferred outcome may influence how the problem is framed. See Example 3.8.

Example 3.8: Interpretation and Analogy

Assuming that there is no criminal provision against computer intrusion, can the old criminal provision regarding "unlawful break in to a house, safety box or *other locked object*" be applied to computer intrusion? This requires that the computer can be deemed to be an "other locked object." What do you think?

The suspect has unlawfully deleted computer data on a computer system. Can he be criminally charged for "vandalism against an object"? Does it make any difference (1) if the *computer went dead* because its software was deleted; (2) if the system still *kept functioning*; or (3) if the deletion only affected *user-generated content*?

3.2.5.2 Application of Old Criminal Provisions to New Modes of Conduct

The restrictions on interpretation described above do not, by themselves, rule out the application of old criminal provisions to new modes of conduct. The law is *inherently flexible and develops over time*. It can absorb new phenomena that were nonexistent and not even originally imagined by the legislator when the law was written. For example, it is clear that the word *object* includes a computer system in its physical manifestation, notwithstanding the fact that computers (at least as we know them today) did not exist when the criminal provision originated. Doubtlessly, a smartphone can be subject to theft.[36]

Moreover, one may generally assume that crime committed *in the form of speech* is equally criminal online as offline. The web and social media are all about

---

36 A smartphone is a computer system within the meaning of the Cybercrime Convention article 1. Theft is a crime from time immemorial.

communication. So, fraud by deception; identity infringement (by presenting oneself as another person, by image, text, or sound); the marketing of illegal drugs, weapons, or child sexual abuse material; and the dissemination of hate speech are offenses that are equally criminal on the Internet as in physical space.[37] Old provisions may therefore be applicable.

Finally, criminal provisions concerned with the *outcome regardless of the manner in which it was achieved* are applicable to digital crime. Such provisions tend to be technology-neutral. For instance, homicide is homicide regardless of whether the victim was stabbed in the heart or her pacemaker paralyzed by online interference. Likewise, burglary is burglary regardless of whether the entrance door was smashed with a crowbar or the electronic door-lock disabled by hacking the online computer system.

3.2.5.3 Interpretation of Procedural Provisions Authorizing Coercive Measures

The points already discussed in this chapter are also relevant to interpretation of procedural rules that authorize coercive investigation methods. Notably, the traditional distinction between fixed phenomena on the one hand and communication between individuals (suspects of crime) on the other has broken down with respect to methods regarding digital evidence.

Formerly, digital evidence was computer data stored on a physical medium, and was conceptually similar to physical objects. This concept has broken down due to user accounts on cloud services where the computer data resides without any clear permanent location. Search as a method is strictly limited in time. Search is permissible only for the time necessary to look for evidence at the search location. A new permission is necessary should a new search of the same spot be required. Search as a procedural concept is hardly reconcilable with the act of accessing a computer over the network, over time, repeatedly and secretly. Moreover, monitoring of computer activity over time (e.g., capturing keystrokes) is conceptually irreconcilable with traditional interception, which targets communication under transmission between endpoints.

Thus, the concept of *computer surveillance as a distinct method* has been developed. One may assert that there is a legal basis for computer surveillance *by combining the legal authority to perform computer search with the legal authority for interception*, making a separate regulation superfluous. But no; computer surveillance makes it possible to capture *data that is not even intended* to be transmitted (and could not be intercepted) and has not yet been stored (volatile data such as passwords and encryption keys) (and could not be seized).

In addition, surveillance of an object so personal as a person's computer (including user accounts on cloud services) can be deemed as being qualitatively more intrusive in relation to the right to private life (ECHR article 8) than other methods. For instance, according to Kerr (2013), US courts have "generally concluded that personal computers deserve a high degree of privacy protection under the Fourth Amendment." He provides an example from 2007, where the court states, "For most people, their computers are

---

37 Due to the fundamental right to freedom of speech, the regulation of hate speech may differ between states. But the issue does not turn on the use of digital media, but whether hate speech is treated as a criminal offence or a matter for civil litigation.

their most private spaces" (Kerr, 2013, p. 392 et seq.).[38] Hence, also a *qualitative assessment* of the invasiveness may indicate that lawful application of computer surveillance requires new legislation. In the legislative debate in the Norwegian Parliament on June, 8 2016, a representative claimed that computer surveillance "brings state surveillance one step closer to the soul" (MP Iselin Nybø (V) at 10:47:46 AM, The Parliament's Agenda 89/2016 Case 1).

Using computer surveillance as an example here serves only to explain the implications of the principle of legality to procedural criminal law [ECHR article 8(2)]. The exact scope of procedural provisions, and understanding the methods they authorize, must be determined according to national procedural law in the relevant jurisdiction.

3.3 Digital Crime – Substantive Criminal Law

The criminal offenses of the Cybercrime Convention are categorized as follows: "Offences against the confidentiality, integrity and availability of computer data and systems" (articles 2 through 6); "Computer-related offences" (articles 7 and 8); "Content-related offences" (article 9); and "Infringements of copyright and related rights" (article 10). Article 11 concerns *aiding, abetting,* and *attempt to commit* the offenses. Article 12 concerns *corporate liability;* the parties must secure that *legal persons such as corporations and organizations* may be held liable for committing the criminal offenses (not further dealt with here).

Pursuant to article 13, the parties must secure that the crimes are "punishable by effective, proportionate and dissuasive sanctions, which include deprivation of liberty." The national legal provisions prescribe the maximum penalty for each criminal offense. *This is the theoretical (or formal) level of punishment.* Thus, the scope for sentencing ranges from the mildest reaction generally prescribed in national criminal law to the maximum prescribed for the individual offense. Occasionally, the criminal provision specifies a minimum level considerably higher than the general one. This reduces the judge's scope of discretion with respect to the leniency of the sentence for that particular offense. The theoretical level is relevant to more than sentencing; for example, it is relevant *to the scope for application of coercive investigation methods* (see section 3.4.3.3) and as a *criterion for determining whether an offense is "serious,"* thus falling under the scope of international arrangements for cooperation against transnational organized crime. Pursuant to article 2(b) of the UN Convention against Transnational Organized Crime of 15 November 2000, a crime is "serious" if it is punishable with imprisonment for a maximum of 4 years or more. This is relevant to cybercrimes that take the form of transnational organized crime.

The actual level of punishment for offenses of the same kind can vary quite a bit between national jurisdictions. The explanations are that the *legal principles* applicable to sentencing may be different, and that *social and cultural traditions* particular to a nation have an impact on the court's sentencing practice. However, the occurrence of such differences *within a single jurisdiction* challenges notions of equality and fairness; for instance, should a court in the north apply a more severe sentencing practice than a court in the south? To prevent this, national sentencing guidelines are developed in the case law of that jurisdiction. Some states do also appoint advisory expert bodies

---

38 The quote cited by Kerr is from *United States v. Andrus* (10th Cir. 2007).

designated to suggest "standard rates" for certain criminal offenses (e.g., for youth crime, domestic violence, and drunk driving).

3.3.1 General Conditions for Criminal Liability

In order to be convicted for a criminal offense, the following conditions must be fulfilled:

1) The act must be rendered criminal according to law (see Section 3.2.3.5). The legislative technique is to *specify the conditions that an action must fulfill* in order to fall under the scope of the criminal provision (see Definition 3.1). These are *the objective conditions* of the criminal offense. The objective conditions relate to the When, Where, and How of the 5WH.
2) The individual must have acted with intent (*dolus*), which means that she must know what she is doing. *Intent is the main rule* (negligence is sufficient only when clearly expressed in relation to the criminal provision). Intent is indicated by words such as *knowingly, intentionally, forsett, Vorsatz,* or *uppsåt*.[39] This is the *subjective condition* of the criminal offense. Intent concerns the *facts of the crime* and *must cover all of the objective conditions.* It relates primarily to the Why of the 5WH, but naturally, intent may also be inferred from the objective circumstances of the criminal act.
3) The individual must be *criminally capable,* meaning that she must be above a minimum age determined by law, and not be mentally incapacitated. This relates primarily to the Who of the 5WH.
4) There must not be *circumstances that render an otherwise criminal act lawful,* such as emergency or exigent circumstances. This relates to the When, Where, How, and Why of the 5WH.

The conditions must be fulfilled by the perpetrator *at the moment when the act (crime) was committed* (the When of the 5WH). A *moment* can be everything from a fraction of a second (as when pressing a computer key) to years (e.g. possession of child sexual abuse material). The crime is *completed* when all of the objective conditions are fulfilled.

The *subjective condition* – which is just as important as the objective – involves multiple issues. First, the suspect *is not criminally liable* if she acted unintentionally. For example, one who deletes data on purpose by entering the Delete key has acted intentionally and can be convicted for vandalism. But if she entered the Delete key *by accident,* the act was unintentional, and she is not criminally liable. Second, *good intentions* do not exclude criminal intent; for instance, one who unlawfully accesses a computer system in order to alert about inadequate security is still guilty of intentional computer intrusion. Third, a perpetrator *who is in error with respect to relevant facts* lacks intent. For example, the criminal provision of computer vandalism requires that the data belongs to somebody else. The condition must be covered by the perpetrator's intent. If she erroneously thinks that the data is hers, then there is lack of intent with one of the conditions of the criminal offense, and she is not criminally liable. Finally, if the perpetrator acted intentionally, she still *cannot be held criminally liable* if this cannot be proved.[40]

---

39 *Forsett* is Norwegian and Danish, *Vorsatz* is German, and *uppsåt* is Swedish.
40 See Example 3.7 about digital evidence that proved planned (intentional) homicide.

Intent is required with respect to the offenses of the Cybercrime Convention; see paragraph 39 in Council of Europe (2001). If the national criminal provision extends criminal liability to include negligence as well, this is a secondary option for investigation. *Negligence* means that the individual can be blamed for having acted *contrary to how a prudent person would have acted in the same situation.* The personal characteristics of the individual (young/old, skilled/experienced/"newbie," well-functioning/vision impaired, etc.) are relevant to the assessment. Negligence can relate to *lack of sound judgment* (she is aware of the facts yet willing to take the risk) and/or *lack of attention* (she can be blamed for not having thought of the risk).[41]

Attempt, aiding, and *abetting* are usually criminalized in national legislation, but nevertheless explicitly mentioned in article 11 of the convention. *Attempt* requires that the perpetrator *has taken action with the intent to complete the crime.* Fantasizing about committing a crime, thinking of it, and even planning and preparing for it (e.g., by buying necessary equipment) do not amount to criminal attempt. Instead, such activities may be criminalized as *individual offenses* per se (though with an exception for "thinking of it," as the concept of *thought crime* is not generally recognized). Notably, pursuant to article 6 ("Misuse of Devices") of the Cybercrime Convention, the parties must criminalize certain actions that are regarded as potentially harmful to computer security. The acts would not, as a rule, be regarded as attempts, but they could, depending on the circumstances, be regarded as aiding or abetting (discussed in the next paragraph). For the sake of clarity of the law, and in order to emphasize the significance of secure and reliable computer systems, the activities are regarded as criminal offenses per se.

Aiding and abetting (ancillary liability) pertains to somebody who *intentionally assists or encourages* the main perpetrator to commit the crime. These are not lesser crimes, as they can be pivotal for the main perpetrator's ability and decisiveness to commit the crime. The main perpetrator may even have been led into it by one who planned and organized it all. Thus, the "organizer" can get a more severe sentence than the main perpetrator.

One may ask whether *causality* is needed between the aid (or abetting) and the perpetration of the crime. The classical example is a person who – on his own initiative – posts himself as guard for one who commits a burglary. If the burglar himself was not aware of the service, is the guard criminally liable for *aiding* the offense? Or is it, perhaps, *attempt to aid* the perpetration of an offense? What if a person urges another to commit burglary, but the latter refuses to do it? Is the first one liable for *attempt to aid* the commission of a crime?

Parallel examples are practical in relation to cybercrime. One example is a malware developer who gives an exploit to one who intends to commit computer intrusion; is the malware developer criminally liable if the other perpetrates the crime *without making use of the exploit*? And what if the malware was tried out, but proved to be unsuitable for the task?

Article 6 comes to the rescue, because development and distribution of such malware comprise an *independent criminal offense*, thus eliminating the need to consider liability for aiding or abetting. Sometimes a person is not helpful at all, even if his intention was to contribute to the commission of the crime. For instance: A, who has very limited

---

41 Different national jurisdictions may operate with different concepts of intent and negligence. Here, only basic concepts are outlined. Modifications must always be expected to occur in national legal systems.

technological skills, sits with his friend B in front of a computer, where B is busy executing a distributed denial of service (DDOS) attack. A means to be of support, but his advice is wholly useless to B. Is A still liable? Does he in fact *have to leave the place* – or *actively object* to B's activity – in order not to be held liable for participation? Again, the solutions in national law may vary.

With respect to *organized crime*, the scope for criminal liability can be more far-reaching (Definition 3.3). Pursuant to article 5 of the UN Convention against Transnational Organized Crime, *participation in an organized criminal group* shall be a criminal offense. It means that one can be held criminally liable without personally having committed or actively contributed to the perpetration of a specific crime. Money laundering and corruption are activities that facilitate and make organized crime grow, and they are criminalized as separate offenses pursuant to the UN convention articles 6 and 8.

Definition 3.3: Organized Criminal Group

"Organized criminal group is a *structured* group of *three or more* persons, existing for a *period of time* and *acting in concert with the aim of committing* one or more *serious* crimes [. . .] in order to obtain, directly or indirectly, a financial or other material benefit." (Emphasis added.)

UN Convention against Transnational Organized Crime article 2(a)

Each suspect shall be judged according to her own actions. This is a fundamental rule regardless of jurisdiction, and it means that the objective and subjective conditions must be proven for each suspect. Conversely, no one can be held guilty for something done by somebody else, *unless covered by the intent* (in which case it is a form of aiding, abetting, or organized crime). Also, the level of punishment is individually determined, but for reasons of fairness – and all things being equal – the punishment will tend to be the same.

As one can see, the Who of the 5WH not only is relevant to the identification of the perpetrator, but also is a *systematic criterion for building a case against each one of the suspects*. A focus on Who leads the criminal investigator to keep control and check that all the conditions for criminal liability are fulfilled for each perpetrator. This may prevent issuance of an indictment for an offense that is not fully covered by the evidence.

The *legal exercise* is to apply the conditions of the criminal provisions, one by one, to the facts of the case. The purpose is to check whether the facts displayed by the evidence match the words of the relevant provisions. If satisfied that the activities and mindset of a suspect (Who) fulfilled the conditions of a criminal provision at the moment when the crime was committed, an indictment may be issued. If not, one must drop the case (provided further investigation is not an option). Then, one may move to the next task. As emphasized already, the applicable criminal provisions form part of the national legal system, and the conditions for the same kind of offense may be (slightly) different in different systems. The consequence is that the themes that must be proved – and the evidence obtained for this purpose – may be (slightly) different, always depending on which jurisdiction tries the case. This has been shown in Example 3.6.

3.3.2 Real-Life Modus Operandi

The structured approach explained above must be applied, albeit that a *real-life modus operandi* is often complex, with several of the offenses occurring in combination, and with motives that cannot always be read from the legal provision. Clearly, the criminal offenses against computer security are often committed for reasons other than interfering with security [this assumption underlies Guidance Notes 2–4 and 6 of the Cybercrime Convention Committee (T-CY), 2014].[42] *Economic gain* is a frequent motive, and in order to attain this goal, a series of computer intrusions, modifications of computer data, ID theft, and manufacturing of malware can be committed. The attacks against the computers are methods to achieve economic gain, not goals by themselves. The scenario is realistic both for a lone perpetrator and for several who cooperate (which can, depending on the facts, amount to organized crime). Criminals can also be hired by others, for instance to commit economic espionage through illegal access to computers. This could take the form of crime-as-a-service.

The scenario is realistic for *other motivations* as well. For example, computer intrusion can be a means to get hold of intimate images, while the ultimate motive is *personal satisfaction*. In Example 3.9, the perpetrator was found guilty of approximately 200 computer intrusions committed for this purpose. Getting control over such images can also be a means to *commit sextortion* (by threatening to distribute the images on social media, unless the victim complies with certain sexually motivated orders) or *take revenge* on an ex-partner by distributing the images on social media.

Things can get complicated when more people are involved; for instance, a malware developer A gives malware to B, who then uses it in order to gain illegal access to a computer system. B has clearly committed computer intrusion (article 2) and acquired malware for this purpose (article 6). With respect to A, the question is whether the liability is limited to the development and distribution of malware to A (article 6), or if he is liable for aiding or abetting to the computer intrusion as well (article 2 in conjunction with article 11).

It is a fact that cybercrime may take the form of transnational organized crime with many participants. Online bank fraud is an example in point: as described in Section 1.3.4.1, the crime pattern involves multiple actors and a long-term commitment, requiring a criminal organization with access to highly specialized competencies and tools. Central actors in such schemes are thus the malware programmers, the command-and-control center managers, the mules, as well as the organization that is recruiting the mules and profiting from the operation. Access to the required botnet, consisting of the command-and-control center and a network of compromised computers with active malware, can be purchased as a service on underground forums. Keeping in mind that each suspect shall be judged according to her own actions, the investigation must be

---

42 The assumption concerns *botnets, DDOS attacks, ID theft and phishing in relation to fraud,* and *new forms of malware*. The notes explain how new forms of cybercrimes are covered by the provisions of the convention, and it turns out that most of the provisions are applicable. The reason why is that the provisions are by default applicable to crime committed through the use of computers in networks, because this affects computer security (protected by articles 2–6 of the convention). It does not matter to the relevancy of the provisions whether the ultimate goal of the criminal activity is more distant.

carefully adapted to this end. An investigation guided by the criminal provisions prepares the ground for individual assessment of each of the suspects as closure.

3.3.3 Offenses against the Confidentiality, Integrity, and Availability of Computer Data and Systems

The offenses mentioned in the Cybercrime convention articles 2 through 6 concern acts that interfere with the security of computer systems and computer data. The legal protection supports the security principles of *confidentiality*, *integrity*, and *availability*, which in turn seek to enhance reliability and trust in computer systems and services. The primary objective of the convention is to secure that national criminal law is adequate to strike down on criminal activity that involves computer technology. The presumption was that the conceptualization of computer data as a protected object was the weak spot in national criminal law. Thus, the protection of *computer data*, not of the physical equipment, is the focus of the convention (see Definition 3.4).

Definition 3.4: Computer Data

Computer data means any representation of facts, information or concepts in a form suitable for processing in a computer system, including a program suitable to cause a computer system to perform a function.

Cybercrime Convention article 1(b)

The definition includes *user-generated data* no matter the kind of content or format (Word files, PowerPoint, images, video clips, music files, and program files). Furthermore, *programs that run on the computer system* are included, as well as all sorts of logs, registries, administrative files, utility files, security software, filters, and so forth.

The convention defines *computer system* as well (see Definition 3.5).

Definition 3.5: Computer System

Computer system means any device or a group of interconnected or related devices, one or more of which, pursuant to a program, performs automatic processing of data.

Cybercrime Convention article 1(a)

The crucial element is the condition "pursuant to a program, performs automatic processing of data." A device that fulfills this condition is a computer system, regardless of its size and purpose [the notion of *computer system* is dealt with by Guidance Note 1 of the Cybercrime Convention Committee (T-CY), 2014]. Consequently, small devices such as smartphones, tablets, and laptops are included, as well as large computer systems utilized by public agencies, by multinational corporations with global reach, and by cloud services that offer storage and processing services or social media. A user account is *part of* a computer system. Obviously, a device can be a computer system in itself (e.g., a laptop) and be part of a larger system (e.g., a laptop placed in a docking station at the workplace, or connected by a VPN). Several of the provisions of the convention permit the condition in national legislation that the computer system "is connected to another computer system." Keeping in mind that the convention dates from 2001 and that network technology and services have developed tremendously since then, the condition is of little significance, and it is not further mentioned as an issue.

Although storage media are not by themselves computer systems, they are covered by the definition provided that they are "interconnected" with a device that performs automatic data processing pursuant to a program. For instance, a memory stick is covered if it is inserted in the USB port of a laptop, but not if it lays in a drawer. There is the option, though, that the stick is "related," but it is not really clear what that means. Computer data and computer systems presuppose each other. Legally, it is not always clear whether the protected phenomenon is computer data *or* a computer system *or* both. Again, taking a USB stick connected to a computer as an example; the question is how to regard the unlawful removal of the stick and the subsequent sifting through of its content (when it is connected to the perpetrator's own computer).

One can probably agree that the removal of the USB stick amounts to *theft of an object*. The question concerns the legal appraisal of the ensuing steps: taking control of the data, and the subsequent search. One option is to consider taking control of the data as an *aggravating circumstance* related to theft. But the question still remains of whether sifting through the data is a separate offense or is consumed by the theft. The parallel is that one is not punished for *reading* a book, only for *stealing* it. However, a USB stick may contain so much data that an analogy to a book may be regarded as patently misguided. This makes a case for regarding the search through the data as illegal access to "part of" a computer system (i.e., a separate offense following the theft). The result of the first approach, which focuses on the physical object (the stick), is *but one offense*, that is, unlawful interference with property rights (theft); whereas the result of the second is two offenses, that is, unlawful interference with property rights (theft of the stick) and with data security (illegal access). The legal solution of a specific case must be determined according to national legal provisions.

The definitions of *computer data* and *computer system* clarify the exact scope and nature of the offenses set out in the convention. A party does not have an obligation to implement corresponding legal definitions. If the scope and nature of the national criminal provisions are such as to cover the offenses, the obligation under the convention is fulfilled.

3.3.3.1 Illegal Access and Illegal Interception

Legal Provision 3.5: Illegal Access

"The access to the whole or any part of a computer system without right."
    National legislation may apply the condition that the offence be committed by infringing security measures.

Cybercrime Convention article 2 (excerpt)

Legal Provision 3.6: Illegal Interception

"The interception without right, made by technical means, of non-public transmissions of computer data to, from or within a computer system, including electromagnetic emissions from a computer system carrying such computer data."

Cybercrime Convention article 3 (excerpt)

Illegal access is the act of unlawfully gaining access to "the whole or any part of a computer system without right" (see Legal Provision 3.5). National legislation may require that the offense is committed by infringing security measures. The rationale is that when security measures have been overcome by the perpetrator, there is not much doubt with respect to the lack of right to access the system or that the act was intentional.[43]

Circumvention of security measures may be divided into two *modi operandi: password intrusion*, whereby a stolen or cracked password is used, and *vulnerability attack*, whereby a vulnerability on the computer system is exploited (see Example 3.9). The vulnerability may have existed on the system previously or be created by the perpetrator, for instance by infecting the system with malware attached to an email.

Example 3.9: Password Intrusion and Vulnerability Attack

A computer engineer had gained illegal access to around 200 computer systems/user accounts. He set out from his own legitimate user account on a commercial cloud service for personal photo and video management. Here, he installed an exploit that enabled him to get access to the system administrator's account (vulnerability attack). He then copied the user registry, which was a database containing the usernames, passwords, and email addresses of the 66 million users of the service. He extracted the personal information of Norwegian users, 120,000 in all, including email addresses and passwords, and finally used this to gain access to and copy intimate images from the accounts.

HR-2012-2056-A

The provision concerning *illegal interception* (Legal Provision 3.6) is there to protect communications for which one has a reasonable expectation of privacy. The right to private communication is at the core of the right to private life (ECHR article 8), and electronic communication is protected regardless of whether it is performed in a private capacity or as part of one's professional duties.[44] Article 3 reaches even further than that, because it protects not only communication between different communication systems (to/from) *but also transmissions within a computer system*. It means that using a Trojan for catching keystrokes to copy passwords or payment card numbers when they are

---

43 Example 3.6 shows this condition as included in the German StGB § 202a(1) and in the Norwegian Criminal Code § 204.

44 *Halford v. UK*, judgment June 25, 1997 (telephone at the workplace); *Copland v. UK*, judgment April 2, 2007 (Internet at the workplace); and *Barbulescu v. Romania*, judgment January 12, 2016 (use of Internet account at work), referral to the Grand Chamber by decision June 6, 2016.

entered by the legitimate user of the system, and the unlawful use of a packet sniffer, fall within the scope of article 3.

Articles 2 and 3 provide protection on different levels. Article 2 protects *the system,* which means that the offense is completed *once access has been gained.* Article 3 protects against *"interception" of the nonpublic data under transmission.* A contravention of article 3 is completed first *when interception has succeeded.* If performed by the use of an external "tapping" device, the crime is completed once the data stream is intercepted by the device. If the data stream is intercepted by use of malware inserted into the computer system, the interception is preceded by illegal access (article 2), and, likely, by a *system interference* as well (article 5). This makes a case for applying both articles 2 and 3 to cover the successive steps of the criminal activity, in addition to article 5. The exact regulation is determined in national law.

Articles 2 and 3 do not protect *property rights* to data, and as mentioned, the concept of *data theft* is controversial. However, this has not prevented information fencing from developing as a legal concept in national legal systems. *Information fencing* means *unlawful dealing in information that is the outcome (spoil, proceeds) of a crime.*[45] Criminal liability is especially relevant for information that has economic value (images, passwords, credit card numbers, etc.). Usually, it is not necessary to prove the exact nature of the predicate offense [i.e., the offense which results in stolen (copied) data]. It is sufficient to prove that the data leakage did not occur by accident or any lawful action.

Article 2, "Illegal access," raises several issues:

First, *password intrusion* has to be distinguished from *ID theft. ID theft* is an interference with the right to private life, and it victimizes the individual (or legal person) whose identity is unlawfully used (see Definition 3.6 Identity theft in relation to fraud; and Harris *et al.,* 2009, p. 367 et seq., about identity within the scope of the private sphere). The interference (victimization) occurs when the identity data is used externally toward a third party, for instance as a means to commit fraud. Thus, the scenario involves *two* victims: the *owner of the personal data* (victim of ID theft), and the *third party who is defrauded* (victim of fraud). *Password intrusion* is committed by "fooling" the authentication procedure that seeks to secure that only the legitimate user accesses the computer system/user account. Thus, it is a breach of *computer security*, not an interference with *identity* protected by the right to private life. The immediate victim is the person who owns the password; there is no third-party victim who has acted in reliance of the password.

Second, the crime is completed when illegal access has been gained. The question is, then, how to assess *subsequent unlawful use of the computer system or service.* Should it be taken into account in the assessment of the access (whether it is illegal or not), or should it be subject to a separate assessment? The question has caused some debate with respect to publicly available websites that are used contrary to the host's guidelines or intentions. For instance, should automatic circumvention of a "captcha" in order to make more extensive use of a service be deemed as illegal access? Is a "captcha" a *security measure* within the meaning of the criminal provision, or a measure to secure *fair use* of the service? And how about ignoring the dropdown menu offered by the host, and rather directly accessing the content of the service because one has succeeded in figuring out

---

45 "Dealing" is for instance sale, purchase, exchange, concealment, storage, etc. of the proceeds of the crime, *in casu* the data.

the technical setup? Yet another example is the use of a website that has been left exposed accidentally by a security flaw, but clearly is not intended for that use. These questions have been analyzed by Kerr (2015) in the context of US criminal law, focusing on the relevance of technical hindrances, contractual conditions, and social norms to the legal assessment. It has been further analyzed in a European context by Gudmundsdottir (2015). In the end, national legal rules determine the outcome.

Third, there is the "catch 22" of the condition concerning *interference with security measures*: it presupposes that the system must be protected, which it in effect turns out not to be, because if it were, the vulnerability attack would not have succeeded. To avoid this problem, some jurisdictions apply the alternative condition, that access must be gained by an "other method without right." The condition is quite vague and prompts the question of whether systems/user accounts that are wholly unprotected can be subject to illegal access. The question is practical, for example for personalized applications accessible from the user's smartphone. The owner's lack of concern of computer security does not make a third party *entitled* to accessing or making use of his or her personal accounts. The outcome seems to hinge on elements relating to context and the personal relation between the third party and the owner of the smartphone. It may for instance be relevant whether the smartphone was lying unprotected on a table or in the owner's handbag, and whether the third party had a close personal relation with the owner or none at all. The digital content as such may be protected against unlawful access pursuant to provisions concerning *personal mail* or *business secrets.* There may also be special provisions striking down on *unlawful use* of an object or device. Such provisions are independently applicable.

Finally, one may ask exactly what constitutes "access"? Computers in a network, including the Internet, are constantly accessing each other as part of the information exchange. According to the Explanatory Report to the convention, "the mere sending of an email message or a file to that system" does not constitute "access" (see Council of Europe, 2001, paragraph 46). This does not clarify much, because as long as the email or file is legitimate, sending it is not "without right." There is much to indicate that "access" must be interpreted to imply that *control* can be asserted over the computer system or user account. Prior to the Internet age, physical login was the routine, which gave immediate control of the user account; the convention is drafted in this modus. Nowadays, remote access and control are common. This can be achieved, for instance, by sending email with a Trojan (spyware) attachment. The implication is that access (gained by a Trojan that provides control of the system) can precede interception, as mentioned above. Malware that causes data deletion or other forms of interference, without enabling the perpetrator to control the target system, does not (according to this view) amount to access within the meaning of article 2.

3.3.3.2 Data and System Interference

Legal Provision 3.7: Data Interference

"The damaging, deletion, deterioration, alteration or suppression of computer data without right." National criminal law may apply the condition that the conduct results in serious harm.

Cybercrime Convention article 4 (excerpt)

Legal Provision 3.8: System Interference

"The serious hindering without right of the functioning of a computer system by inputting, transmitting, damaging, deleting, deteriorating, altering or suppressing computer data."

Cybercrime Convention article 5 (excerpt)

Articles 4 and 5 supplement the traditional provision of vandalism against physical objects. Article 4 protects "computer data," and article 5 "the functioning of a computer system." Physical destruction of a computer system is beyond the scope of article 5, but it is punishable pursuant to traditional provisions of vandalism in the national legislation.

Both articles mention *damaging, deletion, deterioration, alteration,* and *suppression* of computer data. Pursuant to article 4, this is *sufficient* for completion of the criminal offense. Pursuant to article 5, the data interference is a *means to achieve* the "serious hindering . . . of the functioning of a computer system." Article 5 includes the additional alternatives *inputting* and *transmitting* data as well.

As (intentional) *interference with computer data* (without right) is the main condition of both provisions, there seems to be some overlap, and consequently a need to determine their respective scope (see also Legal Provisions 3.7 and 3.8). The analysis starts with article 5 and DDOS attacks.

The purpose of a DDOS attack is "to render a computer system unavailable to users through a variety of means" [Cybercrime Convention Committee (T-CY), 2014].[46] Here, we have in mind the modus of *overloading the target computer with traffic over the network.* Hence, the *modus operandi* is *inputting or transmitting data,* as mentioned in article 5. The attack is directed at the *functioning of the computer system* and constitutes a breach of *availability.* Whether it constitutes a "serious hindering" depends on interpretation in light of the circumstances, and the criteria may be laid down in national legislation (see Council of Europe, 2001, paragraph 67). Aspects of both *capacity* and *time span* may be relevant, and the criteria must be compared with the normal functioning of the computer system. One option is that "serious hindering" is fulfilled once the target computer is entirely brought down (zero capacity). Another option is that also the *time span* must be taken into consideration. The temporal aspect should be significant at least when the system is capable of functioning, albeit on a lower level than normal. Getting precise information about the downtime is important to the assessment of the completion of the offense, as well as to its gravity, which in turn has a bearing on the measurement of punishment.

Insertion of a self-replicating malware can cause the system to slow down and eventually stop. This is also covered by article 5 (see Council of Europe, 2001, paragraph 67).

---

46 Guidance Note 3.

We now turn to article 4: Its scope seems quite far-reaching as its words include any interference with computer data. However, in the event that the data interference has an *effect on the computer system as such, it could be regarded either as vandalism against the computer system pursuant to the traditional provision, or as serious hindering of the functioning of the target system* pursuant to article 5. The exact legal appraisal depends on the circumstances. The following examples show acts that are covered by the words of article 4, but have an effect on the system: the deletion of a user registry on a cloud service (deletion), change of passwords (alteration), moving an HTML file to an inaccessible place on the server and replacing it with a defacing webpage (suppression and alteration), encrypting all the files on the computer system (as a means of extortion) (i.e., deterioration and/or suppression). If the hindering of the functioning of the system is not serious, a secondary option is to apply the traditional provision of vandalism, as this provision does not necessarily require the damage to be serious. The computer system is an object, and there is no reason why the legal assessment of unlawful interference should be regarded differently than, say, tampering with the engine or the lock of a car (which surely amounts to vandalism).

In the end, the independent scope for article 4 seems to be interference with user-generated content, such as Word files and PowerPoint presentations. In this case, neither article 5 nor the traditional provision of vandalism is applicable.

Finally, *malware* come in different forms: logical bombs cause damage to the system sometime in the future. Spyware may be remotely controlled by the perpetrator, but the exact point in time when it becomes exploited may be uncertain. Back doors implemented on the target system may be used off and on. And it goes for all malware that it may be detected and removed before it has had any impact on the functioning of the system.

This brings up the question of when the system interference is *completed*. Attempted crime gets a milder sentence than an offense that has been completed, and for malware there can be a time span between its insertion on the system and when it is activated (causing damage). If the later point in time is deemed to be crucial, then an interruption of events caused by the detection and removal of the malware leads to the result that the perpetrator is liable for attempt. It seems unfair that the perpetrator shall benefit because the owner of the computer system has implemented adequate security measures. In addition, the *integrity* of the system, which is a protected interest underlying the provision, is interfered with already at the stage when the malware is inserted. The subsequent unfolding of events depends much on happenstance. The critical point in time for completion of the system interference should for these reasons be when the malware is inserted.

Nowadays, it is often hard to distinguish the computer system from the enterprise that makes use of it, because services often are the very product of the computer system. To illustrate: in the aforementioned case of deletion of the user registry of a cloud service, one may claim that the computer system as such is in good standing, despite that it is emptied of data. The occurrence is only detrimental to the economic business, but that is another story. The scope of article 5 is not clear, and, again, national law is in any case determinative. However, the seamless integration of technology and enterprise promises a steady flow of legal challenges.

3.3.3.3 Misuse of Devices

Legal Provision 3.9: Misuse of Devices

"The production, sale, procurement for use, import, distribution or otherwise making available of [and possession of]:

litra a:

i. a device, including a computer program, designed or adapted primarily for the purpose of committing any of the offences [mentioned] in articles 2-5, and

ii. a computer password, access code, or similar data by which the whole or any part of a computer system is capable of being accessed."

Cybercrime Convention article 6 (excerpt)

Pursuant to article 6 "Misuse of devices," the parties have an obligation to secure that intentional dealing with items as mentioned in litra a (i) and (ii) (see Legal Provision 3.9) is a criminal offense. The rationale for the provision was explained in Section 3.3.1. There is no obligation to criminalize if the motive is something other than committing one of the offenses mentioned in articles 2–5 [article 6(2)]. It means that the provision does not represent an obstacle to, for instance, security personnel and computer scientists to make use of the items for legitimate purposes. The national legislator may opt for a less specific motive requirement than that set out in article 6. For instance, pursuant to § 201 of the Norwegian criminal code, it is sufficient that dealing with the items is performed with the motive *to commit a crime*, which more or less equals the condition "without right." In this manner, it has been sought to make the provision more effective in practice, as it can be very hard to prove a motive nailed down to a specific offense.

Article 6 specifies the offense as *production, sale, procurement for use, import, distribution, or otherwise making available* of the items. *Possession* may be included as well, but this is optional [article 6 (1)(b)]. The items specified in litra a (i) are "devices," both physical (e.g., a keystroke logger) and computer programs (i.e., malware, exploits, root kit, ransomware, spyware, etc.); and the items in (ii) are "password, access code, or similar data by which the whole or any part of a computer system is capable of being accessed." This alternative is almost self-explanatory, but one can ask if *credit card information* is included. Illegitimate dealing in such information is a well-documented problem and justifies a need to strike down on it. The information enables access to a bank account, which certainly today is "part of" a computer system (article 2). This should lead to the conclusion that credit card information is included among the items mentioned in litra a (ii). Alternatively, the provision concerning (information) fencing should be applicable (information fencing is explained in relation to data theft in Section 3.3.3.1).

The difference between physical and "informational" items, in litra a, has a bearing on the interpretation of the various alternatives of dealing. As regards *physical items*, their production, sale, and so on must be deemed as self-explanatory. However, with regard to *informational items*, such as passwords or credit card numbers, the interpretation needs some thought. May criminal liability be incurred by *guessing* a password (procurement for use), by *remembering* it (possession), or by *telling* it to a third party (otherwise making it available)? Recalling that "thought crime" as a concept is not generally recognized (Section 3.3.1), *guessing* and *remembering* are beyond the scope of the provision.

However, *technically assisted password cracking* (brute force/dictionary attack) is "procurement for use," and *oral information* about passwords (simply telling it to somebody else) is covered by "otherwise making available."

3.3.4 Computer-Related Offenses

Legal Provision 3.10: Computer-Related Forgery
"The input, alteration, deletion, or suppression of computer data, resulting in inauthentic data with the intent that it be considered or acted upon for legal purposes as if it were authentic, regardless of whether or not the data is directly readable and intelligible." **Cybercrime Convention article 7 (excerpt)**

Legal Provision 3.11: Computer-Related Fraud
"The causing of a loss of property to another person by: (a) any input, alteration, deletion or suppression of computer data, (b) any interference with the functioning of a computer system, with fraudulent or dishonest intent of procuring, without right, an economic benefit for oneself or for another person." **Cybercrime Convention article 8 (excerpt)**

Basically the offenses of computer-related forgery and fraud are interferences with computer data and systems as mentioned in articles 4 and 5, with some additional conditions attached. These are, with respect to forgery, the condition of *inauthentic data*, and with respect to fraud, standard conditions concerning *loss of property* and *fraudulent or dishonest intent* of procuring an economic benefit.

Thus, *computer-related forgery* (see Legal Provision 3.10) can be explained by starting with traditional document forgery, which is the creation and use of an *inauthentic (fake) document* under the pretense that it is *authentic*. Usually, the offense requires that the document is of such a nature that reliance upon it by a third party has legal consequences, and article 7 includes this condition as well. To illustrate: presenting a copy of a postcard claiming that it is authentic can hardly have legal consequences, but presenting a fake passport does. Article 7 was needed in order to secure that the condition of authenticity did not pose a problem, given some incertitude caused by the phenomenon of digital duplicates. At present, the important point is that the act that causes inauthenticity is data interference (article 4). It does not matter whether the data is directly readable and intelligible. Hence, electronic certificates applied in the authentication procedures of computer systems may be subject to forgery.

Similarly, *computer-related fraud* (see Legal Provision 3.11) is committed by the *modus operandi* of article 4 (data interference) or 5 (causing an interference with the functioning of a computer system), supplemented with the *additional conditions* mentioned above, thus distinguishing fraud from interference. The reason for including a provision concerning computer-related fraud was that the traditional concept of fraud was based on *deception* of another person. Computer-related fraud is simply a manipulation of information or processes of a computer system, not deceiving any person.

As noted in the Explanatory Report, articles 7–10 relate to the digital perpetration of ordinary crimes that most states have criminalized (see Council of Europe, 2001, paragraph 79). Thus, the situation in the national legal systems with respect to fraud is that there are *two basic concepts of fraud*; one based on *deception*, the other relating to *misuse or manipulation of a computer system*. One may assume *fraud by deception* nowadays to be at least as practical in a digital context as so-called *computer-related fraud*. Internet fraud perpetrated by providing false or materially misleading information to others is widespread. Examples are sale of products that will never be sent to the buyer, or that are substantially different from that which was ordered and paid for; and the sale of fake tickets, for instance to Premier League soccer games. Computer fraud may be more practical in an "insider" context, for instance in financial institutions where accounts can be manipulated to skim profits. It may also be practical in the digital interface between public agencies and the citizens, typically when personal information relevant to getting social benefits or a tax deduction is provided by checking "boxes" in a digital form, which is then automatically processed. (This form of digital interaction with the citizen is known as *e-government*.)

Payment cards may be forged and fraudulently used. If an individual is deceived by the fake card, it is an instance of forgery and fraud by deception. If an authentic card that is stolen or a fake card is used as a means to manipulate the transaction system, this is computer-related fraud against the *card issuer* that backs the transaction (e.g., VISA or MasterCard). There are also situations where no person is defrauded despite that the card obviously is fake, such as when the card is used in "unmanned" situations, for instance on an ATM, or the personnel at the user place act in complicity with the criminal user of the card. In such a case, the personnel are liable for aiding or abetting computer-related fraud. Finally, the fraudulent use of the payment card is ID theft; the owner of the card is the victim. (See Definition 3.6.)

Definition 3.6: Identity Theft in Relation to Fraud

Identity theft in relation to fraud may entail the misappropriation of the identity (such as the name, date of birth, current address, or previous addresses) of another person, without their knowledge or consent. These identity details are then used to obtain goods and services in that person's name.

T-CY Guidance Note 4

Phishing may involve a combination of criminal offenses. First, the pretension of representing a well-known financial institution or other corporation of good repute is ID theft. This may be performed in an email soliciting personal information of the "customers" or, similarly, by false information on a website closely resembling the official website of the real corporation. If the information sought is encompassed by article 6, the *information harvesting* is a contravention of this article. The *subsequent use* of the information may be password intrusion (article 2) and forgery and fraud (including computer-related fraud). Insofar as the information is used for committing forgery and fraud, it is *ID theft* against the rightful owner of the personal information. Finally, if the information that has been harvested *is made available to others*, this is a contravention of article 6, and can be regarded as information fencing as well. (See Example 3.10 for more information.)

Example 3.10: Online Bank Fraud – Articles 2 through 8

The case has been described in Section 1.3.4. However, chronologically the events are as follows (simplified):

Step 1, the *development phase*: The development of malware that can be remotely controlled (article 6).
Step 2, the *distribution phase*: Vulnerable computers are infected, and the criminal comes in position to take control with the connection to the Internet bank [illegal access (article 2) and system interference (article 5)].
Step 3, the *exploitation phase*: The perpetrator exploits the vulnerability. The *authentication procedure* is circumvented by forging the electronic ID associated with the login credentials of the account owner (article 7). The access to the bank account (article 2) is succeeded by a *payment order* [computer-related fraud (article 8)]. In addition, the facts include that the account owner was *tricked unwittingly to confirm* the payment order by a repeated fake login request. This is *deception*, which could justify application of the traditional fraud provision. The "mule" who cashes the money and secures the proceeds of the crime commits money laundering. As the whole scheme fulfills the criteria for organized crime, there can be convictions for taking part in it. Those who are found guilty of planning and organizing it get a more severe penalty. There are also several issues concerning aiding and abetting. The proceeds of the crime should be confiscated (UN Convention against Transnational Organized Crime, article 12).

Example of confiscation: In June 2016, Australian police auctioned 144,000 Bitcoin confiscated from the founder of the "online drug bazaar Silk Road." According to the exchange rate at the time, the amount equaled USD 13 million ("Australian Police," 2016).

3.3.5 Content-Related Offenses

Definition 3.7: Child Sexual Abuse Material

Child sexual abuse material "shall include pornographic material that visually depicts:

a) a minor engaged in sexually explicit conduct;
b) a person appearing to be a minor engaged in sexually explicit conduct;
c) realistic images representing a minor engaged in sexually explicit conduct.[47]

   The term 'minor' shall include all persons under 18 years of age. [A lower age limit may be required, but] not less than 16 years."

Cybercrime Convention article 9.2 and 9.3 (excerpt)

---

47 "Sexually explicit conduct" covers "at least real or simulated: a) sexual intercourse, including genital-genital, oral-genital, anal-genital or oral-anal, between minors, or between an adult and a minor, of the same or opposite sex; b) bestiality; c) masturbation; d) sadistic or masochistic abuse in a sexual context; or e) lascivious exhibition of the genitals or the pubic area of a minor. It is not relevant whether the conduct depicted is real or simulated"; Explanatory Report to the Cybercrime Convention, paragraph 100.

Production and subsequent *dealing* with child sexual abuse material shall be criminalized in the national legal system pursuant to article 9(1) (not cited in Definition 3.7, but confer with article 6, which includes largely similar alternatives). Article 9 is a supplement for the event that national criminal law does not adequately address dealings with such material in digital form. As mentioned in Section 3.2.4, several other international legal instruments are relevant as well. The result is a *global ban* on such material. Interpol and Europol have made digital signatures (see Section 2.3.5 and 5.4.3), which makes it possible to quantify known illegal material on a server without having to look at it. Newly produced material must be legally assessed by other methods. The main problem, however, is hardly the legal appraisal, but the enormity of the illegal material that falls within the scope of article 9 by good measure.

Production means the photographing or video recording of the material. The criminal who physically forces himself on the child, or threatens or entices it to partake in the production, is criminally liable for sexual offenses against the children as well. The photographer ("producer") can be liable for aiding and abetting the physical offense. *Production and distribution* are the most serious forms of dealing, because of the causation of the everlasting availability of the material on the Internet. The investigation should have strong focus on these alternatives of article 9.

Currently, streaming of sexual abuse on demand is an increasing phenomenon. This form of criminal conduct was not so practical when the convention was made, due to lack of bandwidth. Many jurisdictions have included criminal provisions that explicitly make such streaming an offense as well, since it may be unclear if the word "material" covers it.

In the present context, the significance of criminal investigation and prosecution of such offenses may be illustrated by the words of the Norwegian Supreme Court in Example 3.11. As children lack the means to protect themselves from such abuse, the *positive obligation to secure respect for their private life* must weigh heavily as priority for law enforcement agencies (see Section 3.2.3.7).

Example 3.11: The Everlasting Violation of the Child

"In addition to the enormously widespread distribution which is the result of making the images available on the Internet, it is not practically possible to delete them. Children who over years have suffered sexual abuse may therefore experience that they are recognized for years to come. This is properly to be regarded *as an everlasting violation.* . . . One has to take into account the risk that others may be exposed to the images, *which constitutes a considerable extra burden on the victim [displayed on the image] later in life.*" (Emphasis added, translation from Norwegian by the author.)

HR-2001-1545

3.3.6 Offenses Related to Infringements of Copyright and Related Rights

---

Legal Provision 3.12: Offenses Related to Infringements of Copyright and the Like

The article confers an obligation to criminalize acts that impinge on the rights laid down in a number of treaties concerning the protection of copyrights and related rights, where such acts are committed willfully, on a commercial scale, and by means of a computer system. The international instruments mentioned in article 10 are:

- The Paris Act of 24 July 1971, revising the Bern Convention for the Protection of Literary and Artistic Works
- The Agreement on Trade-Related Aspects of Intellectual Property Rights
- The WIPO Copyright Treaty
- The International Convention for the Protection of Performers, Producers of Phono-grams and Broadcasting Organisations (Rome Convention)
- The WIPO Performances and Phonograms Treaty.

Cybercrime Convention article 10 (excerpt)

Copyright means that the creator of the works has a sole right to determine whether it shall be publicized. The creator can transfer or sell its rights to a publishing house, and get royalty for each copy sold, the number of clicks on Spotify or Netflix, the number of broadcast transmissions, and so forth.

Infringement of these rights is a considerable problem to the right holders. The legal approach can be civil litigation and criminal prosecution. Pursuant to article 10, criminalization is only required with respect to infringements committed *willfully, on a commercial scale and by means of a computer system*. Both the *IP content* and the *access control system* applied in order to control distribution of the content are protected by the law.

File sharing in combination with *torrent technology* challenges the business models of the entertainment industry and causes a series of legal problems. This has been demonstrated in high-profile cases against services such as the Pirate Bay, Megaupload, and Popcorn Time.

Naturally, the IP right holders would prefer to take down the illegal service and punish those behind it, who get the economic gain from commercial advertisements on the service and the subscriber fees (if any). Without a closer look at the legal obstacles, they are the *organizers* of copyright infringements on a commercial scale, which amounts to *serious organized crime*. However, legal problems may be encountered despite that criminal provisions in accordance with article 10 are implemented. These can briefly be summarized as follows.

First, pursuant to EU regulation as well as the US Digital Millennium Copyright Act (DMCA), *service providers* are protected from liability arising from unlawful usage of the service by the subscribers or users. The insulation from liability applies to providers of services of *a passive or technical nature*, such as providing broadband connection or a caching service. As regards providers of *hosting services*, there is a notice and takedown procedure that must be complied with. The fact that causes a problem to the law is that the provider of a *torrent service* only provides the torrent files, which enables the users to locate the entertainment files on other computers. The actual file sharing goes directly between the users, so the provider does not host illegal material *per se*. But of course, rules of aiding and abetting are applicable here just as in other cases.

Second, while the legal rules conceptualize a hosting service as having a special location – a site – on the Internet, a *torrent service* might take the form of an *application* that can be downloaded from anywhere, even if the developers behind it can be located. So the genie is out of the bottle, and the service can hardly be taken down.

In Belgium, IP rights holders were able to implement deep-packet filters that blocked peer-to-peer file sharing of IP-protected material. The arrangement was struck down by the ECJ in two judgments from 2011 and 2012 (the *SABAM* cases).[48] The court said that, while the need for respect for IP rights could not be overlooked, it was not overriding in light of other competing interests, especially the right to privacy and freedom of speech (the risk of a chilling effect). Hence, the filters had to be disabled.

On this backdrop, the easy case – in terms of the law – is to prosecute one who has downloaded and stored a large number of pirated files, provided that the case is sufficiently serious to amount to a criminal offense. This depends upon national legislation. Predefined hash signatures may be used to analyze the files, similarly to the material mentioned earlier in this chapter.

3.3.7 Racist and Xenophobic Speech

The additional protocol to the convention confers an obligation on the parties to criminalize "acts of a racist or xenophobic nature committed through computer systems."

Definition 3.8: Racist or Xenophobic Material

"Racist or xenophobic material means any written material, any image or any other representation of ideas or theories, which advocates, promotes or incites hatred, discrimination or violence, against any individual or group of individuals, based on race, color, descent or national or ethnic origin, as well as religion if used as pretext for any of these factors."

Additional Protocol to the Cybercrime Convention article 2(1)

The parties must criminalize (1) dissemination of racist and xenophobic material to the public through computer systems (article 3); (2) threatening individuals or groups of individuals with the commission of a serious criminal offense against them, which is racist or xenophobically motivated (Article 4); (3) insults made in public that are racist or

---

48 Case C-70/10, November 24, 2011, *Scarlet Extended SA v. Société belge des auteurs, compositeurs et éditeurs SCRL (SABAM)*; and Case C-360/10, February 16, 2012, *SABAM v. Netlog NV*.

xenophobic motivated (Article 5); and denial, gross minimization, approval, or justification of genocide or crimes against humanity (Article 6).

Violent threat is generally criminalized in national legal systems, and the theoretical level of punishment is usually raised for threats motivated as described in article 4. However, there are differences in the national legal policy when it comes to criminalization of the forms of speech mentioned in Articles 3, 5, and 6. This has to do with different approaches as to how the fundamental right to freedom of speech shall be protected (ECHR article 10; the First Amendment of the US Bill of Rights). The additional protocol has not gained the same kind of support as the convention itself.[49]

If the material or speech mentioned above is criminalized, the legal assessment may still be difficult. The content must be interpreted, and contextual information taken into account. Incitement to violence against a minority group and grossly dehumanizing speech are indicators to look for, and there is extensive case law in relation to ECHR article 10 to guide the legal assessment. To a digital investigator, the most important task is to secure the content and any contextual information, and then hand the material over to a lawyer who is trained to assess the legality of such speech.

3.4 Investigation Methods for Collecting Digital Evidence

The procedural part of the Cybercrime Convention (articles 14 through 21) sets out coercive investigation methods for the purpose of collecting digital evidence.[50] The parties have an obligation to implement the methods in national legislation. The motivation is to secure that computer data can be sought after and collected as evidence, to the same extent as can physical objects. The improvement of national legislation enhances the legal framework for international cooperation (see Section 3.5). A nation state may authorize such methods without necessarily being party to the convention. The international framework is still improved.[51] This section is focused on the investigation methods set out in the convention, while taking account of the digital forensic methods explained elsewhere in this book. Rules of national procedural law are not dealt with.

3.4.1 The Digital Forensic Process in the Context of Criminal Procedure

The main activity performed in a criminal investigation is the *collection of evidence in order to identify the suspect and prove or disprove the alleged crime* (remember 5WH from Definition 1.4). Pursuant to the rule of law, each investigative step *must be justified* in light of the nature of the crime and the concrete circumstances. Put differently, the professionals working on the case *must be able to state the reason why* they do what they are doing. The obligation to justify one's actions prevents arbitrary

---

49 As of September 2016, 24 states have ratified, and 15 signed without following up with ratification.
50 See Definition 3.2, "Coercive Investigation Method."
51 See further notes on this point in Section 3.2.2.

interference with private matters, and the waste of public resources on matters irrelevant to the task.

By implication, the steps to collect evidence should be limited to computer data *that can be deemed to be relevant* given the purpose and context of the specific investigation. Hence, the *legal principle of relevancy* is applicable to every criminal investigation method. There is a problem with computer data as evidence: that the data must be collected more or less in bulk, before one has had the chance to look into its contents and identify relevant parts. Thus, only a *preliminary relevance assessment* can be made at the initial stage. This gives rise to some *legal* and *terminological* issues of which professionals in multidisciplinary teams should be aware.

The starting point is that a digital investigation should adhere to the *digital forensic process* in order to secure that the investigation or, rather, the digital evidence is *forensically sound*. The principles of *evidence integrity* and *chain of custody* (as defined in Section 1.2.3) should be complied with at all phases of the digital forensic process (as discussed in Chapter 2). In a criminal investigation, the digital forensic process must be fitted into the framework of *procedural criminal law*, which is concerned with *relevancy*, *legality*, and *right to fair trial*. Consequently, two procedures are at play, one a *de facto standard* and the other *legally determined*.

We now turn to the expression *data that is secured*, which is commonly used in digital investigation; but what does it mean? Within the context of the *digital forensic process*, it may conceivably refer to steps taken in the *collection phase*. Data that is collected may be deemed to be secured, in which case any subsequent steps, for instance in the *analysis phase*, concern something else. The phases of the process are consecutive (see Section 2.1.4), so the digital investigator moves onward once a phase is completed.[52] *In a legal context*, things may look different. Legal rules have *legal effects*. If we know what the rules say, we can look for the facts that trigger the legal effects. This is now explained in relation to *search* and *seizure* of digital evidence. The methods are very practical and applicable to most criminal investigations. Search means *to look for*, whereas seizure means *to take control over*.[53]

On first glance, *seizure* seems to correspond with *collection* in the digital forensic procedure, and *search* with *analysis*, because in this phase one actively tries to single out computer data that is relevant as evidence. Alternatively, search could take place in the *identification phase*, because that is when one *tries to figure out where* potential evidence *may be located* ("look for"). Besides, in the analogous situation of physical evidence, search normally precedes seizure. However, the significant point is that one cannot by looking at the digital forensic process determine whether an activity amounts to search or seizure, as these are *legal* concepts defined by *conditions laid down in procedural law*. In the end the point is that the legal effects of the *activities* conducted in the process can only be determined according to a concrete legal assessment.

The *scenario* is that the criminal investigators want access to the suspect's laptop, which she keeps in her house. Police investigators arrive, enter her house, and take her

---

52 The phases are also iterative, in which case the digital investigator moves to a preceding phase. However, the identification phase that precedes collection is obviously not the phase in which the data is secured.
53 These are working definitions meant as guidelines in the present context. The exact legal definitions are laid down in national procedural law.

laptop with them. The question is: is the *computer data* thus seized, or what is the crucial point in time? The question is important because seizure as well as search trigger *effects* in the form of *rights* of the suspect and *obligations* of the professionals in charge of the investigation.

Now, the focus is on seizure, and the suspect's *legal right to challenge it.*[54] The suspect may request that a court reviews the seized material in order to determine whether it is relevant to the investigation or not. If the court agrees with the suspect and concludes that the material is not relevant, then the police must return her material. This is problematic to the criminal investigation, which is concerned with securing *forensically sound evidence.* The digital forensic process may require the data to be secured by an image copy, which implies that mere control of *the digital storage media* does not count as *collecting the data.* Unless the procedural rules are in alignment with the digital forensic process, the suspect's right to a court review may come into effect prior to the relevancy assessment of the data (i.e., if the data is regarded as being *seized simultaneously* with the storage media). Thus, the digital investigators may not be in a position to effectively rebut the suspect's claim, and the equipment (with the data) must be returned. This shows a possible tension between the digital forensic process and the legal rules.

Alternatively, if taking control of the storage media *does not amount to seizure* of the *computer data*, the suspect's right to challenge is not yet triggered, and the digital investigation may pursue the phases of the digital forensic process undisturbed by any judicial intervention. It could well be that *seizure of computer data* legally first takes place in the *analysis phase*, when relevant data is identified and picked out as evidence.

In multidisciplinary investigation teams, terms and expressions such as *securing data* may be used in different meanings. This can cause misunderstandings, especially when having a breach of procedure in mind. So, to pick up on points mentioned in Sections 3.2.3.8 and 3.2.3.9: whether a deviation from the digital forensic process affects the right to adduce the evidence at trial is contingent on national legal rules in light of the principles of fair trial.

3.4.2 Computer Data That Are Publicly Available

Pursuant to the territoriality principle, the investigation methods included in the Cybercrime Convention must be carried out *within the territory of the state.* In order to collect digital evidence located abroad, assistance from public authorities in that state is necessary (Section 3.5). However, computer data that is publicly available can freely be collected. This is expressed in article 32(a) of the convention.[55]

---

54 See, for instance, the Norwegian procedural Criminal Code § 208.
55 The territoriality principle reflects the principle of sovereignty. Article 32(a) seeks only to give a limited solution to the problem of territorial limitation of investigation powers. Other rules not dealt with here may also be relevant to the situation, such as *data protection rules* that regulate the legality of collecting, storing, and analyzing personal data for the purpose of crime prevention or investigation. Rules as mentioned address the individuals' right of private life, in the balance with the societal need for safety and reasonably effective crime preventive measures.

3.4.2.1 Transborder Access to Stored Computer Data Where Publicly Available

---

Legal Provision 3.13: Transborder Access to Stored Computer Data Where Publicly Available

"A Party may, without the authorisation of another Party . . . access publicly available (open source) stored computer data, regardless of where the data is located geographically."

Cybercrime Convention article 32(a)

The crucial phrase is "publicly available (open source) stored computer data." Pursuant to Guidance Note 7, "Transborder access to data (Article 32)," it is "commonly understood that the law enforcement officials may access any data that the public may access, and for this purpose subscribe to or register for services available to the public. If a portion of a public website, service or similar is closed to the public, then it is not considered publicly available in the meaning of article 32a" [Cybercrime Convention Committee (T-CY), 2014]. It follows that a criminal investigator may freely subscribe to a service offered by a host or provider in another state, and make use of the information thus gathered, in order to investigate and prosecute crime.

Article 32(a) mentions computer data that is "stored." This excludes *real-time* methods such as interception. The exclusion can also be inferred from the condition that the computer data must be "publicly available." However, both expressions may be deemed to be vague.[56] In light of the increasingly dynamic technical development, one may ask how strictly the word *stored* shall be interpreted. For the technically skilled, collection of geolocation data can be gathered from social media, but are they "stored"? And are they "publicly available" when not everyone has the skills to collect them? Technically educated persons and lawyers may differ on these issues. Article 32(a) should in any case be interpreted in light of its purpose, which is to sort out questions regarding the territorial limitation for investigation. Specifically, as regards the protection of the individual's right to respect for private life in the Internet environment this should be determined pursuant to national legal rules as interpreted in light of the fundamental human rights.

3.4.2.2 Online Undercover Operations

Article 32(a) does not authorize, nor does it prohibit, the use of *fake identity* in order to conceal one's professional status as criminal investigator. Methods for *infiltration and undercover operations* are generally not dealt with by the Cybercrime Convention, but the procedures for international cooperation set out in its third part can be utilized in order to organize and coordinate such operations (see Section 3.5). Some online undercover operations are well known, for instance the FBI investigation against the people behind Megaupload, Megavideo, and Megaclick.com (the "Mega Sites"; see Example 3.12).

---

56 Vagueness is explained in Section 3.2.5.1, and followed up with respect to procedural law in Section 3.2.5.3.

Example 3.12: Online Undercover Activities against Mega Sites

"The FBI has conducted online undercover activities involving the Mega Sites. These undercover activities include identifying, viewing, and down-loading copyright-infringing materials on these websites; opening "premium" accounts on these websites to analyze how these websites operate from a customer viewpoint; and performing network analysis to further analyze how these websites operate."

Summary of evidence (Criminal No. 1 : 12CR3), paragraph 4,
US District Court for the Eastern District of Virginia, November 22, 2013

3.4.3   Scope and Safeguards of the Investigation Methods

The Cybercrime Convention includes the following investigation methods: preservation and production order (articles 16–18), search and seizure (article 19), and real-time collection of traffic data and interception of content data (articles 20–21).

3.4.3.1   Suspicion-Based Investigation Methods

The methods must be implemented in national procedural legislation "for the purpose of specific criminal investigations or proceedings" [article 14(1)]. The methods are suspicion based. The convention does not authorize methods solely for general crime-preventive purposes. Collection in bulk from cloud services or other digital sources falls beyond the scope of the convention, as well as the procedures for subsequent data mining, which eventually may lead to targeted analysis regarding certain individuals.

As a main rule, there must be *probable cause* for the suspicion, and the assessment must be based on some external facts (albeit of a preliminary nature), not merely a gut feeling.[57] The legal conditions are subject to independent court control. The suspect is also entitled to be informed about the steps taken against her, if not exactly when they are performed, and within a certain time thereafter.

3.4.3.2   The Scope of the Investigation Methods (Article 14)

Scope means *the situations (purposes) for which the methods can be applied.* The main rule is specified in article 14(2) (see Legal Provision 3.14).

Legal Provision 3.14: The Scope of the Investigation Methods

"... each Party shall apply the powers and procedures ... to:

a) the criminal offences established in accordance with Articles 2 through 11 of this Convention;
b) other criminal offences committed by means of a computer system; and
c) the collection of evidence in electronic form of a criminal offence."

Cybercrime Convention article 14(2) (excerpt)

---

57 National legal systems may make use of a scale with different degrees of suspicion, such as, in the United States: *reasonable suspicion, probable cause,* and *a preponderance of evidence;* and in Norway: *grunn, rimelig grunn, skjellig grunn,* and *overveiende sannsynlig.*

While litra a specifies a list of criminal offenses, litra b and c are more broadly construed. The obligation flowing from litra c effectively makes the coercive methods potentially applicable to every criminal offense, the only condition being that the investigation or procedure necessitates "the collection of" digital evidence. There has been a tremendous development in the use of digital evidence over the years that have passed since the convention was signed in 2001. Litra b and c may have been regarded as radical solutions at the time, but now they are taken for granted.

The convention does not limit the investigation methods to specific phases, as long as the suspicion requirement is fulfilled. Investigation is an *activity* that may be carried out in several phases (depending on the rules in national procedural law). Imagine a witness who, during trial, comes up with information that calls for an additional search in secured data. This could lead to a time-out in the proceedings, granting opportunity to conduct the search, plus sufficient time for the defense lawyer to go through new material, whereupon the proceedings may resume. For this reason, the description of the investigation methods does not pay any attention to the procedural stage.

3.4.3.3 Conditions and Safeguards (Article 15)

The Cybercrime Convention article 15 expresses the procedural principles of legality and proportionality (the principles are described in Section 3.2.3.6). Pursuant to article 15(1), the parties "shall provide for the adequate protection of human rights and liberties" while making use of the investigation methods.[58] The second paragraph explicitly sets out specific control measures (see Legal Provision 3.15).

Legal Provision 3.15: Conditions and Safeguards Concerning Coercive Methods

"Such conditions and safeguards shall, as appropriate in view of the nature of the procedure or power concerned, inter alia, include judicial or other independent supervision, grounds justifying application, and limitation of the scope and the duration of such power or procedure."

Cybercrime Convention article 15(2)

The *strictness* of conditions and control measures are relative to the *invasiveness* of the investigation method. Taking Norwegian procedural law as an example: interception may be applied provided that the criminal offense can be punished with imprisonment for 10 years or more. It means that *interception* may be applied in investigations concerning, for instance, homicide, armed robbery, and profit-motivated organized crime, but not for investigation of computer intrusion, as the theoretical level of punishment is a maximum of 2 years.[59] *Seizure* is traditionally considered as much less invasive and can be applied with regard to all criminal offenses, as is the case for *search*, as long as the theoretical level of punishment is imprisonment (no matter how short).

Traditional notions – for instance, that *interception* is more invasive than *search and seizure* – are challenged by technological developments. Digitalization, compression

---

58 Article 15 also makes a reference to international legal instruments, mentioned in Section 3.2.3.
59 The theoretical level of punishment is explained in the introduction of Section 3.3.

technology, and huge storage space at low cost lead to the accumulation of massive amounts of computer data, which can be subject to search and seizure. Under such circumstances, one has to question whether search and seizure are less intrusive than, say, interception of a telephone line for a 2-week period. Rational differentiation is difficult because the interferences cannot be compared along the same scale (it is like asking what is worst: losing a driver's license for 3 months or spending 3 nights in jail?). Likewise, it is hard to compare the invasiveness of collecting vast amounts of metadata to interception.

The questions put forward illustrate problems *de lege ferenda* with which the politicians have to struggle. In a *de lege lata perspective*, what matters is, above all, that the methods are described in law, with a specification of the criminal offenses for which they can be put into use. Independent control mechanisms must be in place, primarily in the form of independent judicial review. Moreover, the technological development may have an impact in relation to the *proportionality assessment*. As regards investigation methods that can be performed over time, the law requires limitation to a specific period. Within the limits of the law, the exact period is fixed according to a proportionality assessment; for instance, permission to intercept the suspect's cellphone for 2 weeks, and extension pursuant to judicial review. Proportionality considerations may limit *search and seizure* of *stored data* as well. The large amounts of data that are available for seizure in a *technical* sense are therefore not always *legally* available (see Example 3.14).

It has become increasingly clear that the *temporal limitation* is relevant to every investigation method that seeks to collect *evidence that materializes in the future*. Traditionally, *production order* and *seizure* were applied to evidence that already existed at the time when the order was issued. This has changed. For instance, a production order may be granted for financial records from a historical date until a future date, and the bank is compelled to hand over records of future transactions to the police on a running basis. In effect, this is *account monitoring*, carried out under the label *production order*. Another example is (computer) *search*. Search as a method is performed at *a certain point in time*, not on a running basis, in which case it would amount to (computer) surveillance. However, it can be conducted *repeatedly* (see Example 3.13). Hence, the period granted for repeated search must be stated in the court's permission, specifying the dates in both ends of the period. It may even be required to specify the number of searches. This is contingent on national legal provisions.

Example 3.13: Repeated Search in Danish Procedural Law

"The court can permit repeated search [to be conducted within a specified period]. The court shall decide the number of searches. If supported by special reasons, the court can decide that the number of searches may be unlimited."

Danish Procedural Code (Retsplejeloven) § 799(3)
(author's translation from Danish)

The *proportionality principle* may also lead to limitations back in time (see Example 3.14).

Example 3.14: Search and Seizure in Relation to a Charge of Securities Fraud

The Norwegian national fraud agency conducted search and seizure of the computer system of a bank, on a charge of securities fraud. According to the criminal charge, the relevant period went 3 years back in time, but the police claimed that data for a longer period – 10 years – was needed. This was rejected by the court, as not proportionate in relation to the period specified in the criminal charge. Thus, digital material for 7 years had to be returned to the bank.

LB-2009-7217

3.4.3.4 Considerations Relating to Third Parties

Article 15(3) includes an obligation to "consider the impact of the powers and procedures . . . upon the rights, responsibilities and legitimate interests of third parties." The background is that *third parties unrelated to the crime* may be affected by the investigation. The problem is very practical, but too variegated to lend itself to a single rule. Article 15 only requests the parties to be aware of it, without prescribing a concrete solution. (See Examples 3.15 and 3.16.)

Example 3.15: Megaupload.com

In January 2012, the site Megaupload.com was seized and shut down by the US Department of Justice, charged with criminal copyright infringement and racketeering. The site had 66.6 million users, whose accounts thus became inaccessible. US officials claimed that the investigation was not directed at individual users, but at 12 individuals who had offered and made profits from the services. Still, millions of users were affected by the measure. What do you think about the position of the subscribers? Do you consider them to be "third parties" within the meaning of article 15, on the ground that they were not formally declared suspect? Or do you think they should be treated in light of their activities, which undeniably, for many, was participation in unlawful file sharing of copyrighted material?

Example 3.16: Evidence and Excess Information - Balancing Different Rights

In a criminal investigation concerning serious economic crime, the police had seized *16 million computer files* from defendant A. The files were secured by an image copy, whereupon the computer equipment was returned to A with the source files intact. The secured data was assumed to contain excess information about third parties. In the analysis phase of the digital forensic process, the digital investigator applied an automatic search using keywords. Matches were picked out and included in the case file.

Both defendant A and co-defendant B asserted that pursuant to the rights of *contradiction and equality of arms*, they were entitled to go through all of the 16 million computer files. The Norwegian Supreme Court rejected the claim made by A, stating a lack of need as he already was in possession of the source files.

Concerning B, the court set out by acknowledging that the technological development had brought about situations not contemplated by the legislator in 1981 (the year of the Procedural Code), and that even small digital devices could store large amounts of potential evidence. In the opinion of the court, the procedural provisions had to be interpreted in light of basic principles, in conjunction with the need for practical solutions, without jeopardizing the right to private life of third parties.

The court held that the *right of contradiction* encompassed the computer files identified by the automatic search. In addition, the search criteria had to be disclosed, as well as the report that described the actual circumstances of the search.

Thus, B got access to the files that the police had looked into, and the *equality of arms* was maintained. The solution enabled B to assess the quality of the search, and request new investigation steps, if need be. This secured the *right of contradiction* and to prepare the defense. Finally, concerning the interests of the *third parties*, the *duty of confidentiality* regarding excess information was maintained, and their *right to private life* respected.

HR-2011-1744-A

3.4.4   Search and Seizure (Article 19)

Article 19 of the Cybercrime Convention regulates search and seizure. The provision emphasizes that the methods must be confined within the territory. This poses a practical problem, because once a computer system has been accessed in order to conduct a search, it can be hard to know if, when, and where a geographical border is transgressed. But for the purpose of explaining the rules, we merely *assume* that the methods are conducted within the territory. The *defining features* of the methods are set out in the first and third paragraph of article 19, as shown in Legal Provision 3.16.

Legal Provision 3.16: Search and Seizure

"The competent authority shall be empowered to

1) search (a) computer system or part of it and computer data stored therein; and (b) a computer-data storage medium in which computer data may be stored.
2) . . .
3) seize or similarly secure computer data accessed [by a search pursuant to (1)]. These measures shall include the power to (a) seize or similarly secure a computer system or part of it or a computer-data storage medium; (b) make and retain a copy of those computer data; (c) maintain the integrity of the relevant stored computer data; (d) render inaccessible or remove those computer data in the accessed computer system."

Cybercrime Convention articles 19(1) and (3) (excerpt)

3.4.4.1   Main Rules

To make sense of article 19, one must *distinguish* between the *physical equipment*, including storage media, and the *computer data* (bits and bytes). It is clear that a computer system or part of it (e.g., a user account) can be searched [article 19(1) litra a].

In addition, a computer-storage medium can be searched [article 19(1) litra b]. This is, for instance, a USB stick, a CD or DVD disk, a hard drive, as well as every little chip or memory card that can contain data. The kind of device is legally irrelevant.

Consequently, *when one looks into* the contents of a computer system, *one conducts a search*. For instance, a criminal investigator who looks into the computer system of a corporation, in order to determine which parts of it to secure, performs a search of the computer system. Similarly, a criminal investigator who looks into a laptop or a smartphone performs a search of the device (a smartphone is a computer system that resembles a phone). In the USA, a computer is compared with – or regarded as – a container, which can be searched. (See Kerr (2013) regarding search under the Fourth Amendment of the US Bill of Rights).

Digital devices and storage media can be small and easily taken away by the criminal investigators before they have been looked into. Going back to the scenario described in Section 3.4.1, the initial step when one got access to the digital equipment was a *house search*. The *equipment* was then *seized* (taken out of the suspect's control). To maintain the chain of custody, two reports are needed: one that describes the house search, and one specifying the seized objects.[60] Seizure of digital devices is mentioned in article 19(3) litra a.

We now assume that the above-mentioned *equipment* does not have any particular relevance to the investigation, other than storing data that is potentially relevant as evidence. Once the data has been copied to an evidence file, or differently secured pursuant to a forensically sound method, *the seizure of the digital equipment must be lifted*, and the equipment returned to the owner (suspect). This follows from the rule that investigation steps must be justified in light of the purpose and relevance (Section 3.4.1). As the *potential evidence* has been secured, seizure of the equipment cannot be upheld for evidentiary purposes. There can be other reasons for keeping the equipment, however, such as securing a claim of confiscation, or because the content was digital contraband (which should lead to the destruction of the storage media).

3.4.4.2 Special Issues

Search and seizure raise some issues which are not clearly solved by article 19. The first question is *whether at all computer data can be seized*. This must be performed by making a copy to the criminal investigator's storage media. Article 19 does not explicitly confirm this, but makes it brilliantly clear that national procedural law must, in any case, provide for solutions that permit computer data to be *secured* as evidence *independent of the digital equipment*. This is expressed in litra b–d, which effectively acknowledge steps of the digital forensic process, by mentioning the power to (b) "make and retain a copy of [the] computer data," to (d) "remove [data] in the accessed computer system," and to (c) "maintain the integrity of the relevant stored computer data."

US law in relation to the Fourth Amendment seems not to have arrived at a clear conclusion so far, but Kerr (2013) argues that the suspect's *informational property interest* entails that copying *amounts to seizure*, because *the suspect is deprived of her exclusive control* of the data. This does not change even if she keeps the source data.

---

60 The obligation to document the investigation steps can be deemed to flow from the right to fair trial, as it is necessary in order to prepare the defense and control the performance of the police (see Section 3.2.3.8). As one can see, the chain of custody as part of the digital forensic process supports fair trial.

Kerr's view has support in *US v. Ganias* (755 F.3d 125 (2nd Cir. 2014). In this case, the police held copies in custody for over two years, which the court regarded as a *continuing Fourth Amendment seizure* of the data. Kerr's point relates to copies made without the investigators having looked into the files. In the context of Norwegian procedural law, the Supreme Court has simply concluded that computer data *can be subject to seizure*, as it must be regarded as a "thing" within the meaning of the rules of seizure of the procedural code (HR-2011468-A; 2011-1744-A and 2013-1383-A).

The next question is, *when is the data seized?* Is it when they are copied, or sometime later? This has partly been answered already with respect to US law (i.e., at the time when the copy is made, because the suspect is deprived of her exclusive control of the data). As related to the digital forensic procedure, it means that a copy made during a house search is seizure and takes place in the *collection phase*.

The Norwegian Supreme Court seems to go down a different avenue: data that is copied without the police looking into it beforehand is deemed to be seized first *when relevant files are picked out as evidence*. The reason is that this is the moment when the relevancy assessment, required by the legal provision, is made. Only then are the legal conditions for seizure of the data fulfilled. Obviously, this occurs in the *analysis phase* of the digital forensic procedure. Moreover, the analysis that is conducted in search of digital evidence is a *continued search* pursuant to the procedural rules, as interpreted by the Supreme Court. Hence, *both search and seizure* of the digital evidence take place *in the analysis phase*. It further means that excess information not looked into by the digital investigator *is not considered seized*. Thus, the suspect's right to challenge the seizure is pushed out in time until the investigators have had a fair chance to analyze the data (the time is not unlimited pursuant to the "reasonable time" condition in the fair trial doctrine; see Section 3.2.3.8).

The third question is: do the police have *an obligation to seize computer data by making a copy*, because this is less burdensome to the suspect than taking her equipment (and source data) away? One can argue that the *principle of proportionality* implies that the police have this obligation. On the other hand, bearing the burden of proof justifies a wide discretion for the police to decide the manner in which to conduct the investigation. There are different priorities to be made, and while the proportionality principle is generally relevant, the assessment must be made in light of the concrete circumstances of the individual case.

The fourth question is: can the digital investigator *routinely apply a hash analysis*[61] of the material? This must depend upon the purpose; that is, whether the search is suspicion based or not. If the hash analysis is performed for a purpose covered by the criminal charge, it should be deemed lawful. Conversely, if it is carried out without concrete grounds for suspicion, perhaps as a routine search for child sexual abuse material, the method seems to lack legal basis.

The fifth question is whether a separate permission to search is needed for a digital device that has been lawfully seized. The alternative is that the permission to seize the device is deemed as sufficient, because it follows by implication that a device seized for evidentiary purposes must also be examined. This mirrors the discussion concerning computer intrusion and data theft in Section 3.3.3, where application of an analogy between searching through the contents of a memory stick and a book was rejected. As

---

61 See Section 5.4.3 regarding hash analysis.

small devices can contain large amounts of data, a search is a clear interference with private life and needs clear legal basis. It indicates that a separate permission for the search is needed. This was also the conclusion of the Icelandic Supreme Court in the case mentioned in Example 3.17.

Example 3.17: Search of a Smartphone

A person arrived at the airport with fake ID documents. Icelandic police officers seized his smartphone, reckoning that it contained information that could reveal his identity. The seizure was lawful, but search of the smartphone could not lawfully be conducted without a new permission by the court. It was relevant that a smartphone contains content stemming from communication, which is at the core of the protection of the ECHr article 8. The judgment was followed up with a second judgment the same season (spring 2016). The need for explicit permissions both for seizure and search is thus settled Icelandic law.

H. 291/2016 and 297/2016

Finally, the criminal investigators may have problems with getting access to the relevant computer system. Article 19(4) thus confers an obligation on the parties to empower the criminal investigators to order "any person who has knowledge of the functioning of the computer system" to provide login information. It is uncertain if this encompasses an obligation to decrypt content. Access data can take the form of biometrics, such as reading fingerprints. In this context, the Norwegian Supreme Court has taken the view that the obligation to provide access data does not mean that a police investigator may press the suspect's finger onto the seized computer in order to gain access. Physical coercion needs a separate legal basis, so far not provided for in Norwegian procedural law (HR-2016-1833-A).

3.4.5 Production Order

Production order is a means for getting access to digital evidence in possession of a third party that is cooperative with the law enforcement agency. Article 18 imposes an obligation on the parties to authorize this method in national legislation. The method is traditional, so article 18 only clarifies its application to computer data. The order can concern historical data and future data (see Section 3.4.3.3).

There are several reasons why an order may be needed despite that the third party is cooperative (or at least not inclined to subvert the investigation). First, the third party may be under a legal duty of confidentiality. Information about financial transactions, or relating to electronic communication, is often relevant to criminal investigations and subject to such protection. This prevents the financial institution and the e-com service provider from disclosing the information without an order that lifts the duty of confidentiality and orders disclosure to the police. Example 3.4 illustrates this with respect to e-com data. Second, data protection rules require *a specific legal basis* in order to expose personal data to a third party (*in casu* to the police). Merely a *request* from the police may not suffice despite that general data protection rules do not impose a duty of confidentiality. Third, commercial enterprises may prefer having to comply with a clear order instead of facing their customers with the fact that they "voluntarily" provide the police with information.

A production order is suitable when the data is not readily accessible for seizure. If the data is immediately accessible, it may be more practical (and within the law) to apply seizure. This could for instance be the case with respect to a CCTV recording that is accessible on the spot where the robbery took place.

Article 18(3) mentions *subscriber data*, which is identity data about subscribers to e-com services (something "other than traffic or content data"). These are fixed data usually found in a subscriber registry. The intention is to make such data more readily available to the police, also with wider scope for international exchange through police cooperation. But again, this depends on national legislation. Furthermore, the issue really belongs to the field of data protection law (with respect to law enforcement and international police cooperation), which tends to be steadily regulated in more detail internationally.

3.4.6   Expedited Preservation and Partial Disclosure of Traffic Data

Articles 16 and 17 concern expedited orders to preserve stored data. It is in the nature of this method that the formal procedure shall be more expedited (less formal) than for the other methods. The procedure shall be determined by national law.

Article 16 concerns stored data regardless of content, while article 17 concerns traffic data and situations in which more than one service provider is involved. An expedited preservation order can be used as a means to secure data until they can be taken under control pursuant to a production order or, as the case may be, seizure. Article 16 thus states that the law enforcement agency must demonstrate that "there are grounds to believe that the computer data is particularly vulnerable to loss or modification."

As computer data is inherently vulnerable to loss or modification, the "grounds to believe" must be specified in more detail. Possible grounds could be that national e-com regulation or data protection rules impose an obligation to delete data within a short time. Notably, this could be the case for traffic data that is vital to an investigation. Taking Norwegian law as an example, IP-logs must be deleted after 3 weeks. With a preservation order, the period can be extended for a period not exceeding 90 days [article 16 (2)], with an option for renewal. Another reason could be that a corporation transfers its data to a storage service abroad as a daily routine, and is not in a position simply to keep them without a formal preservation order. This scenario may be practical to subsidiaries in global corporations.

Article 17 takes measure of the situation that traffic data is vital to *identifying the source* of a communication. If it becomes clear in the course of complying with a preservation order that the source originates from a different service provider, who should rightly be contacted by the police, this information shall be disclosed expeditiously to the police.

3.4.6.1   Real-Time Investigation Methods (Articles 20 and 21)
Articles 20 and 21 are *real-time methods* for the purpose of collecting traffic data (article 20) or intercepting content data of electronic communications (article 21(1)). The conditions are largely similar; see Legal Provision 3.17.

Legal Provision 3.17: Real-Time Investigation Methods

"The Parties shall . . . empower its competent authorities to

a) Collect or record through the application of technical means on the territory of that Party, and
b) Compel a service provider, within its existing technical capability:
   i. To collect or record through the application of technical means on the territory of that Party; or
   ii. To co-operate and assist the competent authorities in the collection or recording of

[article 20]: Traffic data, in real-time, associated with specified communications in its territory transmitted by means of a computer system.

[article 21]: Content data, in real-time, of specified communications in its territory transmitted by means of a computer system."

Cybercrime Convention articles 20 and 21(excerpt)

As interception of content data has been regarded as more intrusive than real-time collection of traffic data, the parties are permitted to limit the scope for interception to "a range of serious offenses to be determined by domestic law" [article 21(1)], whereas this limitation is not introduced for real-time collection of traffic data.

The methods are suspicion based and limited to "specific communications." This means that the methods must be limited to traffic or content data relating to a *specific communication address*. The address can be specified by a *unique number*, typically a dial number, a SIM card number, IMSI and IMEI numbers, or a fixed IP address. The convention does not limit the range of persons whose communications can be subject to the methods. Thus, the parties may decide if the methods shall be limited to target communication addresses that are registered on, or otherwise associated with, the suspect, or if a third party can be target of the method as well. This could, for instance, be family members or friends whom the suspect is likely to contact. National jurisdictions may apply different scope for the methods in this regard.

Article 20 concerns *traffic data*. The definition of traffic data in article 1(c) does not include location data, which is important to investigations today, but this can be dealt with in national legal rules. *Communication* pursuant to article 21 refers to the *transmission between end points*. Thus, the provision does not impose an obligation to authorize computer surveillance, but a party is free of course to authorize this method on its own initiative. Furthermore, communication devices can be activated in order to perform audio recording; for instance, in order to secretly listen in on a meeting. This is beyond the scope of article 21, which only concerns collection of the electronic transmission as such. All forms of electronic transmissions may be intercepted, regardless of content (voice or other forms of content).

The features of communication services may be exploited in various manners, such as *IMSI catching, silent SMS,* and bulk data from a mobile base station (see Section 6.1.3 for additional details). The convention does not regulate this, but it can still be authorized in national legislation.

On the backdrop of transnational organized crime, nation states often cooperate in joint investigations, and they have entered into agreements that enable *direct transfer* of real-time collection of traffic data and the intercepted data stream to the state that requested it.

3.5 International Cooperation in Order to Collect Digital Evidence

This section concerns the principles and procedures for international cooperation in order to collect digital evidence in a criminal investigation. First, a reminder of a point mentioned a few times in this chapter: the legal power of law enforcement agencies to investigate and prosecute crime is limited to the territory of the nation state. This rule follows from the principle of sovereignty in international law. The official authorities of the state in which the digital evidence is located *have exclusive powers* to access and secure the evidence. When a law enforcement agency accesses and secures evidence located within the territory of another state, it exceeds its powers and violates the sovereignty of the other state.[62]

It is not uncommon that digital evidence is located abroad. The question is, then, how to secure the evidence without interfering with the sovereignty of the other state. The simple answer is that the law enforcement in charge of the criminal investigation *has to request assistance* from the other state.

3.5.1 Narrowing the Focus

There are many formal procedures for international cooperation against crime, covering different aspects of investigation and prosecution, such as assistance to seek, arrest, and extradite a suspect, and obtain witness or expert testimony and other forms of evidence for the benefit of a criminal investigation in another state. Procedures have also been developed in order to transfer the responsibility for a criminal investigation to another state. Computer attacks perpetrated over the Internet provide a practical case. As the investigation proceeds, it may become clear that the attack originated from a computer located in another state. Unless the suspect can be extradited for prosecution in the "victim state," it may be necessary to transfer the case to the state where the individual resides. The alternative is that the crime is left unpunished.

All of these measures can be relevant in a criminal investigation. However, this section is focused on the cooperation procedures for the purpose of collecting evidence through the application of *coercive measures* as described in Section 3.4. It should be noted that the procedures are not required for collecting information from "publicly available" (open source) Internet sites (see Section 3.4.2).

Basically, international cooperation must proceed along *procedures for mutual legal assistance* and/or *procedures for international police cooperation*. As a main rule, the procedure for mutual legal assistance must be applied when evidence is sought to be obtained by coercive measures. Police cooperation can be useful in order to prepare for such requests. The formal parties involved are nation states [i.e., the state of the law

---

62 Rereading Section 3.2.3.3, "A Special Note on Transborder Search and Surveillance," before reading this section is recommended.

enforcement in need of assistance (the *requesting state*) and the state that receives the request (the *requested state*)].

Not all information in digital form (which may contribute to an investigation) is regarded as digital evidence, at least not in the present context. Testimony that is audio or video recorded is not digital evidence. *Testimony* is a form of evidence qualitatively different from *objects*, and it is governed by a different set of procedural rules. *Digital evidence* falls in the latter category as an object. This also includes evidence collected in real time by application of computer surveillance or interception of electronic communications.

Information in *national or international police registries* is not digital evidence either. Some examples are information in fingerprint or DNA registries, in a registry of convicts, or in an intelligence database. The information is generally governed by *data protection rules*, which also regulate international data exchanges between law-enforcing agencies.[63] These rules are beyond the scope of this chapter.

3.5.2 A Special Note on Transborder Access to Digital Evidence

Digital evidence may be *technically accessible* for law enforcement globally, due to transnational communication networks and the use of cloud services. Thus, *accessibility* – or, essentially, *controllability* of computer data – seems to be more relevant than *geographical (territorial) localization*, as criteria for international cooperation procedures. The problems of determining the exact location of stored computer data support this view. However, which criteria to apply in the future is subject to an ongoing discussion in international fora. On this backdrop, the present section describes article 32 (b) of the Cybercrime Convention. The provision addresses transborder access to stored computer data *pursuant to consent* (see Legal Provision 3.18).

Legal Provision 3.18: Transborder Access to Data Pursuant to Consent

"A Party may, without the authorization of another Party . . . (b) access or receive, through a computer system in its territory, stored computer data located in another Party, if the Party obtains the lawful and voluntary consent of the person who has the lawful authority to disclose the data to the Party through that computer system."

Cybercrime Convention article 32(b)

There are some difficulties that make the provision less effective than perhaps intended. The issues are addressed at some length in Guidance Note 7, "Trans-border access to data": the condition "stored computer data located in another Party" is deemed to be fulfilled only *if it is known* where the data is located. The provision "would not cover

---

63 This point is expressed in Section 3.2.3.6 as well, where the rules governing coercive measures in order to collect digital evidence are distinguished from data protection rules. Data protection rules governing law enforcement activities emanate – in a European context – from Council Framework Decision 2008/977/JHA of November 27, 2008, on the protection of personal data processed in the framework of police and judicial cooperation in criminal matters, and Directive 46/95/EC on data protection. The European legal framework on data protection is developing in light of the agenda of the Single Digital Market and the General Data Protection Regulation (GDPR) (EU 2016/679).

situations where the data are not stored in another Party, or it is uncertain where the data are located" [Cybercrime Convention Committee (T-CY), 2014]. However, there is a risk that the aforementioned problem with determining the *exact location of stored data* makes the provision impracticable as a legal basis for accessing data.

There are also problems regarding the condition "lawful and voluntary consent." The guidance note mentions that "many Parties would object – and some even consider it a criminal offense – if a person who is physically in their territory, is directly approached by foreign law enforcement authorities who seek his or her cooperation." It is further claimed that "the standard hypothesis is that the person providing access *is physically located in the territory of the requesting Party*" (emphasis added). Service providers are moreover "unlikely to be able to consent . . . to disclosure of their users' data [as they] will only be holders of such data; they will not control or own the data." Finally, it is emphasized that law enforcement authorities must apply "the same legal standards under Article 32b as they would domestically. If access or disclosure would not be permitted domestically it would also not be permitted under Article 32b."

As search of a user account is a coercive measure, there is narrow scope for relying on consent, at least from a suspect.[64] In the end, the practical significance of article 32(b) is that transborder search is permitted provided that the owner of the user account gives a free and voluntary consent and is present in the territory of the law enforcement agency that conducts the investigation.

3.5.3 Mutual Legal Assistance

To begin with, we assume that the requesting and requested states have not entered into any convention that imposes obligations to provide legal assistance to one another. The assumption is not unrealistic. Global Internet reach may lead states, which hardly have had any direct formal contact, to cooperate, and they may have to do so without the guidance of a binding treaty.

3.5.3.1 Basic Principles and Formal Steps of the Procedure

Absent a cooperation treaty, the starting point is that no nation state has any *obligation* to provide assistance to another nation state in order to secure digital evidence. However, it can do so as per its own volition, thus adhering to the *principle of comity*. This can be translated into *expressing a civil, peaceful, or polite attitude*. As the requesting state must be equally civil, its formal request for assistance (formally, the *letter rogatory*) must offer *reciprocity*. Thus, it has to demonstrate that it is willing and able to serve a similar request from the other state, should the need arise.

The formal request must *describe the crime under investigation* and *cite the relevant provision of the criminal code*. Next, it must *cite the relevant procedural provision* and show that a legal permission would have been granted in its own jurisdiction, had the evidence been located there. One way to do this is to obtain permission *in abstracto*, regarding the coercive measure requested. The permission must be granted by the

---

64 See Section 3.2.3.6 about the procedural aspect of the principle of legality, and Section 3.4.4 about search and seizure of computer data.

competent authority (usually the magistrate court or the public prosecutor). It must be demonstrated that the conditions of legal basis, necessity, and proportionality of the coercive method are fulfilled.

The request for assistance, supported by the required documentation, is then submitted through official channels. This could involve the Ministry of Justice and even the Ministry of Foreign Affairs, in both the requesting and requested states. Once the requested state has received the request for assistance, it is submitted to a law enforcement agency in the area where the digital evidence is located, or, rather, where the *method* can be carried out. Then the digital evidence must be obtained according to standard procedures applicable in the requested state. After the investigative step has been performed, and the evidence gathered (hopefully), formal channels must be used in reverse, in order to transfer the evidence to the requesting state. To speed up the procedure, exchange of the request, documents, and evidence may be carried out directly between the law-enforcing agencies in the requesting and the requested states. This parallel procedure, however, cannot entirely substitute the formal procedure between nation states.

To illustrate: there is often a need to collect digital evidence from user accounts on social media such as Facebook and Google. The corporations that own the services are located in California, USA. For a nation state to get *content data* from user accounts on these services, the above-mentioned procedure must be applied (absent a cooperation treaty with the USA).

The *principle of dual criminality* operates to secure a nation state's level of protection for its citizens, as per the principle of legality. Thus, the requested state may set as conditions for providing assistance that: (1) the conduct described in the request is regarded as a criminal offense in its own jurisdiction; and (2) the conduct (offense) qualifies for application of the requested coercive method.

Finally, a nation state may legitimately refuse to cooperate when it considers assistance to put its national interests or security at stake, if essential principles of that state are contravened (*ordre public*), or when there is a risk of capital punishment.

3.5.3.2 International Conventions Concerning Mutual Legal Assistance

International conventions seek to build on the *principle of comity*, by requiring the parties to cooperate and assist "to the widest extent possible." This is laid down as a general principle in the Cybercrime Convention article 23, and in article 25(1) specifically with respect to "the collection of evidence in digital form of criminal offences." Initiatives have also been taken to reduce the scope for invoking *absence of dual criminality* as ground for refusal. Harmonization of substantive and procedural criminal law ensures that the condition is fulfilled, because (1) the underlying conduct that motivates the investigation is a criminal offense in both the requesting and requested states, and (2) the coercive methods are legally authorized in both jurisdictions.

Article 25(5) states that the dual criminality condition "shall be deemed fulfilled, irrespective whether [the law of the Requested Party] place the offence within the same category of offence or denominate the offence by the same terminology as the requesting Party, *if the conduct underlying the offence for which assistance is sought* is a criminal offence under its laws" (emphasis added). The provision seeks to limit the condition to "clear-cut" instances, so what matters is that the *actual conduct is criminalized.* The systematic classification of the criminal offense or the name it goes by in the legal systems does not matter.

The practical outcome is that a party to the Cybercrime Convention has an obligation to assist another party with respect to collection of digital evidence, when the investigation concerns the criminal offenses mentioned in the convention articles 2 through 11. The convention also seeks to level the ground for reciprocal assistance with respect to requests concerning investigation of "other criminal offences committed by means of a computer system" and, generally, "the collection of evidence in electronic form of a criminal offence" [article 14(2)(a–c) in conjunction with articles 23 and 25(1)]. As each party has implemented the coercive methods mentioned in articles 16 through 21, assistance may generally be expected, although reservations can be made in order to uphold a certain level of protection against gravely intrusive methods (articles 14 and 15 in conjunction with article 25 *et seq.*).

The Cybercrime Convention is a *supplement* to other international instruments regarding mutual legal assistance in criminal matters (article 23). It makes a contribution to international cooperation particularly by specifying the obligation to assist with expedited preservation and disclosure of stored traffic data (articles 29 and 30). Moreover, it requires each party to designate a 24/7 point of contact "in order to ensure the immediate assistance for the purpose of investigations and proceedings concerning criminal offences related to computer systems and data, or for the collection of evidence in electronic form of a criminal offence" [article 35(1)]. Usually, it is the National Central Bureau of the law enforcement that is designated for the task. This agency also represents the party in Interpol and Europol. Importantly, article 35(3) requires that "trained and equipped personnel are available, in order to facilitate the operation of the network."

From a European perspective, the 1959 European Convention on Mutual Assistance in Criminal Matters (ETS 30) has played a significant role in order to develop formal procedures for such cooperation. The additional protocols from 1978 and 2001 limit the scope for invoking conditions in cases concerning *fiscal crime*, and introduce more efficient procedures for cooperation *in case of urgency*. This is correspondingly reflected in the Cybercrime Convention article 25(4) (fiscal offenses), and articles 25(3) and 27(9) (a) (urgency).

Considerable efforts have been made over several decades in order to speed up the efficacy of international legal cooperation in the investigation of crime, while maintaining respect for fundamental rights and the rule of law. The aforementioned UN Convention against Transnational Organized Crime is an example in point, and article 18 concerns mutual legal assistance. Many international instruments include procedures for expedited preservation and disclosure of traffic data (in the same fashion as the Cybercrime Convention), and there are arrangements for expedited interception of electronic communications and transmissions, which enable *direct transfer of the data stream to the designated law enforcement agency of the requesting party.* The practical facilitation of such assistance is conducted by the National Central Bureau.

The EU plays an increasingly significant role in this respect. Notably, in the year 2000 a convention regarding mutual assistance in criminal matters was entered into between the member states of the EU.[65] In 2003, the EU entered into a corresponding agreement

---

65 EU Mutual Legal Assistance Convention (2000/C 197/01).

with the USA (in force 2010), and in 2009 with Japan (in force 2011).[66] The conventions build on the principles described here, while at the same time trying to implement and thus benefit from new technology. Practical cooperation procedures on the level of prosecutors and courts have developed within the Eurojust system (2002).[67]

The Nordic countries have a history of trust and close cooperation. The Nordic cooperation treaty from 1974, with later supplements and amendments, reduces bureaucracy and increases cooperation even more than described above. However, once a non-Nordic state is involved, other procedures must be applied.

3.5.4 International Police Cooperation and Joint Investigation Teams

Police officers have traditionally been able to cooperate rather informally through Interpol, or simply by a direct phone call to a familiar colleague abroad.[68] Many nations also have *liaison officers* stationed abroad (by permission of the other state) who may be of assistance. Europol and its "EC3 center" (European Cybercrime Center) have had a growing role in Europe, because of their efforts against serious organized crime, including cybercrimes.

The informal character of this kind of international police cooperation is inadequate to support the requests for the application of coercive methods as described in this section. Instead, the formal procedures of mutual legal assistance must be utilized. However, it may be practical to request assistance from police officers abroad in order to explore viable options for assistance, in preparation to a formal request. In some jurisdictions, *subscriber data* (as different from traffic data) may be directly disclosed to criminal investigators in the police. In such cases, the data can be made available to a criminal investigator in another state pursuant to a routine for police cooperation (observing data protection rules applicable to international police cooperation). As regards the procedure for *expedited disclosure of traffic data* (which indicates that a request should properly be directed to a third state; see Section 3.4.6), the procedure is formal. The extent to which it can be performed on the police level is contingent on the procedural law of the national jurisdiction.

Finally, within the EU, the Schengen Information System (SIS) is a system for rapid assistance and transfer of information. This follows a separate set of rules and is managed by the National Central Bureau of each Schengen member.

The territorial limitation along with the complexity of the international cooperation procedures have led to meetings (so-called *consultations*) to identify the practical

---

66 Mutual Legal Assistance: Agreement between the USA and the EU, signed in Washington June 25, 2003 (entry into force February 1, 2010); Agreement between the EU and Japan on Mutual Legal Assistance in Criminal Matters, signed November 30, 2009 (entry into force January 2, 2011).

67 Council Decision 2002/187/JHA, consolidated version July 15, 2009 (14927/08 COPEN 200 Eurojust 88 EJN 66).

68 Interpol is an international police organization. Membership is held by the nation state, which is represented by its National Central Bureau (National Central Intelligence Service, or NCIS), for instance Germany's *Bundeskriminalamt* (BKA) and the Norwegian *Kriminalpolitisentralen* (Kripos). Participation by the USA is performed through the National Central Bureau in Washington, DC. Interpol is a truly global organization, consisting of 190 members; see INTERPOL is the world's largest international police organization, with 190 member countries.INTERPOL is the world's largest international police organization, with 190 member countries.http://www.interpol.int/About-INTERPOL/Overview.

steps that actually must be taken, by whom, in which form and sequence, and so on, for lawfully obtaining evidence abroad. Consultation is a practical measure that aims to convert the conventions into practical means of cooperation. In this spirit, the setting up of Joint Investigation Teams in Europe is supported by both Europol and Eurojust.[69]

A Europol/Eurojust-sponsored Joint Investigation Team consists of law enforcement representatives of at least two states, one of which is in the lead. Nonmembers of the EU and states outside Europe may participate. Formally, a team is set up with a mandate concerning a specific criminal investigation. The team can get support in the form of tactical, technical, and legal advice from Europol and Eurojust, which also help out with practical steps such as identifying the relevant legal provisions and drafting a criminal charge. Necessary equipment may also be provided along with a budget to cover travel costs and document translation. A manual advising how to create a Joint Investigation Team is available online on Eurojust and Europol websites.

3.6 Summary

This chapter has described cybercrime law from different perspectives. The principle of territoriality limits the powers of law enforcement (to investigate and prosecute crime) to the territory of the state. Close international cooperation is needed in order to counteract transborder digital crime and, generally, collect digital evidence (which is relevant in most criminal investigations). However, data stored on publicly available Internet sites may be collected for the purpose of a criminal investigation, regardless of where the data is stored. Harmonization of national substantive and procedural criminal law is a precondition for effective international cooperation, along with recognition of the fundamental human rights and the rule of law. Thus, principles of legality, proportionality, relevance, and fair trial are applicable to cybercrimes, as well as to other crimes. Notably, a national procedural system is in compliance with the fundamental conditions, as long as *the system as a whole* is satisfactory. International cooperation in the form of mutual legal assistance must comply with formal routines. Joint investigations set up in a formalized manner are encouraged. Finally, activities performed as part of the digital forensic process may have legal effects determined by rules of procedural criminal law. The exact rules and legal effects are determined by the national jurisdiction that is in charge of the criminal investigation and prosecution.

3.7 Exercises

1 Explain why criminals too, have fundamental rights.

2 Restate the principle of legality in the context of crime (ECHR article 7).

---

69 Joint investigation is recommended by the UN Convention against Transnational Organized Crime article 19.

3 Why is the principle important, who does it protect, and against what kind of risk does it protect?

4 Describe the characteristics of an investigation method that is "coercive."

5 Explain the conditions that must be fulfilled for lawful application of a coercive investigation method that interferes with the right to private life (ECHR article 8).

6 State the reason why an official may not conduct a criminal investigation on the territory of another state, wothout permission from that state.

7 Assuming that digital evidence has been secretly secured from a user account on a cloud service: is it lawfully obtained? If the answer is negative, who is the aggrieved party? Is the consequence that the evidence must be excluded from being adduced at trial? Which rule (principle) is relevant in this respect, and who decides?

8 Mention the five criteria that determine the relevancy of investigation steps and of the evidence.

9 Why is it important that a digital investigator is able to justify the reason why she does what she does?

10 Does seizure of computer data take place in the collection phase of the digital forensic process? Explain the relation between the digital forensic process and the rules of search and seizure.

11 What should a digital investigator do if she commits a real blunder while dealing with the digital evidence? Should she try to conceal it and repair the damage, or act differently? Mention the legal principles at stake in this situation.

4

Digital Forensic Readiness

Ausra Dilijonaite

Cyber Risk Services, Deloitte AS, Oslo, Norway

> *By failing to prepare, you are preparing to fail.*
>
> —Benjamin Franklin

4.1 Introduction

Many television series with forensics subject matter depict gadgets and amazing hackers who can expose tiny, revealing details to investigators. These details then lead to breakthroughs in their cases. With the spice of drama and suspense, digital forensics seems truly exciting. But while the television series makes it seem convenient, exciting, and easy, real-life investigations require far more effort and preparation. This chapter examines the preparation part of the digital investigation process, which is called *digital forensic readiness*.

This chapter details the definition and rationale for digital forensic readiness, lays down main components to be included (people, processes, procedures, and technology), and discusses the difference between corporate and law enforcement digital forensic readiness. The chapter is based on the research performed in Dilijonaite (2014).

4.2 Definition

Digital forensic readiness is defined by answering the question "What does it mean to be ready?" Simply put, it means being prepared. The goal of digital investigation is to reconstruct the incident and find supporting or refuting evidence. Ultimately, the collected digital evidence can be used in a court of law. Thus, it follows: to be forensically ready means to be prepared to efficiently execute digital investigations and then present evidence to the intended audience (such as auditors or legal advisors in enterprise settings) or in a court of law.

In an ideal situation, we would be able to seize all digital devices, collect and thoroughly analyze all possible data, and quickly come up with a conclusion. Unfortunately, we have

Digital Forensics, First Edition. Edited by André Årnes.

limited resources and time. We must finish the investigation within a reasonable period of time, by focusing on the artifacts that give the most value to the investigation based on the specific incident.

J. Tan has insightfully noted the two objectives of digital forensic readiness (Tan, 2001): "Maximizing the usefulness of incident evidence data, and minimizing the cost of forensics during an incident response."

Summing up all of the above, we define digital forensic readiness, focusing on the digital forensic readiness objectives by Tan (see Definition 4.1).

Definition 4.1: Digital Forensic Readiness
The ability to perform digital investigation with minimal cost, while maximizing the usefulness of evidence.

4.3 Law Enforcement versus Enterprise Digital Forensic Readiness

Who is performing digital investigations? The first thought is usually law enforcement. The common view of forensics (like fingerprints or ballistics) is that of a crime scene where law enforcement personnel conduct an investigation and perform forensics as needed. The same conception applies to digital forensics as well, where law enforcement personnel conduct an investigation and collect digital evidence.

More recently, enterprises have found new application areas for digital forensics. For example, finding the root cause of incidents, providing due diligence (compliance to the normal standards of care in the industry or taking reasonable precautions), supporting disciplinary actions, and more. This led to the birth of a new subarea within digital forensics, enterprise digital forensics.

A mix of law enforcement and enterprise forensic analysts involved in an investigation is also possible. The enterprise can perform its own initial digital forensic investigation as part of the incident response procedures before deciding whether to contact law enforcement and handing off the evidence to a criminal investigation.

Even if enterprises do not initially plan to use the gathered evidence from an investigation of an incident in a court of law, the investigation might reveal criminal activity. Additionally, the loss of personally identifiable information (PII) or intellectual property belonging to a third party may result in lawsuits or other civil action. Whether the ultimate goal of the digital forensic investigation is to present digital evidence for an enterprise audience or to a court of law, the same methodology applies. In both cases, digital evidence must be collected in a forensically sound manner, by following forensic principles (see Section 1.2).

However, unlike law enforcement, enterprises are more likely to be required to ensure business continuity during forensic investigations and limit the potential disruptions to business operations. In addition, different laws and regulations may apply between investigative activities performed by private investigators and forensic professionals in enterprise and regulations that apply to law enforcement.

Accordingly, enterprise digital forensic readiness is defined in Definition 4.2.

Definition 4.2: Enterprise Digital Forensic Readiness

The ability in an enterprise to perform digital investigations with minimal cost and disruption to business operations, while maximizing the usefulness of evidence.

In addition to enterprise digital forensic readiness, you might encounter other terms: enterprise forensic readiness, computer forensic readiness, proactive digital forensics enterprise digital forensics, corporate forensics, and so forth. All these terms are considered synonymous with each other, and here we will use the terms *digital forensic readiness* and *enterprise digital forensic readiness*.

4.4   Why? A Rationale for Digital Forensic Readiness

Generally, everyone agrees that preparation is important for successfully completing any task. Based on the definition of digital forensic readiness and objectives defined by Tan (2001), we will discuss two main reasons for considering digital forensic readiness: cost and the usefulness of the digital evidence that has been collected.

4.4.1   Cost

Based on the objectives (Tan, 2001) and definition of digital forensic readiness (see Definition 4.1), the first important aspect of digital forensic readiness is *minimizing the cost.*

It is easy to get the impression from television series with forensics subject matter that incidents occur one at a time, and that the investigation team has all the resources needed to solve them within the given time period. Real life is not that generous. The attackers do not stand in the line and wait for their turn to act. There are times when the forensic team has to juggle between several investigations at the same time. The number and scope of the forensic investigations are constrained by resource limitations.

What "cost" components are we discussing here? The cost of the investigation involves time spent on the investigation (which can be measured by hours or investigators' fees) and level of effort required, equipment costs, and other costs directly related to conducting the investigation.

J. Tan (2001) provides the following estimate for the costs involved of a forensic investigation *after* the evidence has already been collected. A two-hour intrusion resulted, on average, in the forensic investigator spending 40 hours to perform an analysis and write a report. This assumes that the evidence has already been collected beforehand and the investigators can dive straight into the analysis; a more accurate estimate must also include the costs related to collecting and handling the digital evidence.

Let us look at a few more estimates. Endicott-Popovsky *et al.* (2007) analyzed and compared two cases. Both of the investigations were performed in an ad hoc reactive manner requiring a considerable amount of time and resources:

- The estimated investigation time in a New Zealand hacker's case, characterized as a typical intrusion scenario, was 417 hours, resulting in investigation cost of $27,800 (one victim only).
- A Russian hacker's case (automated online auctions using a stolen credit card) that resulted in prosecution took 9 months of investigators' time. A partial estimate of the cost was $100,000.

In addition, we need to think about indirect costs as well, like resources taken out of daily business operations to support investigation, disruption of restoration operations due to investigation requirements, and legal counseling.

Most decisions in enterprises are based on cost–benefit analysis. The cost of an activity should not outweigh the benefits. The same approach is valid for the digital forensic investigations. If the enterprise does not have a legal obligation to inform law enforcement about the incident, it might choose not to do so in cases where the cost of informing outweighs the compensation it might receive. Finally, if the incident is too expensive to investigate fully, the victims or plaintiffs might choose to withdraw the charges or dismiss the case, like in Example 4.1.

Example 4.1: The Armando Angulo Case

"The usual route to beating the DEA in a case is arguing that the evidence is insufficient. But for Armando Angulo, the win comes from the opposite. . . . A federal judge in Iowa dismissed the charge last week at the request of prosecutors, who want to throw out the many records collected over their nine-year investigation to free up space. . . . Continued storage of these materials is difficult and expensive."[1]

The successful prosecution of Armando Angulo was unlikely, and storing nine years' worth of evidence was too expensive; thus, cost was greater than the benefit, resulting in dismissal of charges.

4.4.2 Usefulness of Digital Evidence

Recall the goals (Tan, 2001) and the definition of digital forensic readiness (see Definition 4.1). One part of the definition deals with "maximizing the *usefulness of incident evidence data.*" What is "useful" digital evidence? The usefulness can be defined through the intended purpose or the situation in which the evidence will be used. Grobler *et al.* (2010) suggest a definition of *comprehensive digital evidence* that captures the components of usefulness, namely:

- evidentiary weight in a court of law,
- relevant and sufficient for
- determining root cause,
- linking the attacker to the incident.

---

1 https://blog.simplejustice.us/2012/08/17/dea-crumbles-under-the-weight-of-evidence/.

To sum up, digital evidence is useful when it can be captured and preserved, contributes to solving the incident or crime, is relevant, is sufficient, and has evidentiary weight in a court of law.

4.4.2.1 Existence of Digital Evidence

Digital evidence is difficult to collect and easy to destroy. The required evidence might not be available. Some digital data (e.g., network traffic) exists only for an instant, unless it is captured and preserved. If activities or actions are not logged, it might be impossible to retrace them. Order of volatility also plays a role (see Section 2.3.6), and we may be changing some types of data in the process of extracting other types of data.

The story in Example 4.2 illustrates one way to destroy or lose potential evidence data in enterprises or on personal devices.

Example 4.2: An Illustrative Story

A user notices that there is something wrong with his computer. The first thing he does to improve the situation is to restart the computer. Then he asks a colleague for help. The colleague suggests it is malware. The user calls IT support all stressed and impatient: "I need to have this up and running now! I have work to do." The helpful IT support staff cleans up the malware. If at this point you were called to do a forensic investigation, how successful would you be?

Include advanced hackers or targeted attack scenarios in the mix, and the investigators' task becomes extremely difficult, because the attackers may also employ anti-forensic techniques. The variety of attack tools and ways of destroying traces introduces additional obstacles to effective and successful investigations.

Digital forensic readiness deals with identifying different scenarios, considering potential evidence sources, and preparing beforehand to increase the probability of finding and properly preserving the digital evidence relevant for the investigation.

4.4.2.2 Evidentiary Weight of Digital Evidence

How much evidentiary weight does digital evidence carry? This can be expressed through degrees of trustworthiness, relevance, sufficiency, and validity.

4.4.2.2.1 Relevance and Sufficiency of Digital Evidence

Relevancy is described as demonstrating that the evidence collected contains information of value and helps to prove or disprove an element in the incident being investigated (see ISO/IEC 27037.2012; ISO/IEC, 2012).

Sufficiency is defined as having enough material to allow the elements in the investigation of the incident to be adequately examined (see ISO/IEC 27037.2012; ISO/IEC, 2012).

4.4.2.2.2 Trustworthiness of Digital Evidence

Even if you manage to collect the digital evidence, how trustworthy is the evidence? Is it accurate? Did it come from sources that you can trust? Was it collected and handled appropriately? How do you know that the evidence has not been changed or forged? Is the evidence complete, or are there attributes or parts of digital evidence missing? What impact did the investigator's tools have on the digital evidence? All of these questions point to various aspects of trustworthiness, namely authenticity, integrity, and reliability. See Example 4.3 and Example 4.4 for illustrations of real-life situations.

Example 4.3: An Obliging Legal Assistant

"An attorney had custody of a client's computers. Information technology staff from the opposing counsel's office insisted on knowing the size of the plaintiff's drives. An obliging legal assistant booted the systems and reported the disk sizes. When the drive was subjected to a proper forensic investigation, 192 files had been changed and the 'last modified' dates corresponded to the time the assistant started the machines."[2]

Example 4.4: Missing Surveillance Footage

"Attorneys for accused double-homicide defendant, Jeffrey Lepsch, are moving for dismissal or, in the alternative, suppression of video-recorded surveillance evidence reportedly depicting Lepsch inside the crime scene at May's Photo between 1:53 and 2:58 p.m. on the date of the gruesome murders. Apparently, missing is surveillance footage after 3:30 p.m. This footage is critical to Lepsch because a witness reportedly saw another person in the store behind the counter between 4:15 to 4:30 p.m."[3]

If we cannot trust the evidence, then it is equivalent to not having evidence at all. Defining and implementing evidence-handling procedures, identifying potential evidence sources, and testing and validating tools are vital components of digital forensic readiness.

4.4.2.2.3 Validity of Digital Evidence

Whether or not digital evidence will be accepted in a court of law depends upon the legal system and regulations related to the digital investigation and the digital evidence (see Chapter 3). Different countries have different definitions of digital evidence, including admissibility requirements in some countries. Thus, for a specific incident, the jurisdiction and legal basis must be considered. However, we can apply a rule of thumb when thinking about the validity of evidence: evidence not collected in a forensically sound manner reduces the evidence quality and credibility in the court. The actual cases in Example 4.5, Example 4.6, and Example 4.7 illustrate the importance of proper evidence collection.

---

2 http://www.electronicevidenceretrieval.com/preserving_protecting_evidence.htm.
3 http://www.onalaska-law.com/onalaska-law-blog/la-crosse-police-accused-of-destroying-digital-evidence-again-jeffrey-lepschs-attorneys-ask-for-dismissal.

Example 4.5: Eliminated Evidence

"In 2003, an Illinois U.S. District Court Judge granted a defendant's motion for sanctions against the plaintiff and recommended that the case be dismissed with prejudice after it was discovered that the plaintiff had attempted to delete relevant evidence from his computer by running the Evidence Eliminator™ software, which claims to defeat forensic analysis software."[4]

Example 4.6: Controlled by Spyware

"In 2007, Julie Amero, a substitute teacher at a Connecticut middle school, was wrongly convicted on four counts of felony charges of risk of injury to a minor and impairing the morals of a child by showing pornography on a school computer. The conviction carried a maximum prison sentence of 40 years. The conviction was eventually overturned, after appeal, when computer experts at a second trial showed that the NewDotNet spyware program, injected into the system days prior to the crime, spawned uncontrollable pornographic pop-ups." See Endicott-Popovsky and Horowitz (2012).

Example 4.7: The Justice System and Digital Evidence

"There are a few examples where the justice system has properly handled the admission of digital evidence. We transition from an example of glaring misunderstandings and lack of knowledge of digital evidence (Amero case), to an analysis of a competent judicial opinion regarding digital evidence, the case of Lorriane v. Markel American Insurance Company." See Alva and Endicott-Popovsky (2012).

Digital forensic readiness examines what is needed and deals with setting up processes, procedures and tools to collect digital evidence in a forensically sound manner.

4.5   Frameworks, Standards, and Methodologies

There is no single answer to "how to become digital forensic ready." Various standardization bodies and organizations propose frameworks and methodologies to address that question, but there is no "one size fits all" or generally accepted practice to follow. In addition to standards and methodologies, the research community also explores the topic and proposes guidelines or frameworks. Digital forensic readiness is still evolving as a discipline, so we only look at the most relevant frameworks, standards, and methodologies that are available at this time.

---

4   http://www.electronicevidenceretrieval.com/preserving_protecting_evidence.htm.

4.5.1 Standards

Two of the most well-known standardization bodies, ISO[5] and NIST,[6] have issued several standards that relate to the digital forensic investigation process and digital forensic readiness.

4.5.1.1 ISO/IEC 27037

The ISO/IEC 27037 standard gives a definition of digital evidence and describes its three main governance principles: relevance, reliability, and sufficiency. General requirements for the handling of the digital evidence based on those principles are provided. They include "auditability, justifiability, and either repeatability or reproducibility depending on particular circumstances" (ISO/IEC 27037.2012; ISO/IEC, 2012). The initial digital evidence-handling processes (identification, collection, acquisition, and preservation) are also detailed through descriptions of key components within the process.

4.5.1.2 ISO/IEC 17025

The requirements for a forensic laboratory are provided in ISO/IEC 17025 (ISO/IEC, 2005). They encompass both management and technical requirements; however, the emphasis is placed on technical requirements. These include, for example, requirements related to methodology, equipment handling, sampling, and quality assurance.

4.5.1.3 NIST SP 800-86

SP 800-86 (NIST SP800-86; NIST, 2006) discusses the phases of the digital forensic process: collection, examination, analysis, and reporting. This standard includes general recommendations as well as more detailed technical guidelines for evidence collection and examination from data files, operating systems, networks, applications, and other sources.

4.5.2 Guidelines

Guidelines for digital forensics were developed in parallel and in addition to the standards. They typically address practices and methods for performing digital investigations and handling of digital evidence. As such, they help to implement digital forensic readiness for private enterprise as well as law enforcement.

4.5.2.1 IOCE Guidelines

The International Organization on Computer Evidence (IOCE) Guidelines (IOCE, 2002) are used for implementing digital forensic examination procedures. They provide general descriptions of the practices for the digital investigation and some specific principles. Most of the requirements are rather high level, for example the competence requirements and proficiency testing. However, the requirements related to digital evidence handling are more detailed and focus on preservation of the evidence integrity and chain of custody.

---

5 http://www.iso.org/iso/home/about.htm.
6 http://www.nist.gov/public_affairs/nandyou.cfm.

4.5.2.2 Scientific Working Group on Digital Evidence (SWGDE)

The Scientific Working Group on Digital Evidence (SWGDE, 2013) lists the primary types of errors found in the implementation of digital forensic tools: incompleteness, inaccuracy, and misinterpretation. The focus of the guidelines is to understand the limitations of tools and techniques, as well as to discuss error mitigation techniques, including tool testing, verification, procedures, and peer reviews.

4.5.2.3 ENFSI Guidelines

The European Network of Forensic Science Institutes (ENFSI) has published a *Best Practice Manual for the Forensic Examination of Digital Technology* (ENFSI, 2015). The manual provides guidance for forensic laboratories and encompasses the framework for procedures, quality principles, training processes, and approaches.

4.5.3 Research

Researchers have worked on digital forensic readiness for the last few decades, and several frameworks have been proposed. We will discuss the most authoritative ones, upon which many other frameworks and methodologies have been built.

4.5.3.1 Rowlingson's Ten-Step Process

Rowlingson (2004) considers the objectives for forensic readiness introduced by Tan (2001) and proposes a framework for digital forensic readiness consisting of ten steps. He highlights the benefits of collecting the evidence in a business context and considers system forensics a part of overall enterprise forensic readiness. Rowlingson also implies that forensic readiness in corporate environments should be aligned with business risks and tied with business continuity and incident response. The paper focuses on corporate environments and lists issues, benefits, and costs that an enterprise should consider when deciding on implementation measures for becoming forensically ready. The author does not go into analysis of specific policies, tools, or mechanisms, but gives a general and comprehensive description for each of the ten steps.

4.5.3.2 Grobler *et al.*'s Forensic Readiness Framework

Grobler *et al.* (2010) introduce the notion of *comprehensive digital evidence* (discussed in Section 4.4.2). The idea of comprehensive digital evidence, as compared to the traditional notion of digital evidence, implies that in addition to using information to support or refute hypotheses, it has to carry evidentiary weight; thus, organizations have to be aware of the risks and legal requirements that they face when collecting useful data as the evidence.

In addition, Grobler *et al.* (2010) propose a framework for the implementation of forensic readiness within organizations. The forensic readiness activities described in the paper are similar to the steps proposed by Rowlingson (2004), but they are presented in a different manner. The activities are grouped, and the groups are called *dimensions*. The grouping of forensic readiness activities into dimensions gives a better overview on how specified activities depend on and relate to each other. The paper also includes suggested deliverables for each of the dimensions.

4.5.3.3 Endicott-Popovsky *et al.*'s Forensic Readiness Framework

Endicott-Popovsky *et al.* (2007) propose a framework for network forensics. The framework consists of several layers to aid enterprises in implementing forensic readiness.

The first layer is the theoretical base that covers information security governance and discusses embedding forensics in an enterprise as a component of its information assurance elements. The second layer of the framework analyzes a "3R" strategy model (resistance, recognition, and recovery) for survivable systems and introduces the notion of a fourth R – redress: "ability to hold intruders accountable in a court of law." The last layer is based on the information systems development life cycle and notes changes to be made to incorporate forensic capabilities (like chain of custody procedures) within the networks. While the first two layers can be applied to more general cases, the third one is mostly concerned with network forensics.

4.6 Becoming "Digital Forensic" Ready

How do we become ready for digital forensic investigations? What activities and requirements are parts of digital forensic readiness? Rephrasing from the digital forensic readiness definition, how do we minimize the cost of the forensic investigation and increase the chance of acquiring relevant digital evidence in a forensically sound manner? This chapter looks into different forensic readiness dimensions: legal, policy, processes and procedures, people, tools and infrastructure.

The story described in Example 4.8 illustrates the challenge for enterprises and serves as a basis for discussion of enterprise digital forensic readiness.

Example 4.8: An Illustrative Story

Wednesday. A regular working day. The sky is gray, and the cloud formations promise heavy rain. The hero of our story, Alex, is responsible for security in the organization. He is drafting an incident response procedure. It has been due for quite a while, but there are always some "fires to extinguish" that take priority and end up eating all the available time. Not today. Today is gray, cloudy, and peaceful. Within the third sentence of the procedure, the phone rings: "There's some unrecognized information in the file." The stressed voice continues: "It is suspicious and no one knows who entered it. What do we do?"

Alex sighs; so much for finishing that draft. At this point, it is not clear how serious the incident is; nevertheless, he has to address it. There are many questions and considerations going through Alex's head. "Did someone make a mistake or was it intentional? Maybe it's a system's error? Do we have a backup? Is the one who updated the file an insider or outsider? Does this affect other systems? Is it a breach? Is the intruder in the organization's networks?" On and on . . .

To add to his worries, the organization is criticized for insufficient focus on information security; management does not want any security issues to be known outside of the organization. "Whom do we inform about it? How to make sure there are no rumors going around? Do we contact our organization's legal counselor? Do we contact the law enforcement? Can we handle it ourselves? Since we don't have forensic experts in house, whom do we hire for the task?"

When Alex reaches the office of the caller, he gets a headache. The IT administrator was passing by the stressed caller just some minutes ago and decided to help to restore the file to the last good version, so that the caller can continue with her work.

"Will we be able to figure out what happened?" Alex asks, while losing hope.

Consider yourself in Alex's situation (Example 4.8). Would you be able to figure out what happened?

The following sections of this chapter are structured to first discuss the enterprise perspective. We will look into the elements of getting ready for forensic investigations as well as complications specific to enterprises. While this also covers many elements of law enforcement's digital forensic readiness, there will be some differences. Those differences or additional elements are further outlined in Chapter 4.8, which discusses considerations for law enforcement.

4.7 Enterprise Digital Forensic Readiness

Enterprises can be very complicated organizations that exert high pressure to keep operations running smoothly. When an incident occurs, there isn't enough time to ask questions; rather, it is time to act. Thus, planning and preparations are crucial.

4.7.1 Legal Aspects

The legal basis of the country (area) where an enterprise operates is an important factor for planning digital forensic readiness. Collecting, analyzing, and presenting digital evidence in an appropriate manner for legal proceedings require compliance with local laws and regulations. Legal aspects differ in various jurisdictions, and this becomes especially tricky for international organizations spanning the borders of multiple countries. The enterprise should carefully consider whether it is allowed to collect the digital evidence at all.

As a starting point for identifying when digital evidence is required, the enterprise can consider a list of cybercrime types (see Example 4.9). When deciding upon scenarios in which digital evidence will be collected and to which extent, the enterprise has to juggle between the need to collect digital evidence, due diligence, admissibility requirements, and regulations related to privacy and data retention.

When preparing for a digital investigation, some important questions the enterprise should ask and evaluate in a legal context include:

- Which scenarios require the enterprise to exercise due diligence and collect digital evidence?
- What is considered to be the digital evidence, and when it is admissible in a court of law?
- Which information and data can be collected as digital evidence, and under what circumstances?

- What are the requirements or procedures required for collecting, preserving, and presenting digital evidence in court?

Example 4.9: SpyEye Online Banking Fraud

Bank Trojans or banking malware campaigns comprise one of the incident scenarios that banks would consider investigating because they potentially involve several crimes: computer intrusion, data and system interference (computer virus), and unlawful dealings (hacker tools). The potential incident evidence sources (see Example 2.4) that can be mapped for collection were listed in Chapter 2.3.1, and Chapter 3.3 provides further descriptions of the crimes.

To illustrate the conflict an organization might encounter, consider a case where data retention requirements have the enterprise retain the data for 90 days, but privacy requirements specify that the data must be discarded after 30 days. Which requirement should the enterprise comply with? Thinking about a digital investigation, it would be more beneficial to keep data for longer periods, as this would allow better tracking of incidents. However, the enterprise must also stay compliant with privacy regulations. It can get even more complicated for international enterprises with a wide geographical coverage that brings it under several jurisdictions.

4.7.2 Policy, Processes, and Procedures

To complement the legal requirements, the enterprise should also identify generally accepted evidence management practices to guide its processes and procedures. In addition, the goal of digital forensic readiness is to align digital forensic investigation policies with the other existing frameworks and practices within the enterprise. That is, the digital forensic investigation policies should follow a risk-based approach; align with the business's goals and objectives; define policies, processes, procedures, roles, and responsibilities; identify skills, competencies, awareness, and training needs; and also utilize infrastructure and tools in the same manner as the rest of the enterprise.

4.7.2.1 Risk-Based Approach

The digital forensic investigation process can be considered a part of the general information security framework within an enterprise. Following recognized security management standards, such as the ISO 27000 family, the enterprise should assess the risk and choose the risk-handling options appropriate and proportional to the risks it faces. How do digital forensics relate to the enterprise risks? To answer this question, we will examine the components that comprise information security risk and how that risk can be assessed.

In enterprises, all types of risk assessment, including IT and information security, should be done with a focus on business operations. Decision makers can better evaluate and choose the measures to implement (including decisions to commence forensic investigations) when weighing business risks against business benefits. Thus, we will consider operational risks related to information security (as derived from the operational risk definition of COSO ERM)[7] as:

- those that are related to information and
- are focused on breach of confidentiality, integrity, and availability.

We will write up information security risks based on how general incident scenarios can progress into damaging incidents that have serious consequences for the enterprise, like financial losses, legal exposure, health hazards, and operational failures.

In particular, we will focus on incident scenarios that are related to information security. "An incident scenario is the description of a threat exploiting a certain vulnerability or set of vulnerabilities in an information security incident" (ISO/IEC 27005; ISO/IEC, 2008).

Example 4.10: SpyEye Online Banking Fraud Risk Scenario

A simple risk scenario related to SpyEye online banking fraud that the financial institution might consider: unauthorized or fraudulent transactions (breach of integrity) made by an attacker lead to loss of clients' money, resulting in financial losses and damage to reputation of the financial institution.

"What does this have to do with digital forensics?" you might wonder. Consider Example 4.10. The incident part of the risk scenario (unauthorized or fraudulent transactions) can be mapped to cybercrime types as illustrated in Example 4.9, identifying the cases when an incident might become the cause for a criminal investigation. Thus, the forensic team in the enterprise can argue for the need to perform investigations rather than just to restore operations, especially when a digital investigation is likely to be initiated due to legal requirements.

Furthermore, with limited time and resources, priorities can be set based on the risk assessment: the incidents leading to a heavy loss or having high impact on the enterprise can be given high priority when performing digital investigations. Getting back to the story of Alex (see Example 4.8), if Alex can map the incident that happened within the different risk assessment scenarios, he can make a better judgment on whether to focus on simply restoring enterprise operations or to escalate into a full-scale investigation. Ideally, we would like to perform an investigation for each incident to get at the heart of the matter. However, it is practically impossible, and so we need to prioritize.

Additionally, the enterprise needs to consider the allowable extent that a business's processes can be interfered with when performing a digital investigation and collecting evidence. Risk assessment results may give us insight into the criticality of a process and its allowed downtime. This will influence the type of digital investigation that we will be able to perform as well as the investigative infrastructure and technology chosen (for further discussion on tools and infrastructure readiness, refer to Section 4.7.5).

Legal obligations and cost–benefit analysis (as part of the risk assessment handling options) help enterprises evaluate which scenarios are worth incorporating into the enterprise forensic readiness plan. In addition to legal and risk-related considerations, an

---

7 http://www.coso.org/-ERM.htm.

enterprise might consider other business scenarios that can benefit from digital forensic investigations, for example demonstrating due diligence for insurance cases, compliance with industry standards, or contractual agreements.

4.7.2.2 Incident Response versus Digital Forensics

A digital forensics investigation within an enterprise is likely to start as part of an incident response. For example, a digital forensic investigation can be initiated when criminal activities are suspected or identified during the investigation of the incident. The incident categories, as well as when the incident response process escalates into a digital investigation, can be defined as part of the incident management or response plan.

The ISO 27001 standard (ISO/IEC, 2013), which is a widely accepted standard related to information security management, also lists the controls related to evidence collection under the incident management group of controls: "Where a follow-up action against a person or organization after an information security incident involves legal action (either civil or criminal), evidence shall be collected, retained, and presented to conform to the rules for evidence laid down in the relevant jurisdiction(s)."

However, although a digital forensic investigation will likely start as part of an incident response, incident response and digital forensics sometimes have conflicting goals. Incident response is concerned with restoring operations as soon as possible, while digital forensic investigation requires the preservation of relevant evidence, which might delay restoration (for further discussion, refer to Grobler & Louwrens, 2007). An important part of digital forensic readiness is to reconcile those goals and ensure proper collection of the evidence with minimal impact on business services restoration. As part of this exercise, new types of incident categories, or new procedures and tools for conducting a proper digital forensic investigation, can be identified.

4.7.2.3 Policy

The organization and relationships between policies, processes, and procedures will depend upon the enterprise. For example, a process-oriented enterprise with a high level of workflow automation might choose to have a high-level policy, implemented through automated processes. Inside the automated processes, the workflows might be defined and used to replace the procedures, paper forms, and checklists. That is, instead of having a documented procedure defining how, for example, the chain of custody is preserved, supported by paper checklists, the workflow within the process could automatically request a user (or assign a user) to acquire the evidence, note where the evidence is located, and so on.

Let's assume that an enterprise decides to define a high-level digital forensics policy, supported by processes and procedures. The enterprise management or governance body should approve the policy in the same manner as other policies within the enterprise. At a minimum, the policy should contain:

- a brief explanation of the purpose of the policy;
- its scope of applicability (what is affected by the policy, and to which extent the policy applies);
- a list of identified judiciary requirements, laws, and regulations related to digital forensic readiness, digital forensic investigation, evidence handling, and similar;

- the relation of digital forensics to the other existing enterprise frameworks and management systems, like risk management and incident response; and
- the policy's relation to the other enterprise policies.

If an enterprise decides not to have a policy specific to digital forensics, then the above-mentioned aspects can be incorporated into other policies, for example incident response or information security, or be covered through procedures. The high-level policy can further contain subpolicies, guidelines, or procedures that detail how the policy or some aspects within the policy should be interpreted or implemented in the enterprise.

Law enforcement will most likely not have a policy for digital forensic investigations. Instead, guidelines, processes, and procedures, similar to those defined in the enterprise, will be followed.

4.7.2.4 Processes and Procedures

The digital forensic investigation process is described in Chapter 2. To support each stage in the digital investigation process, the enterprise digital forensic readiness process can generally be described as follows:

1) Identify relevant laws and regulations related to digital forensic readiness, digital forensic investigations, and digital evidence.
2) Perform risk assessments, or obtain the results of existing risk assessments.
3) Identify incident scenarios that require digital evidence, based on laws and regulations, as well as risk assessment.
4) Identify the relationship of digital forensic capabilities with existing frameworks and processes within the enterprise.
5) Define the general enterprise digital forensic policy, or update existing policies with aspects related to digital forensics.
6) Set policies regarding outsourcing or the use of third parties, and describe the service levels utilized, if needed.
7) Define subpolicies and procedures based on the general policy to support digital forensics capabilities.
8) Establish an organizational structure that specifies allocation of authority and responsibility.
9) Describe the roles and responsibilities, and specify the required skills and competencies.
10) Define the requirements for performing operational and awareness training, conduct the trainings.
11) Prepare tools and infrastructure; specify validation, verification, and calibration requirements.
12) Evaluate and measure the effectiveness and quality of processes and activities concerning digital evidence and investigations.

The enterprise might define different process steps depending on the legal requirements or good practices it chooses to follow, or in relation to other existing enterprise processes and procedures. To support the digital forensic policy and investigation process, the enterprise at a minimum should consider the following aspects in its subpolicies or procedures:

- standard operating procedures for evidence handling;

- monitoring policy;
- privacy protection policy and requirements;
- monitoring requirements to detect the incidents defined in the incident scenarios;
- incident escalation into digital investigation;
- handling specific types of investigations, for example child pornography;
- reporting to external parties, law enforcement, and the release of data;
- outsourcing and involvement of third parties in the digital investigation;
- preparation of the digital forensic laboratory and/or tools;
- training and awareness; and
- roles, responsibilities, and competence requirements.

Guidance provided by standards, for example ISO/IEC 27037 (ISO/IEC, 2012; for other examples, refer to the discussion in Section 4.5), can be used in defining policies, procedures, and routines.

4.7.3 People

People are an important aspect of a digital forensic investigation. For a successful digital forensic investigation, it is necessary to define roles and responsibilities and gather the team with the right skillset and competencies. However, one should not forget others in the enterprise who may potentially play a role in the process. Remember the helpful IT administrator from the story about Alex (see Example 4.8) who restored the files before the forensic investigators could get to the scene? Awareness training for all staff is an essential step in implementing policies, processes, and procedures.

This section examines the three main aspects in the people dimension:

- roles and responsibilities;
- skills, competencies, and training; and
- awareness training.

4.7.3.1 Roles and Responsibilities

The definition of roles and responsibilities usually depends on the size of the enterprise and the maturity of its forensic capabilities. The enterprise can establish a digital forensic investigation organization as a team or a unit. However, for small companies this option might not be feasible. They can dedicate only one or a few persons, or assign forensic responsibilities to other existing roles, often in addition to their usual tasks. Alternatively, the forensic investigation capabilities can be partly or fully outsourced (see Section 4.7.6).

Regardless of how the forensic specialists' roles are organized, their authority (what the roles are allowed to do) and responsibilities (what they are expected to do) need to be clearly defined. It can be done in a separate policy, mandate, or charter; as part of the job description; or as part of existing policies, mandates, or charters (e.g., as part of the incident response plan).

It is important to note that forensic specialists must remain impartial to internal operations and ensure objectivity during the investigation. Thus, the role, team, or unit should have autonomy and not report to the enterprise IT support organization, other units within the enterprise, or anywhere that conflicts of interests might arise. This includes enterprises with limited resources for forensics.

The roles and responsibilities in the digital forensic investigation process can be defined as follows:

- *First responder*: This role is responsible for the initiation of the digital investigation, securing the scene of the incident, primary identification of the digital evidence, securing the evidence, and identifying the digital investigation procedures that should be followed for the specific type of incident. These roles might also be part of the incident response team or security operations center (SOC).
- *Digital forensics specialist*: This role is responsible for identification and collection of the digital evidence ensuring the forensic principles are followed. This role can have a responsibility to perform live forensics.
- *Digital forensics analyst/examiner*: This role is responsible for analysis of different types of digital evidence and reporting the results. This role can also have a responsibility for performing live forensics.
- *Digital forensic investigator/lead investigator*: This role is responsible for directing the investigation, coordinating the activities, interpreting the findings, and reporting the results.
- *Data retention specialist*: This role is responsible to ensure the evidence is retained according to the retention policy or requirements.

The list is not comprehensive and serves just as an example of how the roles can be defined and organized. As mentioned in this chapter, there are several options for distributing responsibilities among the different roles, and all of the above responsibilities can be assigned to one role that is responsible for the entire digital investigation process. Though considering the diversity and complexity of technologies, the enterprise will more likely need to gather several analysts responsible for different types of technologies, for example, computer forensics, mobile forensics, and so on.

If the organization responsible for digital forensic investigation becomes too complex, a RACI matrix can be utilized to clarify the division of accountability and responsibility for the activities in the process.[8] Each role is assigned the letter matching the activity for each step in the process:

- *R* stands for *responsibility* (role performs the activity).
- *A* stands for *accountability* (role is accountable for the success of the activity and has approval authority).
- *C* stands for *consulted* (role provides input for the activity).
- *I* stands for *informed* (role receives information related to activities, decisions, or deliverables).

If the digital forensic investigation is fully or partly outsourced, or if third parties are involved in the processes, the responsibility for contacting and coordinating with those parties needs to be clearly defined. When establishing roles and assigning responsibilities, the enterprise should consider whether the staffing for the roles is sufficiently robust in the event of illnesses, vacations, and other staff absences. That is, backup staff should be assigned for critical roles.

---

8 http://project-management.com/understanding-responsibility-assignment-matrix-raci-matrix/.

4.7.3.2 Skills, Competencies, and Training

One of the core requirements for any of the roles related to digital forensics is knowledge and understanding of digital forensics investigation processes, principles, and methods (see Chapter 2). In addition to the digital forensic methodologies and procedures, any unit acting within the enterprise should be familiar with the enterprise frameworks related to their area of operation. For digital forensics, this would be incident response, information security management, and risk management. Strong reasoning skills are required for defining and testing hypotheses, finding patterns and associations between artifacts, and analyzing and drawing conclusions from the available information.

For most of the digital forensic roles, it is essential to have strong technical skills and competencies. Knowledge of operating systems (including architecture, implementation, and administration), networking protocols and services, various information systems, and applications are just some of the items on the list.

The personnel occupying roles within the team or unit must be able to identify and specify requirements for the digital forensic tools and infrastructure, select the appropriate tools, and set up, configure, and use them. Validation, verification, or testing of tools should be conducted as needed. Thus, appropriate training for using digital forensic tools is required for all team members. Everyone involved within digital investigations should be trained on how to properly prepare investigation-related records and documentation.

The personnel who will be involved in reporting and presenting results, for example to managers or in court, must have excellent communication skills. They should be able to document, present, and explain findings as well as investigation procedures to various groups in language (terminology) those groups can understand.

Like with any other profession, the requisite level of skill and expertise can be acquired through education, training, certification, and work experience.

4.7.3.3 Awareness Training

Awareness training should be conducted with everyone involved in the process of incident response and digital forensic investigations, including IT staff. Furthermore, all employees should know what might be considered an incident, whom to call, and how to behave during the incident response or when a forensic investigation is initiated. Thinking back on Alex's story (Example 4.8), both employees – the stressed caller and the helpful IT administrator – should have known to wait for a decision from Alex before proceeding with other actions (ideally, they would follow defined policy or procedure).

The training material should cover the actions that different roles are expected to take or things not to do during the incident response and the digital forensic investigation. In addition, it should clarify how actions of the participants affect the admissibility or use of digital evidence.

Examples of employees (including those who might not be an active part of the investigation) who should be part of awareness training:

- incident response and forensic team(s),
- IT and information security,
- legal department,
- human resources,

- media contacts and public relations, and
- other employees (e.g., those reporting incidents, and people under investigation).

Awareness training for digital forensics need not be a separate program. It can (or rather should) be integrated into a general awareness program. The awareness training should also present the code of conduct and ethical guidelines (how to behave ethically and professionally) related to a digital investigation.

4.7.4 Technology: Digital Forensic Laboratory

The enterprise needs to decide whether to develop a full-scale digital forensic laboratory, outsource the digital evidence analysis, or acquire and validate digital forensics tools. This section covers the preparation of a laboratory (elements that are needed to establish, operate, and maintain the laboratory), while the aspects of tool validation and verification are discussed later in this chapter. The guidance for a laboratory's preparation is based on:

- the ISO 17025 (ISO/IEC, 2005) standard,
- the ISO 27001 (ISO/IEC, 2013) standard,
- the ISO 9001 (ISO, 2008) standard,
- the ILAC-G19:2002 (ILAC-G19, 2002) guidelines, and
- other general good practices.

4.7.4.1 Accreditation and Certification

The digital forensic laboratory can be established, prepared, accredited, and/or certified according to industry-accepted or international standards, such as ISO 17025 and ISO 9001, and by following guides to good practice. We will focus on two international standards – ISO 17025 and ISO 9001 – as they can be applied across various countries and industries.

Which option to select: accreditation based on ISO 17025, certification for ISO 9001, or both? It will depend on several factors, such as requirements and expectations from the clients, stakeholders, or other interested parties. The ISO 9001 standard is more generic and provides requirements for quality management systems. While there are some overlapping areas or requirements, ISO 17025 contains more technical requirements. If an enterprise already has a quality system based on ISO 9001, then the laboratory might be required by internal policies to follow the requirements from that standard.

The International Laboratory Accreditation Cooperation (ILAC) notes the following reasons for accreditation based on ISO 17025 (ILAC, 2002):

- "A recognition of testing competence,
- a benchmark for performance,
- a marketing advantage, and
- international recognition for your laboratory."

Thus, the accreditation can later on serve as proof of a laboratory's technical competence and be provided to interested parties.

While in this chapter we focus on only two ISO standards, other international or national standards might be applicable and should be evaluated by the enterprise. The enterprise might also choose to refrain from being certified or accredited. One of the main reasons to choose to refrain from certification or accreditation, when it is not required by stakeholders or clients of the laboratory, is the associated costs of running a laboratory in a particular manner and providing required documentation or proving compliance.

4.7.4.2 Organizational Framework

Each laboratory should have a mandate that describes what are its roles, functions, services, clients (who are the functions aimed at?), stakeholders, authorities, and responsibilities. The mandate is part of a laboratory's organizational framework, which is further supported by more detailed descriptions of services, roles, and responsibilities. The mandate or additional documentation will also specify the laboratory's intent for accreditation or certification.

The laboratory's mandate should be derived from and approved by the enterprise's management. Management will assign a certain level of authority to the laboratory or the laboratory's managers: what the laboratory is allowed to do to deliver services, where in the organizational structure (hierarchy) it is placed, and whom the laboratory's manager (s) will report to.

The responsibilities and services also need to be specified. What is the laboratory expected to deliver? In addition to a high-level service description in the mandate, it should specify the specific types of services and service levels that the laboratory offers and the deliverables provided by these services.

After agreeing on what the laboratory will offer, the roles and responsibilities of the personnel required to ensure the laboratory's functions and service deliveries need to be described. For discussion on roles and responsibilities related to digital forensic investigations, refer to Section 4.7.3.1.

Finally, the mandate or supporting documentation should specify how it will integrate with other enterprise structures, external entities, or organizations along with other local, regional, or international laboratories.

4.7.4.3 Security Policy or Framework

The security policy or framework can be specific to the laboratory, or the general framework or policy established for the entire enterprise can apply to the laboratory as well. In the latter case, the laboratory can have additional processes, procedures, or controls that will be a part of the general enterprise security framework, but applicable only to the laboratory. The security framework can be established and (if needed) certified based on ISO 27001 (ISO/IEC, 2013).

At a minimum, the security policy or framework should specify the proper and secure manner for handling information in the laboratory, what the security requirements are, and how they will be met. The requirements and controls can include risk management, encryption management, logical and physical access management, handling of equipment, and more.

4.7.4.4 Control of Records

The records related to investigations need to be managed and controlled to ensure evidence integrity and maintain the chain of custody at all times. These measures must be defined and implemented based on the requirements that support the laboratory's mandate as well as the organizational and security frameworks. The goal of the measures is to protect records from "loss, destruction, falsification, unauthorized access, and unauthorized release" (A.18.1.3 "Protection of records," ISO/IEC 27001:2013; ISO/IEC, 2013). The measures will include administrative (e.g., procedures and guidelines), physical and environmental (e.g., protection against fire and flood, locks), and logical (e.g., encryption) controls.

ILAC (2002) provides further guidance for control of records, including:

- maintaining the records related to each case under investigation, reflecting the principles of repeatability, completeness, reliability, and traceability;
- enforcing quality assurance through policies, procedures, and reviews;
- recording operating parameters;
- recording observations and test results (e.g., by photography, scanning, and sketching) as well as reasons for rejecting them; and
- double-checking calculations and data transfers that are not part of validated tests.

4.7.4.5 Processes, Procedures, and Lab Routines

The laboratory should define processes and procedures for handling digital evidence. They are explored in Section 4.7.2. Processes and procedures and can further be supplemented by guidelines and routines. At the minimum, the routines should detail the ways to protect the evidence during collection and transportation: against tampering, physical damage, water, magnets, statics, heat, cold, and more. The routines for taking notes and describing, documenting, and sketching the scene should follow rules for controlling records (see Section 4.7.4.4). It is important to note passwords and the content displayed on the active screens of devices.

Routines should cover both *physical and logical access* to the laboratory. They should also specify controls to protect specific areas in the laboratory if different levels of access controls are needed. If the laboratory is located in the same area as other business functions, it is important to separate the laboratory from the other functions by restricting and controlling laboratory access.

Procedures and routines for *information reporting and disclosure* both internally and externally need to be defined. They should be aligned with the enterprise's general policies and procedures for communication and disclosure of information. They should also follow applicable laws and regulations, and satisfy internal and external reporting requirements, while preserving objectivity and independence.

Configuration, calibration, and measurement procedures and routines should cover:

- Conformity, monitoring, and measurement requirements;
- documentation, tasks, and activities;
- calibration steps;
- results validation;
- exception and disconformity handling;
- adjustment documentation; and
- controls for maintenance, storage, and protection against damage.

The standards and guidelines discussed in Section 4.5 can serve as a good source for defining procedures and routines.

4.7.4.6 Methodology and Methods

Methodology and methods should satisfy the general requirement, as defined in *ISO/IEC Guide 2:2004* (ISO/IEC, 2004): "Most of the activities performed in laboratories should satisfy the definition of the objective test, or have required controls in place." The objective test, as defined in ISO/IEC (2004), is given in Definition 4.3.

Definition 4.3: Objective Test

"A test which having been documented and validated is under control so that it can be demonstrated that all appropriately trained staff will obtain the same results within defined limits. These defined limits relate to expressions of degrees of probability as well as numerical values." See ISO/IEC (2004).

To ensure objectivity, all methods (including tools) should be documented, validated, tested, and verified before using them on actual cases. The need for procedures and routines in handling the methods and tools is covered in Section 4.7.4.5. In addition to the documentation, the laboratory's personnel are expected to undergo training, which is further discussed in Sections 4.7.3 and 4.7.4.7.

4.7.4.7 Personnel

The laboratory needs competent and trained personnel. For each identified role (see Section 4.7.3.1) of personnel to support the laboratory's functions and services, the description of the skillset and competencies required has to be defined. A training and awareness program should be developed to ensure that personnel maintain the required competencies (see Sections 4.7.3.2 and 4.7.3.3).

4.7.4.8 Code of Conduct

The laboratory's personnel are expected to follow a set of rules or guidelines for professional behavior – a code of conduct, practice, and/or ethics. Here are two example requirements that may be listed in such a code of conduct, from the UK Government (2014):

- "Act with honesty, integrity, objectivity and impartiality, and declare at the earliest opportunity any personal, business and/or financial interest that could be perceived as a conflict of interest."
- "Provide expert advice and evidence only within the limits of your professional competence."

4.7.4.9 Tools

The laboratory operations have to be supported by appropriate forensic tools. *Appropriate* means tested and validated, where results produced by the tool are considered forensically sound in a court of law. Tools are discussed in Section 4.7.5.

4.7.5   Technology: Tools and Infrastructure

There are several important points when considering the tools and infrastructure for digital forensics:

- What are the sources of digital evidence? Do they require special tools, considerations, or infrastructure adjustments, or different configurations?
- Will the enterprise establish its own digital forensic laboratory? Will this laboratory be accredited? Will it be certified?
- Will digital forensic tools be developed in-house, purchased as commercial off-the-shelf products (COTS), or something in between – a combination?
- Are the tools accurate and reliable?

The different aspects of these questions are discussed in the following subsections.

4.7.5.1   Sources of Digital Evidence

Sources where digital evidence can be found are discussed, and examples are provided, in Chapter 2.3.1. When preparing for future digital forensic investigations, it is important to consider where the evidence might come from:

- Based on the type of incident or crime scenario, we can save time by focusing first on the most common places for evidence in that scenario.
- We can prepare the infrastructure by considering the possible scenarios that generate potential evidence and how to collect it in a proper manner.

There are several questions to ask when considering potential sources of evidence (Rowlingson, 2004):

- Where is the data generated? In what format? Does it contain personal or sensitive information? How long is it stored or retained?
- How much data is produced? How much is reviewed?
- Who is the owner or responsible party for the data? Who has access? How is it managed and secured?
- How can data be made available to the investigation? What additional sources of evidence can be enabled?

By formulating hypothetical incident scenarios during the risk assessments, the enterprise will be able to identify possible digital evidence sources (see Section 4.7.2.1). After these possible sources have been identified, the enterprise has to consider:

- Is data generated during the normal enterprise operations sufficient?
- Does specific data need to be obtained to support the digital forensic investigation?

In both cases, data will have to be appropriately managed and protected to enable its utilization as digital evidence. When deciding which evidence sources to use, the enterprise has to take into account the balance between the cost of gathering and maintaining the digital evidence and performing the digital investigation versus the cost of the consequences or impact on the enterprise of the defined business risk scenario. The enterprise should also evaluate the cost of the consequence to, impact on, or interruption to normal enterprise processes or services. In addition, the equipment or software used to generate, gather, or manage data might need to be adjusted or specifically configured to enable the collection of digital evidence (see Section 4.7.5.3).

Note that we are assuming that various incident scenarios will have common patterns, thus resulting in similar or identical sources of evidence. By examining possible attacks, their path, and access points, surface, and patterns that constitute a hypothetical incident, it is possible to map sources of evidence. While this is helpful (by saving time and/or enabling the collection of evidence that would otherwise not exist if the infrastructure was not configured to capture it in anticipation of an incident), it will not necessarily cover all the possibilities. Thus, investigators will need to consider other sources that might be incident specific or that were not considered during the original risk assessment, scenario, and source-mapping exercises.

4.7.5.2 Validation and Verification of Digital Forensic Tools

Digital forensic tools must be appropriately tested and validated. If an enterprise chooses to establish a digital forensic laboratory and perform in-house digital investigations with their own digital forensic tools, there is an obligation to ensure forensic soundness.

The National Institute of Standards and Technology (NIST) proposes the use of a function-driven test methodology,[9] which is cheaper, extensible, and more scalable compared to a full tool-testing method. To this end, NIST has performed a set of forensic tool tests and published the results. If the enterprise uses the same forensic tools as those of the NIST tests, then it can use the NIST test results for tool validation (see Definition 4.4) and verification (see Definition 4.5).

Definition 4.4: Validation

"Validation is the confirmation by examination and the provision of objective evidence that a tool, technique or procedure functions correctly and as intended." (See Guo *et al.*, 2009.)

Definition 4.5: Verification

"Verification is the confirmation of a validation with laboratories tools, techniques and procedures." (See Guo *et al.*, 2009.)

The enterprise can also perform testing of tools based on its own defined testing methodology. The purpose of testing is to prove that the tools used are accurate and reliable. Whether testing in-house or relying on test results by external parties, the enterprise needs to consider if the test corpora is sufficient and realistic.

When reporting test results, investigators and analysts should account for errors related to tools and methods. For further guidance, refer to SWGDE (2013). All records related to validation and verification need to be maintained as discussed in Section 4.7.4.4.

---

9 http://www.cftt.nist.gov/Methodology_Overview.htm.

Table 4.1 The digital forensic development life cycle.

Lifecycle phase	Features
Initial phase	Risk assessment, digital forensic requirements, security requirements, and privacy requirements
Acquisition/ development phase	Security review, threat modeling, security principles, design of security controls based on risk and privacy assessment, security review, and forensic requirements
Implementation phase	Testing, verification, calibration, configuration, implementation of security controls (including hardening, monitoring, logging, etc.), and validation of implementation versus security design
Operation/maintenance phase	Verification, calibration audits, evaluation of effectiveness of security controls, remediation, and mitigation
Disposition phase	Chain of custody, evidence integrity, and continuous monitoring and improvement of security controls

4.7.5.3 Preparation of Infrastructure

Security mechanisms are often costlier, limited, and/or less effective if only considered at the end of the development cycle of the product, process, or system. Security needs to be part of every step within the cycle: from secure design and architecture, to secure development and testing.

The same principles should apply when considering digital forensics. The infrastructure, systems, and tools should be compatible with the demands of digital forensic investigations, and digital evidence and investigation requirements should be incorporated into all phases of the development cycle. This approach is well illustrated through the proposed network forensic development life cycle in Endicott-Popovsky *et al.* (2007). The network forensic development life cycle extends the information systems development life cycle (see NIST, *Special Publication 800-64 Revision 2 – Security Considerations in the System Development Life Cycle*; NIST, 2008) and includes features like risk assessment, checklists, calibration tests, audits, and chain of custody.

If the equipment and systems are purchased off the shelf, then the procedures discussed in Endicott-Popovsky *et al.* (2007) on the network forensic development life cycle can be used when evaluating different types of products. For example, vendors might be asked to describe what kind of development methodologies are used, what kind of testing has been performed, and so forth. Furthermore, the purchased products might be verified through design verification and calibration tests or audits.

We have supplemented the life cycle proposed by Endicott-Popovsky *et al.* (2007) with additional features or procedures based on the Security Development Lifecycle[10] and security good practices to increase robustness of the forensic-ready infrastructure. The resulting digital forensic development life cycle for infrastructure readiness is summarized in Table 4.1.

The existing infrastructure can be tested or verified to see if it meets the established requirements. In addition, some configuration options can enable existing infrastructure

---

10 https://www.microsoft.com/en-us/sdl/.

to become digital forensic investigation "friendly." For example, logging or audit functions often exist in the devices or systems, but are not enabled, used, or reviewed. These functions can be evaluated and configured to satisfy digital evidence collection and maintenance requirements. In addition, local or remote forensic investigation or digital evidence acquisition tools can be preinstalled or configured.

Correlation and event management systems can also be used for more effective logging and audit practices, for example by collecting and analyzing log information from various devices and systems in a centralized manner. Intrusion detection or prevention systems or other monitoring systems can also be utilized to gather and maintain digital evidence.

Another important aspect when considering infrastructure is time synchronization on all the relevant devices and systems (Tan, 2001). This will enable easier construction of timelines during the digital investigation as well as correlation of events and data from different devices.

Logging, monitoring, and audit activities must be performed based on the legal requirements and considerations, such as privacy and data retention. The enterprise needs to find the balance between monitoring and privacy requirements when configuring tools and defining the policies. Furthermore, the criticality of the business processes and their allowed downtime will influence the choice of digital forensics infrastructure components, technology, and methods.

4.7.6 Outsourcing Digital Forensic Capabilities

When preparing for digital investigations, the enterprise needs to decide whether the digital forensic capabilities will be outsourced or maintained in-house. In the story about Alex (see Example 4.8), he was facing a challenge: the enterprise does not have forensic experts. Like other operations, processes, or infrastructure, certain digital forensic capabilities can be either outsourced or maintained in-house. There are various reasons why an enterprise may decide to seek external support or help, such as cost or lack of resources and expertise.

The decision regarding outsourcing will influence the procedures to be defined and implemented, the tools and infrastructure developed or acquired, as well as the requirements for roles, responsibilities, and training. The enterprise might consider choosing forensics as a service, or just outsource some parts of the investigation when an internal forensics team does not have the required expertise, for example when performing mobile forensics.

Regardless of the option chosen, the decision should also be supported by service-level requirements and expectations by including them into the service-level and contractual agreements. Service-level descriptions, whether to external or internal parties, at the minimum should include expected services to be delivered, the speed of reaction, and reporting requirements.

The outsourcing or use of third parties for digital forensic investigations should be compliant with the enterprise's general processes and procedures for procurement, outsourcing, and management of third parties. Furthermore, enterprises need to be aware of and follow legal requirements when choosing the service provider.

How can we evaluate whether the service provider is good enough, besides looking into what kind of services they provide? By asking the provider to describe their digital forensic investigation process and capabilities and present supporting evidence of their claims, for example:

- Do they follow a framework, methodology, or guidelines for digital forensics? Are these established based on widely accepted practices and standards, like ISO or NIST?
- What are the steps in their process?
- Which digital forensic principles do they follow? How do they ensure that those principles are followed?
- Do they have standard operating procedures? Are these procedures documented?
- What roles are established in the team? What are the qualifications and references of the team members?
- What tools do they use? Why? How are the tools configured, calibrated, tested, and updated?

This list is not all-inclusive, but rather is a starting point. To summarize, a good way to choose a service provider is to consider all the aspects of becoming ready for digital investigations and evaluate how a service provider can fulfill them.

4.7.6.1 Continuous Improvement

Digital forensic readiness is not a one-time activity, but rather a process. As a process, it can continually evolve and improve based on the maturity of the enterprise as well as the maturity of the digital investigation process. Determining whether or not the enterprise has achieved the desired state in its digital forensic investigation process (and, at the same time, readiness) could be evaluated through different types of feedback, audits, assessments, and measuring mechanisms.

One example could be defining the audit checklist by using legal and regulatory requirements or using a set of controls required by laws and regulations. The internal audit function in an enterprise could then evaluate its processes, controls, or deliverables by using this checklist to determine how well the enterprise is following legal and regulatory requirements.

Another way to address evaluation for the same target is to define metrics to measure whether the collected evidence conforms to the legal requirements and the management practices. One example is by measuring the case or evidence completeness – the extent to which the artifacts (information) are complete, have all the necessary values, and are sufficient for the given task or purpose. This metric can be applied to a specific case or its average can be calculated over all cases in a given period of time, and the metric can be used to indicate whether there are violations of the evidence integrity requirements.

Profiling different types of digital investigations and enumerating them can give insight and feedback about the quality of the laboratory, sources of digital evidence, and incident scenarios. Based on both past events and current trends, the enterprise can consider additional scenarios to update their digital investigation process or remove some of the obsolete ones. Similarly, the list of evidence sources can be updated to reflect most common sources.

Compliance-related metrics, like third-party audits, can show whether vendors are delivering services based on the agreed levels. A compliance audit can verify if policies and procedures were followed as well as assess the gaps between good practices and the adopted principles, policies, and procedures. The controls implemented through policies, procedures, and processes can be tested to evaluate if they are functioning properly and as intended. Any need for improvements can be identified through these activities.

The process can also be evaluated by using a maturity model, by defining the criteria for different maturity levels, identifying the target level for the process, evaluating the current level of the processes and the gaps to the targeted level, and then finally defining the actions needed to reach the target level.

Competency and skills can be assessed by using specially designed exams or proficiency tests, and awareness levels can be tested by giving automated or paper tests and asking the person being tested to identify his role within the process and actions he should be taking. In addition, if analysis of process and procedure violations shows that they happen due to a lack of knowledge or understanding, then this can also be used as an indication for the need of awareness training.

Tool testing, verification, and validation methods can be used to evaluate the reliability, accuracy, effectiveness, and other aspects of the tools. The requirements that are important for the enterprise and acceptance criteria for the tools need to be identified beforehand.

This is not an exhaustive list of all the possible means of evaluation, but it illustrates how evaluations can be implemented.

4.8   Considerations for Law Enforcement

As with enterprises, the same standards hold true for law enforcement activities – the digital investigation procedures depend on national regulations and international agreements. In addition to evidence-handling procedures, law enforcement has additional considerations and requirements related to using coercive measures in digital investigations, for example in the search and seizure of digital evidence. For a detailed discussion of the legal aspects, see Chapter 3.

Law enforcement also requires policies, procedures, guidelines, and routines (either general or specific) to properly handle digital evidence. The roles and responsibilities will have to be defined based on the jurisdiction and function of the unit. Similar to an enterprise setting, training programs for law enforcement employees involved in digital investigation will have to be developed, including tool-specific training and criminal process.

The forensic laboratories providing services for law enforcement can be established on a national or international level. They can be either government owned or private. Besides being accredited or certified against ISO 17025 and ISO 9001, forensic laboratories might need to satisfy additional requirements or obtain specific certifications to provide services for law enforcement.

In criminal cases, it must be assumed that it is not possible to influence the infrastructure or system's configuration or setup before an incident or crime. Law enforcement agencies will consequently have to rely on the infrastructure and systems in place at the crime scene where the evidence is found. Thus, it is important to have a good understanding of where the evidence comes from and which factors can influence the reliability and integrity of the evidence.

4.9 Summary

In this chapter, we have described the typical activities involved in the preparation for a digital forensic investigation. We have defined the preparation activities as *digital forensic readiness* and identified two main objectives in becoming forensic ready, namely maximizing the usefulness of the evidence while minimizing the cost of an investigation.

We have described common readiness activities within the different dimensions:

- legal;
- personnel;
- policies, processes, and procedures; and
- tools and technology.

Examples of cases, stories, and scenarios have illustrated the importance and application of the various activities within those dimensions.

After reading this chapter, you should have a better understanding of what it takes to prepare for digital investigations and why readiness is important.

4.10 Exercises

1 Name the two main objectives of forensic readiness. Why are these objectives important for digital investigations?

2 What should you consider when identifying potential sources of the evidence?

3 What is the purpose of forensic tool testing? Describe advantages and disadvantages of function-driven testing methodology.

4 You are hired as a network security architect at an enterprise. Your task is to implement a set of controls to get the infrastructure *digital forensic ready*. Describe what steps you would take.

5 Give examples of procedures to support a digital investigation process.

6 A security breach was identified in a system supporting a critical business process. The system has a 99.97% availability requirement. Describe the challenges in performing a forensic investigation under these conditions. Consider how you would resolve these challenges.

5

Computer Forensics

Jeff Hamm

Mandiant, Mainz, Germany

Digital forensics at the system level requires the skills to both acquire and analyze data. This chapter will provide information regarding data collection in a forensically sound manner and forensic analysis techniques. Sometimes data will need to be acquired "live" and the collection techniques used will make changes to the system. In years past, digital forensics practitioners argued that changes should never be made to a system. With average users having accessibility to modern encryption such as BitLocker, and with advances in memory collection and analysis techniques, it has become more common to collect live data – memory images in particular.

5.1 Introduction

After data has been collected successfully, analysis is required to develop accurate theories of the significance of the evidence. To do so, one must, as always, take detailed notes of the techniques used and data analyzed. This chapter cannot possibly cover all situations and artifacts. It should instead be thought of as an introduction to using sound methodology to analyze common artifacts.

Before getting into collection and analysis, a note on timestamps is necessary. In an investigation, a single artifact with a single date in time and no corroborating evidence should not be considered conclusive. Digital forensic examiners have long been skeptical of timestamps because of the relative ease that a system clock can be changed, a file system timestamp modified, or other user manipulation of timestamps. However, if the timestamp can be corroborated with additional evidence, then it can prove to be accurate. For example, if a file system creation date for a file "a.docx" is January 1, 2015, at 12:00:00 UTC, the examiner may be able to corroborate that time as accurate if there is a creation of a corresponding LNK file containing the same date and time, or the metadata in the DOCX file itself, and so forth.

The topics that are covered in this chapter include file system and operating system (OS) artifacts. The focus and our examples will be related to the Windows and Linux OSs and related file systems. Delving into the myriad OSs and file systems available would require a much more extensive discussion than we are able to present here.

Digital Forensics, First Edition. Edited by André Årnes.
© 2018 John Wiley & Sons Ltd. Published 2018 by John Wiley & Sons Ltd.

One well-known OS that is not covered in this chapter is Mac OSX. Apple Computers released Mac OSX in 2001. In 2006 the OS introduced support for Intel-based processors, and in 2009 the OS dropped PowerPC support all together. The OS has garnered a following and devotees, but it's still not widely adopted in enterprise deployment. References to Mac OSX forensics include a limited amount of materials. *Mac OS X, iPod, and iPhone Forensic Analysis DVD Toolkit* by Ryan Kubasiak and Sean Morrissey, and *Mac OS X Forensics* by Joaquin Moreno Garijo are two sources[1] (Kubasiak & Morrissey, 2008; Garijo, 2014).

Even though not all OS and file system artifacts can be described or even listed here, the student should be able to use the principles herein to research and understand the inner workings of additional artifacts and how to derive theories from the evidence they leave behind. The continuing addition of new artifacts and applications, security patches, and enhancements of products is not likely to slow down soon. We need the ability to understand the baseline properties and requirements of evidence collection and analysis in order to develop into competent computer forensic experts.

5.2 Evidence Collection

Evidence collection is a critical component of digital forensics. An examiner cannot come up with valid theories if the data is corrupted during the collection process. Collection, as described in Section 2.3, describes processes that must take place during the collection, including evidence handling and maintaining a sound chain of custody. Here, we will examine the technical aspects of collection.

Steps should be taken to assist low-skilled or new employees in data collection. For some operations, such as the routine collection of a SATA drive from a Windows workstation using a write blocker, a checklist or a step-by-step procedure can be developed. Advanced collection that requires memory collection, or an image of a production Solaris server, or live data that needs to be collected, or a myriad of other unique situations that may arise makes this process more complicatedIn complicated imaging tasks, a senior or more skilled analyst may be necessary to ensure the data is collected properly.

Example 5.1: Data Collection

Imagine a scenario where law enforcement is able to seize a suspect's Windows computer that was being used to access a virtual server – perhaps a SpyEye botnet server – hosted in the cloud. The agency may be able to send a trained, less experienced technician or agent to the field along with a checklist of routine tasks to successfully collect the Windows computer, remove the hard disk, and create a forensic image of the system. To collect the SpyEye server, depending on the cloud service of course, may be a much more advanced task, particularly if the hosting service is not cooperative. Additionally, both of these collections may require one or more legal authorities to seize the data. See Chapter 3 for more information on legal requirements and authorities.

---

1 Available at https://www.ma.rhul.ac.uk/static/techrep/2015/RHUL-MA-2015-8.pdf.

The documentation of the process used, the state of the evidence when it was acquired, the media it was transferred to, and the chain of custody of proper evidence handling are considered critical in a case that has the potential for court proceedings. It is always important for the analyst to follow proper methodologies and documentation for any evidence collection activities.

5.2.1 Data Acquisition

Data acquisition is the act of collecting data relevant to an investigation. This data can be live data, including memory captures, or it can be collected in a forensically sound manner as an image or a forensic copy.

The data acquisition should be conducted in a manner that creates the fewest changes to a system. The acquisition of a system that is powered off is the simplest example of collecting data in a forensically sound manner (Kent *et al.*, 2006; Symantec, 2010; SANS, 2012):

1) The analyst removes the system's hard drive.
2) The hard drive is connected to the read-only port of a firmware write block.[2]
3) A target device to store an image or a copy is connected to the read-write port of the write block.
4) The communications port of the write block is connected to a computer or a stand-alone device, or is built in.
5) The analyst then creates an image or a copy by writing to the target device.
6) The original is maintained and documented in a chain-of-custody form.
7) The image or copy can then be examined (or additional copies made) on the analysis platform. This is typically done as a read-only operation as well, which allows for repeatability of any examination or experiments without modifying the data.[3]

An example "flyaway" kit with several write blockers is shown in Figure 5.1.

Example 5.2: Hardware Write Blockers

In Example 5.1, a field agent or technician may be utilized to collect data from a crime scene or remote office. Traditionally, this data collection has been done with a hardware write blocker. The technician removes the drive from the system and connects it to an imaging system through a write blocker. Note that the term *hardware write blocker* is not synonymous with a physical write blocker. A hardware write blocker uses firmware to interrupt write commands, whereas a physical write blocker may, for example, prevent the disk from spinning at all.

Another physical write protection device could be described as the way floppy drives were write protected – such as by placing a physical hole in a diskette at a prescribed location. When light passed through the hole, the system would not allow writes to the diskette.

---

2 As with all tools used by an analyst, a write blocker should be tested in a controlled environment to ensure that changes to a drive connected to it cannot be written to intentionally or unintentionally.
3 Exceptions to examining a system as read only rare. They tend to be done on custom operating systems, file systems unreadable by forensic tools, or on systems with native applications that cannot be installed or executed on an analysis platform. See the section Forensic Copy for creating a bootable copy of evidence.

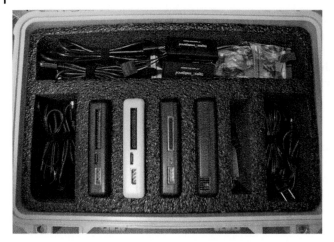

Figure 5.1 Hardware write blockers in a "flyaway" kit.

The list is a straightforward, easy-to-replicate series of steps. Collecting evidence can be more difficult in certain situations as previously indicated. Also, collecting evidence from a live system will certainly create changes on the system. Documenting the steps, tools, and evidence collection cannot be stressed enough – especially where the examiner is forced to make changes to the evidence. These changes can inject doubt about the validity of the collection process if the documentation or collection process is ad hoc or haphazard.

5.2.1.1 Live Data (Including Memory)

Live data acquisition involves collecting data from a running system. This can include memory, mounted files such as Windows registry hives, unencrypted volumes or file systems, security files, or open processes. Live data acquisition has become common in cases where a suspect is believed to have used full disk encryption – which means shutting down the system will remove the decryption key from memory and render the device unreadable without the correct password or key.

5.2.1.1.1 Files

Acquisition of files or mounted volumes can be accomplished by using software such as AccessData's FTK Imager, Mandiant's RedLine, or even custom scripts designed to capture common artifacts gathered for an investigation.

Acquiring files utilizing a forensic tool rather than the Copy command provides better options for accountability of what was acquired, chain of custody documentation, and verification through hashing. And it can allow for acquisition of files that are protected by the OS such as Windows registry hives, the Master File Table, or other metadata files.

Example 5.3: Software-as-a-Service (SaaS) Collection

What if the collection of data were from a cloud-based software as a service (SaaS), such as webmail services? This would have to follow proscribed legal processes, and the collection might be initiated or performed entirely by the hosting company.

In our SpyEye example, the collection of the workstation was completed on site or at an office; the server collection was completed with (or without) the cooperation of the hosting service. Take a third-party server, such as a user communication forum, and you may again add additional required legal process, expertise, and more to the collection of the data. Do you seize the entire third-party service, or will the database files themselves be sufficient for use in legal proceedings – criminal or civil?

5.2.1.1.2 Memory

Memory can be acquired using software tools such as AccessData's FTKImager, Mandiant's RedLine, or a memory dump tool such as LiME. Memory is often acquired from a running system if it's suspected of running malware or encryption. Encryption keys may be located in memory, for example. In many cases, memory has been used to locate attacker command activities on a system as well.

5.2.1.1.3 Volumes

Full volumes can be acquired utilizing a tool such as AccessData's FTKImager. The tool can acquire a mounted volume including unallocated space even if the volume is encrypted.

Example 5.4: Scalability of Live Data Acquisition Instead of Forensic Imaging

In many enterprises, the number of servers and workstations in the environment may number in the hundreds, thousands, or more. When performing an incident response (IR) investigation, the process should include scoping all devices to ensure that an attacker didn't install backdoors, steal data, or otherwise access the device. Traditional forensic imaging of these systems is not practical or efficient. In response, there are several live data IR scripts capable of collecting the most relevant artifacts and their timestamps.

Example 5.5: Scale, Part 2

A case example of an incident response involved over 160,000 Windows systems in an environment. The systems ranged from workstations and laptops to servers. An attacker infiltrated the corporate network and was not detected for over four years. The incident was fully scoped using primarily live response analysis to search for indicators of compromise (IOCs). It was certainly not feasible to do disk-based forensics on 160,000 systems. During the investigation, it was determined that the attacker accessed 80 systems in that environment – less than 0.0005% of the systems in the environment. Even to have performed disk-based forensics on 80 systems would have required significant resources to image and analyze. In this cases and similar cases, the forensic analysis occurred only on systems with evidence of data theft – primarily to analyze unallocated areas to recover artifacts unavailable through live response scripts.

```
---------------------------------------------------------------
Information for C:\Users\user\Desktop\Image:

Physical Evidentiary Item (Source) Information:
[Device Info]
 Source Type: Logical
[Drive Geometry]
 Bytes per Sector: 512
 Sector Count: 125,825,024
[Physical Drive Information]
 Removable drive: False
 Source data size: 61438 MB
 Sector count:    125825024
[Computed Hashes]
 MD5 checksum:    fac41a9fb54197cd213c590db3b77666|
 SHA1 checksum:   476e582cec89d751f26e66cf259e258525ddec27

Image Information:
 Acquisition started:   Thu Aug 04 13:05:57 2016
 Acquisition finished:  Thu Aug 04 13:41:21 2016
 Segment list:
  C:\Users\user\Desktop\Image.E01
```

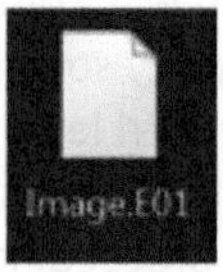

Figure 5.2 E01 example.

5.2.1.2 Forensic Image

A forensic image is the most common way of maintaining evidence from a computer system. In this case, an image file is created from the original source. The image is created in blocks and every byte is copied in the block, including unallocated bytes. This is sometimes slightly inaccurately referred to as a *bit-stream image* or a *byte-for-byte copy*. The image may be stored in a flat file such as a raw "dd" image, or it may be stored in a compound evidence file such as an E01 (see example in Figure 5.2) or AD1. See also NIST (2014).

An advantage to using a raw evidence file is that nearly every tool designed for analysis can read from a raw file or the file can be mounted as a disk image. Disadvantages include the fact that the image is not compressed, it will use as much space as the original device, and linear searching can take longer to perform.

Compound evidence file advantages include the ability to segment the image into "chunks" for backup purposes or for keeping within a file system's file size limitation. Evidence files can also be compressed and encrypted, and segments can contain checksums to help ensure validity.

5.2.2 Forensic Copy

A forensic copy is a copy created in blocks where every byte is copied in the block, including unallocated bytes. This is similar to the way a forensic image is created, but a forensic copy is created on another drive the same size or larger than the original rather than by creating an image file. Common uses of forensic copies include cases where a system needs to be booted for various reasons such as utilizing a password to mount a volume, running software natively, or booting an uncommon OS. The forensic copy can then be used in the system instead of the original evidence.

5.3 Examination

The next phase is the examination phase, in which relevant digital evidence is prepared and extracted from the collected data.

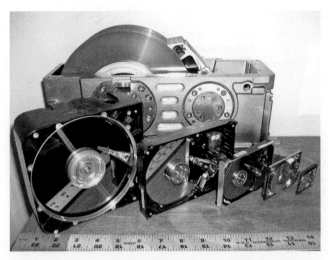

Figure 5.3 Various disk drives (image courtesy Wikipedia, 2015).

5.3.1 Disk Structures

Disk structures, as with most technology, is ever-evolving. A disk is a device used to store and retrieve data readable by a computer system. The means of storing the data on a medium are typically (1) magnetic – as with a hard disk (as shown in Figure 5.3), tape drive, or floppy diskette; (2) optic – as with a CD or DVD; or (3) electronically programmable memory – such as with flash drives or memory cards. Then, of course, there are several subsets of each type of storage device. The scope here is intended to provide a high-level understanding of disk structures for the most commonly examined device in enterprise system forensics – a magnetic disk drive. One cannot begin to understand a file system, unless one understands how that file system is stored on a disk (or other media).

It is important to have a working knowledge of older technology because the examiner may come into contact with older technology for a variety of reasons. For example, the analyst may encounter an old server hosting an application that a business was built upon, and that has never been migrated to a modern OS or hardware.

5.3.1.1 Physical Disk Structures

A physical drive, in general terms, is the entire disk device. This includes the metal housing, platters, read-write heads, motor, and electronics. The electronics in modern hard disks control the drive and send and receive data through an interface that can be interpreted by the computer system.

Interfaces to the storage platters constantly evolve to allow for faster disk access, broader data transmissions, and more storage space. The various drives connect to the computer in different ways, and the common types of connectors the examiner is likely to see include small computer system interface (SCSI), serial attached SCSI (SAS), integrated drive electronics (IDE), and serial AT attachment (SATA). Table 5.1 lists common drive interfaces and key features or limitations.

Table 5.1 Common hard drive interfaces.

Interface	Acronym	Communication	Key features or limitations
SCSI	Small computer storage interface	Parallel	Requires termination, limited to 7 or 15 devices per controller
SAS	Serial attached SCSI	Serial	128 devices, full duplex, hot plugging, can communicate with SATA or SCSI controllers
IDE	Integrated drive electronics IDE is also known as ATA (advanced technology attachment) and now retroactively known as PATA (parallel ATA)	Parallel	18-inch maximum length cable, limited to two devices per controller
SATA	Serial ATA	Serial	Host swapping, one device per channel

Specifications, speeds, versions, and connection methods vary greatly between drives. The analyst performing the imaging task needs to be familiar with the interface being used and the specific limitations, cables, and requirements (such as SCSI devices requiring logical unit number (LUN)[4] assignment and termination[5] at the end of the SCSI chain).

Magnetic disk drives historically stored data in units known as *cylinders, heads,* and *sectors.* These units were then used to assign address to each storage block on a disk. Additionally, concentric circles of storage areas on each side of the drive's platter were known as *tracks.* Tracks were limited to 63 sectors.

As drives evolved, more platters were added internally to create more storage space, which required additional heads for reading and writing. A cylinder is used to refer to all the concentric tracks on the drive. Heads are the read-write devices, and normally there are two per platter on a hard disk drive. Also as drives matured, sector size became standardized as 512 bytes. Physical addressing could then be accomplished by referring to the location in cylinders, heads, and sectors. Maximum size of a drive could also be calculated with the simple formula: the number of cylinders multiplied by the number of heads multiplied by the sector size multiplied by 63 sectors per track, or CHS × 63.

There were additional limitations in the actual implementation that further restricted drive size, based on factors such as maximum number of bits used for addressing, which gave way to LBA (logical block addressing). LBA in its simplest sense points to a specific sector on a disk linearly. In original implementations of LBA, sectors were still standardized at 512 bytes per sector.

It is important to have a basic understanding of physical addressing and how it impacts the way the examiner should approach an analysis. Logical volumes and file systems utilize internal drive electronics to accomplish the physical changes, and a number of limitations of physical devices affected the development and nomenclature of logical structures (and vice versa).

---

4 All devices on a SCSI cable require a unit number assignment, including the controller.
5 Termination at the end of a SCSI cable is required. Some devices are self-terminating.

Although sectors on most drives were 512 bytes, at a strictly physical level, there are additional bytes in use by the drive's electronics that may include metadata such as checksums and block (or sector) number. Sectors (or blocks, depending on the file system) are the smallest unit of data a file system can *write* to (Definition 5.1).

Definition 5.1: Sector
The smallest writeable data unit on a file system.

A cluster is the smallest *addressable* unit on a file system (Definition 5.2). During drive format, cluster size is allocated as a multiple of sectors. On floppy diskettes, normally one sector would equal one cluster. In turn, that indicates one cluster on the same diskette could contain 512 bytes of data.

Definition 5.2: Cluster
The smallest addressable data unit on a file system.

On most modern Windows systems with NTFS (New Technology File System) formatting, one cluster (by default) is often composed of eight sectors (4096 bytes, or 4 Kb). This is further expanded on in the NTFS section (Section 5.3.2.1).

Example 5.6: Creating a One-Byte File
If we created a one-byte file, an NTFS file system would write the single byte and 511 null bytes to the cluster. If the cluster size was equal to one sector, it would be written in the same way. If the cluster size was 4 Kb (eight sectors), then the file system would write the first byte of the file, followed by 511 null bytes into the first sector. The remaining sectors in the cluster would not be written to (or overwritten if they previously contained data from a deleted file). The sectors containing leftover data are commonly referred to as *slack space* or *cluster slack*.

5.3.1.1.1 Logical Volumes, Sectors, and Advanced Format Drives

Formerly, logical volumes could only be created on a track boundary – and the maximum number of tracks on a cylinder is 63, then it can be assumed that a volume can only start on sector 63 and multiples thereof.

Advanced format drives include 4 Kb (4096 byte) sectors and are also known as e512 drives. They were released several years ago, but internal drive electronics interpret storage addressing back to the OS as if they were 512 byte sectors for legacy purposes. They also do away with the limitation of starting a file system on sector 63 – which is messy for computer electronics using binary math. More frequently, a new e512 drive in a Windows 7 or greater system will place the first volume at sector 2048 – which is much easier using binary math (0x 00 08 00 00)

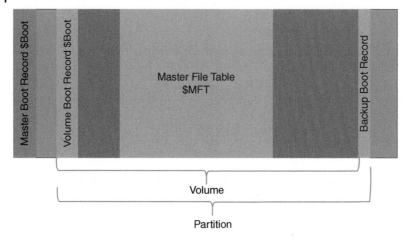

Figure 5.4 Logical drive structure.

than 63. Additionally, it can surprise an examiner that has an old understanding of CHS by changing the expected location of the first (or subsequent) volume (Hamm, 2010).

5.3.1.2 Logical Disk Structures

Logical structures on a physical disk are required for the OS to access the storage space on the physical device. As shown in Figure 5.4, logical structures include partition tables such as an MBR (master boot record) or a GPT (GUID partition table) or an actual partition. A partition can include an entire logical volume or a portion of a volume. A volume in turn typically contains a file system.

On a single-user, single-drive system, when a user attaches a new hard drive that contains no data,[6] the user must follow these steps to access the drive as storage media:

1) Create a partition table – either MBR or GPT – with a tool such as FDISK.
2) Format the partition into a logical volume that contains a file system.
3) Assign the partition a drive letter or mount point.

When installing an OS on a drive, the installation manager or the user at installation will handle these options. In OSs such as Linux, the user can specify multiple mount points or partitions during installation.

Example 5.7: Windows NTFS Recovery Partition

Modern Windows operating systems create a hidden partition with an NTFS volume at installation called the NTFS Recovery Partition by Microsoft. This partition contains information to restore a volume boot sector or perform low-level operations to attempt to access data on a corrupted volume, and it is not a data backup.

Some computer manufacturers will also store data in hidden partitions for OS or software installation, software reinstallation, or other purposes.

---

6 A newly purchased drive today normally already has a partition, volume, and file system formatted on it.

Table 5.2 Simplified MBR data table.

Offset	Length	Data
0x00	446 bytes	Bootstrap code
0x1BE	16 bytes	Partition entry
0x1CE	16 bytes	Partition entry
0x1DE	16 bytes	Partition entry
0x0EE	16 bytes	Partition entry
0x01FE	2 bytes	Boot signature (0x55AA)

As mentioned, a disk can contain portions of a file system. This is true in situations where a RAID (redundant array of independent disks) or LVM (logical volume manager) is used. These technologies take advantage of multiple drives or virtual drives to create file systems that are redundant and/or faster and/or larger than a stand-alone device. Examining RAIDs or LVMs requires individuals with a greater understanding in these areas than the scope of this work covers. For imaging, see Mead (2015).

5.3.1.2.1 MBR
IBM implemented MBR partitioning in 1983. The partitioning scheme is still the most common in use at the time of this writing. Modern OSs can read this style of partitioning, and many create a MBR partitioning scheme on a drive during installation.

The MBR itself consists of one sector – absolute sector zero. This first sector (see Table 5.2) includes the boot code, disk signature, and primary partition definitions, and ends with a signature (a two-byte code represented in hexadecimal as 0x55AA). Additional sectors in the boot record are not typically accessible by the user without tools that have raw access to the drive – such a hexadecimal editor, or *hex editor*. As previously discussed, earlier installations required the first partition to be created on a track boundary (track 63), while newer implementations remove this require- ment and the first volume can be anywhere the MBR defines it (typically, at sector 2048 or 4096).

An MBR-formatted disk, as shown in Figure 5.5, can contain up to four partitions in the boot record (see Table 5.3 for a partition entry and Table 5.4 for common partition types) – all of which can be primary and only *one* of which can be an extended partition. A primary partition can contain one and only one volume, and only one of these volumes can be bootable (an extended partition cannot be natively bootable).

An extended partition, as shown in Figure 5.6, can contain additional logical parti- tions. The first defined logical partition utilizes the volume boot record (VBR) to define

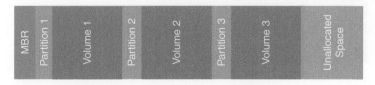

Figure 5.5 Example diagram of partitions on an MBR disk.

Table 5.3 Partition entry.

Offset	Length	Data
0x00	1 byte	Active or bootable partition (only one can be marked active per disk)
0x01	3 bytes	First absolute sector for CHS addressing (legacy)
0x04	1 byte	Partition type
0x05	3 bytes	Last absolute sector for CHS addressing (legacy)
0x08	4 bytes	First absolute sector for LBA addressing
0x0C	4 bytes	Number of sectors in the partition

Table 5.4 Common partition types.

Partition type	Description
0x00	Empty partition
0x07	NTFS, HPFS, exFAT
0x0B	FAT32 with CHS addressing
0x0C	FAT32 with LBA addressing
0x0F	Extended partition with LBA
0x17	Hidden NTFS, hidden HPFS, hidden exFAT
0x82	Linux swap space
0x83	Native Linux file system

itself and the next logical partition. The second defined logical partition defines itself and the next logical partition. This continues as a linked list until the final logical partition defines only itself. In this scheme, specific problems for a digital examiner include:

- A person wanting to hide data could manually edit the partition table and skip a partition by pointing to the next partition in the link.
- If a partition in the chain becomes corrupted, all subsequent partitions have no definition.

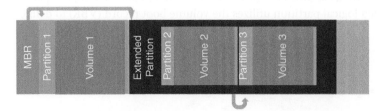

Figure 5.6 Example diagram of extended partitions on an MBR disk.

Example 5.8: Drive Lettering

In Microsoft file systems, access to these partitions is limited to 24. Microsoft uses ASCII drive letters to refer to file systems. The letters A and B are reserved for floppy diskettes whether or not they are present. This leaves available drives C–Z.

5.3.1.2.2 GUID Partition Table (GPT)

To address limitations of the MBR partitioning format, GPT schemes were created. Some advantages of this partition scheme include using GUIDs (global unique identifiers) to reference each partition; not limiting the number of partitions to a defined set of four; using 64 bit LBA for storing sector numbers, thereby increasing the theoretical maximum disk size; and maintaining backups and CRC32 checksums to detect and fix potential corruption.

The GPT partition scheme reserves absolute sector zero and utilizes the same offset as the MBR uses to describe a partition. This first entry describes the entire disk up to 2 TiB (the maximum size definable in an MBR). The next sector contains the GPT header and defines the disk contents, as shown in Table 5.5 and Table 5.6. Contents include the GUID for the disk, partition table location, maximum number of partitions, and location of the backup header.

5.3.2 File Systems

File systems are formatted onto a volume – either a single-partition or a multiple-partition volume in the case of a RAID or an LVM. The file system provides a means by

Table 5.5 GUID partition table (GPT).

Offset	Length	Data
0x00	8 bytes	Signature ("EFI PART")
0x08	4 bytes	GPT revision level
0x0C	4 bytes	GPT header size
0x10	4 bytes	CRC32 of header
0x14	4 bytes	Reserved
0x18	8 bytes	LBA address of current header
0x20	8 bytes	LBA address of backup header
0x28	8 bytes	First addressable LBA for partitions
0x30	8 bytes	Last addressable LBA for partitions
0x38	16 bytes	Disk GUID
0x48	8 bytes	Starting LBA of partition entry array
0x50	4 bytes	Number of partition entries in the array
0x54	4 bytes	Size of a single partition entry
0x58	4 bytes	CRC32 of partition array
0x5C	420 bytes	Reserved

Table 5.6 GPT partition entry.

Offset	Length	Data
0x00	16 bytes	Partition type GUID
0x10	16 bytes	Unique partition GUID
0x20	8 bytes	First addressable LBA
0x28	8 bytes	Last addressable LBA
0x30	8 bytes	Attribute flags
0x38	72 bytes	Partition name

which the OS can access the actual files stored on disk. At its core, a file system can be thought of as a database in the sense that, like a database, data is stored (in this case, somewhere on the volume) and metadata is used to track the data. (See Definition 5.3.)

Definition 5.3: File System

A file system stores data on a device so data can be retrieved by the system or a user. File systems are largely independent of an operating system (OS), and different file systems can be supported on different OSs when necessary drivers are installed.

Modern file systems are largely independent of the OS – Linux can read and write to the Microsoft NTFS, and with the proper drivers, Windows can read and write to Linux EXT (Extended File System). While the terms *operating system* and *file system* are often used interchangeably, this is not technically correct. An OS is independent of the file system and vice versa – for the most part. However, there is a symbiotic relationship between the OS and file system that may be required for functionality – for example, Windows 7 cannot boot to an EXT volume. Table 5.7 provides an overview of OSs and their native file systems.

Table 5.7 Operating systems and their native file systems.

Operating system	Native file systems
Windows 98	FAT16, FAT32
Windows 2000	FAT16, FAT32, NTFS
Windows XP	FAT16, FAT32, NTFS
Windows Vista	FAT16, FAT32, NTFS, exFAT (with SP1 and later)
Windows 7	FAT16, FAT32, NTFS, exFAT
Windows 8	FAT16, FAT32, NTFS, exFAT
Windows 10	FAT16, FAT32, NTFS, exFAT
Linux	EXT2, EXT3, EXT4, XFS
Mac OSX	HPFS, exFAT

Metadata in a file system includes items like a file's location (or address) and the size of the data so the system can retrieve it from the hardware. Typically, a file system will track the location of a file's data location as block addresses. Multiple blocks of data may be necessary for files that are too large to be stored in a single block and/or cannot be stored in consecutive blocks on the device. Each file system, as will be discussed, tracks this information in different ways.

Definition 5.4: Metadata

Metadata is data about data. Metadata can be used to track timestamps, location of data, the exposure setting on a digital image, or any number of arbitrary items that allow a user or the system to locate, sort, or collate data.

Metadata also includes items like a file name and the location of a file in hierarchical directory structures or paths so the user can find the file. File names can be limited like in the FAT16 file system to eight bytes with a three-byte file extension (referred to as 8.3), or they can be long filenames such as is the case with most modern file systems. Of course, even filenames have limitations that can be limited by the file system, or in some cases limited by the OS and the ability to address finite characters in a file's full path.

A file system can store metadata to make retrieval by the user or the system easier or faster, such as by using timestamps or catalog numbers. Early UNIX file systems do not include a creation date (or birth date), while more modern file systems such as NTFS and EXT4 (fourth extended filesystem) have this ability. Other metadata include flags such as telling the user if the file is an archive, if it is a deleted file, if it is read-only, or even if the "file" is a directory.

The format operation creates the file system in a volume. The volume contains a VBR in the first sector of the volume that defines the important structure(s) of the file system, what the size of the data storage units are, and other data about the file system itself.

The storage units on a disk are *sectors*. Sectors are 512 bytes in size (as exemplified in Figure 5.7), or if the drive is an *advanced format drive* (e512) the sectors are virtually reported to the OS as 512 bytes. A sector is the smallest unit that a file system can write to. If one byte is needed for a file, for example, it requires 512 bytes of storage space (one sector). The remaining bytes in the sector are written as NULL value bytes.[7]

Microsoft file systems utilize clusters in addressing, while Linux nomenclature refers to addressing in blocks. A cluster or a block consists of one or more sectors. Formatting options in file systems allow the user to customize the cluster size or allow the OS to automatically customize this. A typical Windows system running an NTFS file system on a one-terabyte drive will likely contain a cluster size equal to 4096 bytes – or eight sectors per cluster. This allows for larger drives to be utilized because the file system only has to address one-eighth the number of sectors. The impact of this, then, is that if a one-byte file is created, it will occupy 4096 bytes – or eight sectors – of space. Most file systems will not write data or NULL values to the sectors that are not necessary to store the file.

---

7 Early versions of DOS did not always use NULL values to complete a sector write. In some cases, DOS wrote portions of memory to bytes not used by a file. This is sometimes referred to as *RAM slack.*

```
00000000  eb 48 90 10 8e d0 bc 00  b0 b8 00 00 8e d8 8e c0  |.H..............|
00000010  fb be 00 7c bf 00 06 b9  00 02 f3 a4 ea 21 06 00  |...|.........!..|
00000020  00 be be 07 38 04 75 0b  83 c6 10 81 fe fe 07 75  |....8.u........u|
00000030  f3 eb 16 b4 02 b0 01 bb  00 7c b2 80 8a 74 03 02  |.........|...t..|
00000040  ff 00 00 20 01 00 00 00  00 02 fa 90 90 f6 c2 80  |... ............|
00000050  75 02 b2 80 ea 59 7c 00  00 31 c0 8e d8 8e d0 bc  |u....Y|..1......|
00000060  00 20 fb a0 40 7c 3c ff  74 02 88 c2 52 be 7f 7d  |. ..@|<.t...R..}|
00000070  e8 34 01 f6 c2 80 74 54  b4 41 bb aa 55 cd 13 5a  |.4....tT.A..U..Z|
00000080  52 72 49 81 fb 55 aa 75  43 a0 41 7c 84 c0 75 05  |RrI..U.uC.A|..u.|
00000090  83 e1 01 74 37 66 8b 4c  10 be 05 7c c6 44 ff 01  |...t7f.L...|.D..|
000000a0  66 8b 1e 44 7c c7 04 10  00 c7 44 02 01 00 66 89  |f..D|.....D...f.|
000000b0  5c 08 c7 44 06 00 70 66  31 c0 89 44 04 66 89 44  |\..D..pf1..D.f.D|
000000c0  0c b4 42 cd 13 72 05 bb  00 70 eb 7d b4 08 cd 13  |..B..r...p.}....|
000000d0  73 0a f6 c2 80 0f 84 ea  00 e9 8d 00 be 05 7c c6  |s.............|.|
000000e0  44 ff 00 66 31 c0 88 f0  40 66 89 44 04 31 d2 88  |D..f1...@f.D.1..|
000000f0  ca c1 e2 02 88 e8 88 f4  40 89 44 08 31 c0 88 d0  |........@.D.1...|
00000100  c0 e8 02 66 89 04 66 a1  44 7c 66 31 d2 66 f7 34  |...f..f.D|f1.f.4|
00000110  88 54 0a 66 31 d2 66 f7  74 04 88 54 0b 89 44 0c  |.T.f1.f.t..T..D.|
00000120  3b 44 08 7d 3c 8a 54 0d  c0 e2 06 8a 4c 0a fe c1  |;D.}<.T.....L...|
00000130  08 d1 8a 6c 0c 5a 8a 74  0b bb 00 70 8e c3 31 db  |...l.Z.t...p...1.|
00000140  b8 01 02 cd 13 72 2a 8c  c3 8e 06 48 7c 60 1e b9  |.....r*...H|`..|
00000150  00 01 8e db 31 f6 31 ff  fc f3 a5 1f 61 ff 26 42  |....1.1.....a.&B|
00000160  7c be 85 7d e8 40 00 eb  0e be 8a 7d e8 38 00 eb  ||..}.@.....}.8..|
00000170  06 be 94 7d e8 30 00 be  99 7d e8 2a 00 eb fe 47  |...}.0...}.*...G|
00000180  52 55 42 20 00 47 65 6f  6d 00 48 61 72 64 20 44  |RUB .Geom.Hard D|
00000190  69 73 6b 00 52 65 61 64  00 20 45 72 72 6f 72 00  |isk.Read. Error.|
000001a0  bb 01 00 b4 0e cd 10 ac  3c 00 75 f4 c3 00 00 00  |........<.u.....|
000001b0  00 00 00 00 00 00 00 00  fb f5 09 00 00 00 80 01  |................|
000001c0  01 00 83 fe 3f 2a 3f 00  00 00 2c 8a 0a 00 00 00  |....?*?...,.....|
000001d0  01 2b 05 fe ff ff 6b 8a  0a 00 a9 60 f5 00 00 00  |.+....k....`....|
000001e0  00 00 00 00 00 00 00 00  00 00 00 00 00 00 00 00  |................|
000001f0  00 00 00 00 00 00 00 00  00 00 00 00 00 00 55 aa  |..............U.|
00000200  52 56 be 03 21 e8 2a 01  5e bf f8 21 66 8b 2d 83  |RV..!.*.^..!f.-.|
```

Figure 5.7 One full sector and 512 bytes displayed in ASCII and Hex.

The remaining sectors may contain data from previously deleted files – this unused space is known as *file slack*.

Figure 5.8 depicts a high-level example of a volume that is laid on 512 byte sectors. Each cluster in Figure 5.8 contain four sectors, or 2048 bytes. The smallest addressable unit on the volume is a cluster, and the smallest writeable unit is a sector. The smallest physical size of a file is therefore 2048 bytes. If a file uses only one sector of a cluster, the remaining sectors are not overwritten and may contain data from a file previously allocated to the cluster. The remaining data in a sector is overwritten with nulls.

To understand file systems, it's essential that an examiner have familiarity with binary systems. In particular, the examiner will need to be familiar with what an *offset* is and what *Endianness* refers to. Much of the analysis and interpretation of metadata in a file system can be conducted at a hexadecimal level.

For the purposes of this work, the reference to an offset will always start at zero. This means that if a byte contains eight values, the bytes are numbered 0–7. The first byte is at offset 0 – zero bytes from the first; and the eighth byte is at offset 7 – seven bytes from the first. Figure 5.9 depicts a representation of offset 0 and offset 8 in the hexadecimal output from an on-disk structure.

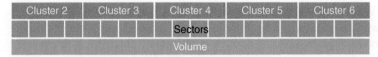

Figure 5.8 Conceptual volume with clusters and sectors.

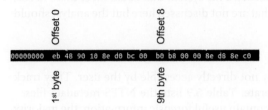

Figure 5.9 Byte offset.

Endianness refers to the way address data is read and stored. Big-Endian data is stored with the most significant bytes listed first. Little-Endian data is stored with the least significant bytes listed first (See Definition 5.5.). The way the data is stored is determined by the technology used in memory arrays. In general, Intel-based processors store data in Little-Endian, while Motorola-based processors store data in Big-Endian.[8] This becomes important when looking at file systems because they store address data in the same manner as the processor.

Definition 5.5: Endianness

Endianness refers to the way address data is read and stored. Big-Endian data is stored with the most significant bytes listed first. Little-Endian data is stored with the least significant bytes listed first.

5.3.2.1 NTFS (New Technology File System)

The NTFS is the most common file system examined in an enterprise environment. To give the analyst a basis for understanding file systems and file system artifacts, it is perhaps the best starting point. It is important to keep in mind that there are many file systems available between OSs, as well as custom file systems that are beyond the scope of this chapter.

NTFS has been the file system of choice for Windows OSs since Windows 2000 was released. Microsoft has developed two more recent file systems: the ReFS (Resilient File System) for primary use in clustered file or database servers, and the exFAT (Extended File Allocation Table) file system for primary use in removable media. The NTFS file system continues to be used as the default file system in Windows 10.

NTFS is released in two major revisions: 1.x and 3.x. There were two minor revisions in Windows NT: 1.0 with NT 3.1 and 1.2 with NT 3.5x. There were also two minor

---

8 *Endianness* is a term derived from Jonathan Swift's novel *Gulliver's Travels*. In his story, there was a dispute between the inhabitants of Lilliput over which side of a hard-cooked egg should be opened first – the big end or the little end.

revisions: from the Windows 2000 release – NTFS 3.1; and the Windows XP release – NTFS 3.5. The file system was derived from the need in a network environment and a need to introduce controls such as ACLs (access control lists) and quotas to prevent users from using all volume space, thereby preventing the OS from functioning. The previous Microsoft FAT file system did not have any of these controls, and with the release of Windows NT 3.1, Microsoft needed a file system that could meet these needs.

Table 5.8 lists several NTFS artifacts that are not discussed here but the analyst should be aware of.

5.3.2.1.1 Metadata Files

Metadata files are files that are generally not directly accessible by the user. They track data required for the file system to operate. Table 5.9 lists the NTFS metadata files.

While many of the metadata files can contain useful forensic information, the majority of them are out of scope to discuss here. The analyst is encouraged to get an understanding of the $MFT as presented here and continue to research the additional metadata files.

5.3.2.1.2 Master File Table (MFT)

The MFT is a collection of file records in an NTFS volume. All objects in the NTFS are tracked in file records – including files, directories, and even the VBR.

The MFT is created during formatting of a volume. The file system determines a place to allocate the MFT on the physical media. It does this by determining things such as

Table 5.8 Some NTFS artifacts that are not covered herein.

Artifact	Description
Encrypted File System (EFS)	EFS allows for a user to encrypt user files on an NTFS volume. This provides additional protections in a multiuser environment to prevent users from reading each other's data. EFS cannot be used on system files and is not a full disk encryption (FDE) technology.
Reparse points	Reparse points are volume-level artifacts that allow for object-level redirects of file or directory lookups. A common example of this would be the "Documents and Settings" directory in the Windows 2000/XP OS, which was changed to "Users" in Windows Vista/7 and later. To maintain backwards compatibility, "Documents and Settings" is a default reparse point to "Users."
BitLocker	BitLocker is a full volume encryption (FVE) solution developed by Microsoft to encrypt an NTFS volume.
Journaling ($LogFile and $UsnJrnl)	NTFS is a journaling file system that maintains redundant change logs so that if a write operation fails, the system can roll back to a previous state. Some research in this area has yielded results that can assist in rebuilding the previous state of a file system and can recover deleted information.
NTFS compression and sparse files	NTFS allows for the use of compression and sparse files to save space on a volume. The analyst should be aware that if a file is reported as 20 GB and contains compressed data or sparse data, it may not physically take up 20 GB in space on the physical media.

Table 5.9   NTFS metadata files.

Filename	Description
$MFT	The $MFT file is the master file table. This file tracks all file records on a file system, including itself. This file is discussed in more detail in this chapter, and knowledge of this file is critical for the analyst to understand the NTFS file system and forensics.
$MFTMirr	The $MFTMirr is a file that contains a copy of the first four MFT records in a file system: $MFT, $MFTMirr, $LogFile, and $Volume.
$LogFile	The $LogFile is a transactional file used for changing log journaling to help maintain file system consistency in the event of write errors.
$Volume	The $Volume file contains volume-specific information, including the volume label, dirty mount flag, and NTFS version.
$AttrDef	The $AttrDef file contains file attribute definitions and associates numeric values with attribute names.
"."	The "." file is the root directory of the volume.
$Bitmap	The $Bitmap file contains a bit for each cluster on the volume. The file system can scan the file for free (0) or allocated (1) clusters.
$Boot	The volume boot record for NTFS is stored in the $Boot file. This file resides at the beginning of the volume and is defined in detail in this chapter.
$BadClus	The $BadClus file tracks all clusters on the volume that contain bad sectors.
$Secure	The $Secure file is a database used to map ACLs to files or groups of files. Unlike EXT file systems, mapping ACLs is not specific to the file and thereby reduces the overhead of storing permissions in every inode/record.
$UpCase	The $UpCase file contains information to ensure compliance between Win32 and DOS namespaces. This is necessary because NTFS is case-insensitive.
$Extend	The $Extend metafile is a directory that contains additional metadata files including: $ObjID, $Quota, $Reparse, and $UsnJrnl.
$ObjID	The $ObjID file contains an index of all of the $OBJECT_ID attributes on a volume (Russon, 2015).
$Quota	The $Quota file is used to track user quota data on a volume.
$Reparse	The $Reparse file is used to track reparse points including mount points in a volume. In NTFS, a volume can be mounted into a nested directory without a drive letter similar to mount points in UNIX and Linux systems.
$UsnJrnl	The $UsnJrnl file is a transactional file that tracks changes on a volume to assist in preventing write errors by allowing the system to revert to a prior state. Therefore, the file can contain metadata about a system's previous state.

allowing more file system stability, providing efficient access time, and decreasing the likelihood of fragmentation. The location of the MFT on the volume is defined in the VBR.

5.3.2.1.3   *MFT File Records*
The MFT consists of sequential MFT file records. While file record size is defined in the VBR, in practice these are 1024 bytes (1 KB). The MFT file records consist of an MFT record header that defines the file record as well as a series of attributes that define data

File Record 0x00 $MFT	File Record 0x01 $MFTMirr	File Record 0x02 $LogFile	File Record 0x03 $Volume	File Record 0x04 $AttrDef	File Record 0x05 .	File Record 0x06 $Bitmap

Figure 5.10 MBR and the first six file records abstract on an MFT.

about a file or directory. Figure 5.10 is a hypothetical diagram of an MFT with file records every 1024 bytes listed in sequence.

The MFT record header always starts with the identifier *FILE*. It contains metadata essential for the MFT record as a whole. The content includes the record's physical and logical size, where the attributes begin in the record, the sequence count for the record, and the MFT record number. It attempts to ensure it is not corrupted by the use of *fix-up arrays*. To examine the individual structures in the NTFS file system, the analyst can determine the offsets to the data through the use of a table defining each byte. For a consolidated quick reference guide, the analyst can use a mobile application or a flipbook such as the Lock and Code Pty Ltd. (2014). Figure 5.11 is an expanded view of the file record for MFT record 0x03 – the VBR.

The $MFT file record data is laid out in the format listed in Table 5.10.

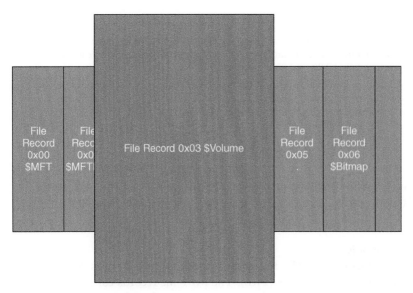

Figure 5.11 MFT file record.

Table 5.10 File record data.

Offset	Size	Data
0x00	4 bytes	Signature
0x04	2 bytes	Offset to fixup array
0x06	2 bytes	Number of entries in the fixup array
0x08	8 bytes	$LogFile sequence number
0x10	2 bytes	Sequence count
0x12	2 bytes	Link count
0x14	2 bytes	Offset to the first attribute
0x16	2 bytes	Allocation status (allocated, directory, or not allocated)
0x18	4 bytes	Logical size of the $MFT record
0x1C	4 bytes	Physical size of the $MFT record
0x20	8 bytes	File reference to the base record
0x28	2 bytes	The next attribute identification (shows a count of the attributes in the record)
0x2a	> 0	Fixup codes and attributes (NTFS 3.0)
0x2a	2 bytes	Zero padding (NTFS 3.1 and greater)
0x2c	4 bytes	$MFT file record number (NTFS 3.1 and greater)
0x30	> 0	Fixup codes and attributes (NTFS 3.1 and greater)

The sequence count of the attribute is used by NTFS to assist in maintaining a clean file system. This sequence count is incremented to 0x00 01 when the MFT record is allocated for the first time. The count is then incremented upon the associated file or folder's deletion. This helps prevent a deleted file from being reactivated in an incorrect directory if the file's parent directory MFT record is reused. For more detail on this, see Section 5.3.2.3, "Orphan Files."

Fix-up codes are used to help ensure that the two sectors of the MFT record (two 512-byte sectors make up one 1024-byte file record) are not corrupt. They contain bytes to be swapped at the last two bytes of each sector.

5.3.2.1.4 Attributes

Attributes track metadata about specific structures in an MFT record. This can include the data, directory content, file timestamps, filename, security information, and more. Some attributes are required: the standard information attribute and file name attribute, and either a data attribute or an index root attribute. Each attribute begins with a header that describes the attribute's physical size and how to find the content of the attribute. Figure 5.12 further expands the file record into the contents of a record header and separate metadata attributes.

Resident and Nonresident Attributes The content of an attribute can be resident or nonresident. Most files are larger than 1024 bytes and will therefore be nonresident attribute data. The standard information attribute, filename attribute(s), and index root attributes are required to be resident. Both types of attributes begin with a 16-byte

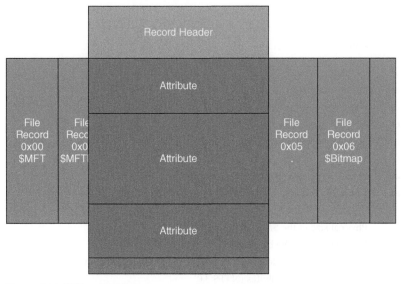

Figure 5.12 MFT and attributes.

header as shown in Table 5.11, which describes the attribute number, its total length in bytes, and if the attribute is resident or nonresident.

A resident attribute, as shown in Table 5.12, then has additional bytes describing where the content of the attribute begins, its length, and a stream name if required (see Definition 5.6). This data, therefore, is variable in length.

Table 5.11 Resident and nonresident attribute headers.

Offset	Size	Data
0x00	4 bytes	Attribute type identifier
0x04	4 bytes	Length of the attribute
0x08	1 byte	Resident or nonresident flag
0x09	1 byte	Length of the "stream" name
0x0A	2 bytes	Offset to the "stream" name
0x0C	2 bytes	Flags identifying if the attribute is "compressed," "sparse," or "encrypted"
0x0E	2 bytes	Attribute identifier

Table 5.12 Resident attribute header.

Offset	Size	Data
0x00	16 bytes	Attribute header information
0x10	4 bytes	Size of the content
0x14	2 bytes	Offset to the content

Table 5.13   Nonresident attribute header.

Offset	Size	Data
0x00	16 bytes	Attribute header information
0x10	8 bytes	Starting VCN of the runlist
0x18	8 bytes	Ending VCN of the runlist
0x20	2 bytes	Offset to the runlist
0x22	2 bytes	Used for compression
0x24	4 bytes	Unused
0x28	8 bytes	Allocated size of the content
0x30	8 bytes	Actual size of the content
0x38	8 bytes	Initialized size of the content

A nonresident attribute has a standard header, as shown in Table 5.13, with information about where the content of the attribute exists on disk. The data also includes virtual cluster numbers (VCNs) for fragmentation tracking if necessary.

Definition 5.6: Named Data Stream

A stream name is the name of the data content that an attribute points to. A stream name does not have to be provided for the attribute's content, and indeed the default stream is unnamed. Common stream names include *$130*, which is the stream of an index attribute. See the subsection entitled "Named and Unnamed Streams" in this section.

Locating nonresident attribute content on disk can be accomplished through the runlist information contained in the attribute header. To track a file on an NTFS file system, at minimum the file system needs the file record header along with the standard information attribute, at least one file name attribute, and the data attribute. Figure 5.13 lists the required attributes and record header core information stored in an MFT record for a file.

Standard Information Attribute   MAC (modified, accessed, changed) times were origi-nally derived from the three UNIX file system timestamps – file content **M**odified, file last **A**ccessed, and inode **C**hanged time. Various tools and OSs often refer to these times differently. Table 5.14 provides a comparison of UNIX MAC file time descriptions to Microsoft Windows file time descriptions.

Understanding timestamps as they relate to an incident response can be critical. To assist the analyst's understanding, there has been research into why timestamps change. Lee (2010) has developed a diagram with quick explanations on these updates. Since a Windows application programming interface (API) can modify these timestamps, it can be relatively simple for an attacker to manipulate these to blend in with normal system files.

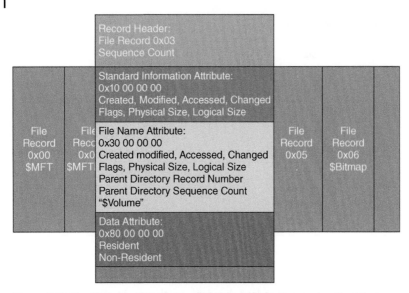

Figure 5.13 The MFT record header and attributes required to track a file object.

Additional information found in the standard information attribute (see Table 5.15) includes DOS file type attributes such as read only, hidden, system, and directory. There is also security and quota information, whose explanation is beyond the scope of this book. See Carrier (2010) and Russon (2015) for more detailed information.

Table 5.14   NTFS file metadata times.

Unix name	Windows name	Description
Birth date (does not exist in most UNIX file systems)	Created date	The time a file was created on the volume.
Modified date	Last written	The time the content of the file was last modified. Note that in many cases, when a file is extracted from an archive or moved from one directory to another on the same volume, this time may be older than the created time because the content of the file was not necessarily changed when the file was "created."
Accessed date	Accessed date	The time the file was last accessed by a user or an application. This timestamp is disabled by default in Windows Vista and later operating systems. The timestamp still exists but is not updated on access.
Inode changed date	Record modified	The time the MFT record for this file was last modified.
Deleted date	N/A	This timestamp does not exist in the NTFS file system. A file sent to the recycle bin in Windows has a "deleted" date associated with when it was sent to the recycle bin. See Section 5.3.2.5.3, "Recycle Bin."

Table 5.15   Standard information attributes.

Offset	Size	Data
0x00	8 bytes	Creation time
0x08	8 bytes	File modified time
0x10	8 bytes	$MFT modified time
0x18	8 bytes	Last access time
0x20	4 bytes	File type flags
0x24	4 bytes	Maximum number of versions
0x28	4 bytes	Version number
0x2c	4 bytes	Class ID
0x30	4 bytes	Owner ID (version 3.0 and greater)
0x34	4 bytes	Security ID (version 3.0 and greater)
0x38	4 bytes	Quota charged (version 3.0 and greater)
0x40	8 bytes	Update sequence number (version 3.0 and greater)

Filename Attribute   The filename attribute contains the MFT record number and the sequence number for the file or directory's parent directory. See Section 5.3.2.3 on "Orphan Files" for an example of how these work to prevent data corruption in directories.

A copy of the four NTFS file timestamps is maintained in the filename attribute. These are not accessible by the Windows API and are not as easily modified by an attacker or normal Windows processes. *If the attacker is suspected of manipulating file dates and time, this attribute's timestamps should be examined.* See Lee (2010) for operations and how they affect timestamps.

The filename is also maintained in the filename attribute in Unicode characters, as shown in Table 5.16.

Data Attribute   The data attribute content contains the data for the file (e.g., the picture, the Word document, or the PDF). There are therefore no NTFS structures to define. The attribute is used simply to point to the file's content. The data attribute is required if the MFT record is associated with a file. If the data attribute is resident, that data will exist in the MFT record itself. If the data attribute contains nonresident data, that MFT record will contain pointers – or runlists – to the location of the data on the file system.

Index Root   The index root attribute, as shown in Table 5.17, is required if the MFT record is associated with a directory. The attribute must be resident. An MFT record for a directory contains attributes for files or subdirectories in the content of the index root attribute. The attribute type is tracked in the index root attribute and is, in practice and observation, the filename attribute for the associated record. *For forensic examiners, this can be another source of a file's four Microsoft timestamps.* See the "Filename Attribute" subsection above.

Table 5.16 Filename attributes.

Offset	Length	Data
0x00	6 bytes	$MFT record number of the parent directory
0x06	2 bytes	Sequence number of the parent directory
0x08	8 bytes	File creation time
0x10	8 bytes	File modification time
0x18	8 bytes	$MFT modification time
0x20	8 bytes	Last access time
0x28	8 bytes	Allocated size of the index (if the record is an index)
0x30	8 bytes	Actual size of the index (if the record is an index)
0x38	4 bytes	File type flags
0x3c	4 bytes	Reparse value
0x40	1 byte	File name length in Unicode characters
0x41	1 byte	File name type
0x42	Varies	File name

The attributes are tracked in nodes and are sorted in a B-tree, as shown in Table 5.18. The full functionality of this structure is beyond the scope of this book. Refer to Carrier (2010) for more information on the index attributes.

Index Allocation Attribute The index allocation attribute, as shown in Table 5.19, is required when the content of a directory becomes too large to be contained as resident data in the index root attribute. The content of the attribute is a header that points to an index node. This content is normally seen as a named data stream: $I30. Some tools such as FTK Imager[9] will display the $I30 records to the examiner in the associated directory for offline examination.

Table 5.17 Index root attributes.

Offset	Size	Data
0x00	4 bytes	Type of attribute stored in the index
0x04	4 bytes	Collation sorting rule
0x08	4 bytes	Size of each index record in bytes
0x0c	1 byte	Size of each index record in clusters
0x0d	3 bytes	Unused
0x10	Varies	Node header

---

9 www.accessdata.com.

Table 5.18 INDX nodes.

Offset	Size	Data
0x00	4 bytes	Offset to the index entry list
0x04	4 bytes	Offset to the end of the used portion of the entry list
0x08	4 bytes	Offset to the end of the allocated index entry list buffer
0x0c	4 bytes	Flags [0x00 = no children; 0x01 = child(ren) present]

Table 5.19 Index allocation attributes.

Offset	Size	Data
0x00	8 bytes	$MFT record number of the entry
0x08	2 bytes	Length of this entry
0x0a	2 bytes	Length of the file name attribute of the entry
0x0c	2 bytes	Flags (0x01 = child node exists; 0x02 = last entry in list)
0x10	Varies	File name attribute of the entry
*	8 bytes	The VCN of the child node in the index allocation attribute (if it exists) will be listed in the last 8 bytes of the entry.

Named and Unnamed Streams Attribute content can be contained in named and unnamed streams. Most attributes, such as the data attribute, will read the data from the unnamed stream unless the stream is specifically called. This can allow an attacker to hide malware in a named stream [also known as an *alternate data stream* (ADS)] or allow a suspect to hide data from casual view.

Windows Vista and later do not allow for execution of PE (Windows binaries) from an ADS directly. Prior to Vista, the author has observed attackers hiding executable malware in an ADS in system-protected areas. An attacker storing malware in C:\Windows\System32 as an ADS was a simple way to prevent antivirus solutions (AVs) from removing the virus as well – System32 is a heavily protected directory, and the AV was unable to quarantine the folder.

Figure 5.14 shows a simple text file named *A.txt*; the file content was the string "File content from A.txt." After the creation of the file, an ADS was embedded in the file. The ADS was named *secret.txt* and contained the content "File content from B.txt." These are examples of both data streams being resident in the $MFT.

5.3.2.2 INDX (Index)

As mentioned in this chapter, directory contents in NTFS are defined in the named data stream $I30. These INDX records can be sources of evidence even if the directory has been deleted. NTFS does not immediately overwrite content, so if a directory has been deleted, the INDX records (content of an index attribute) can still be located on disk. The index always starts with *INDX*, and records that have not been overwritten can be carved with tools – or even viewed with a hex editor.

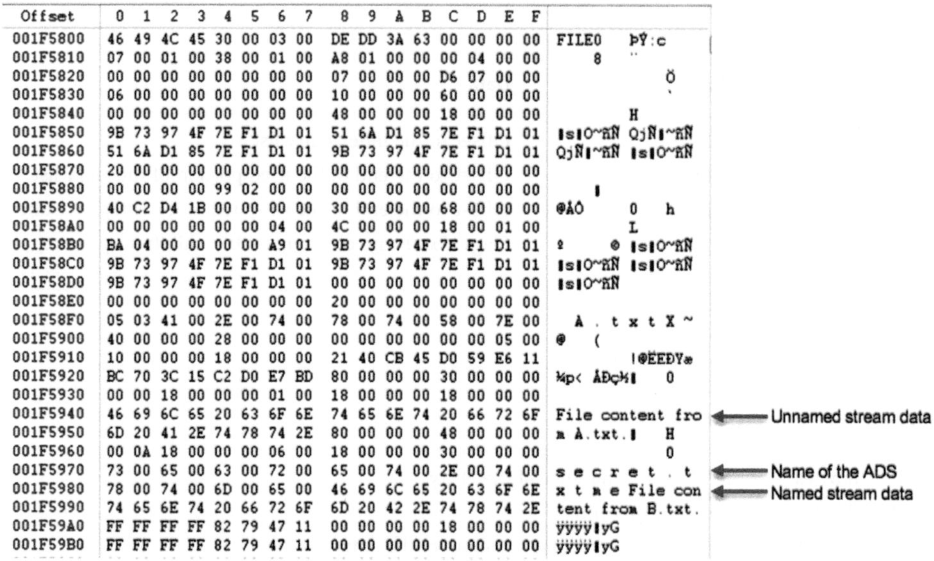

```
Offset     0  1  2  3  4  5  6  7   8  9  A  B  C  D  E  F
001F5800  46 49 4C 45 30 00 03 00  DE DD 3A 63 00 00 00 00  FILE0   ÞÝ:c
001F5810  07 00 01 00 38 00 01 00  A8 01 00 00 00 04 00 00      8   ¨
001F5820  00 00 00 00 00 00 00 00  07 00 00 00 D6 07 00 00              Ö
001F5830  06 00 00 00 00 00 00 00  10 00 00 00 60 00 00 00              `
001F5840  00 00 00 00 00 00 00 00  48 00 00 00 18 00 00 00          H
001F5850  9B 73 97 4F 7E F1 D1 01  51 6A D1 85 7E F1 D1 01  ▮s▮O~ñÑ Qj Ñ▮~ñÑ
001F5860  51 6A D1 85 7E F1 D1 01  9B 73 97 4F 7E F1 D1 01  QjÑ▮~ñÑ ▮s▮O~ñÑ
001F5870  20 00 00 00 00 00 00 00  00 00 00 00 00 00 00 00
001F5880  00 00 00 00 99 02 00 00  00 00 00 00 00 00 00 00      ▮
001F5890  40 C2 D4 1B 00 00 00 00  30 00 00 00 68 00 00 00  @ÂÔ     0   h
001F58A0  00 00 00 00 00 00 04 00  4C 00 00 00 18 00 01 00          L
001F58B0  BA 04 00 00 00 00 A9 01  9B 73 97 4F 7E F1 D1 01  º     © ▮s▮O~ñÑ
001F58C0  9B 73 97 4F 7E F1 D1 01  9B 73 97 4F 7E F1 D1 01  ▮s▮O~ñÑ ▮s▮O~ñÑ
001F58D0  9B 73 97 4F 7E F1 D1 01  00 00 00 00 00 00 00 00  ▮s▮O~ñÑ
001F58E0  00 00 00 00 00 00 00 00  20 00 00 00 00 00 00 00
001F58F0  05 03 41 00 2E 00 74 00  78 00 74 00 58 00 7E 00    A . t x t X ~
001F5900  40 00 00 00 28 00 00 00  00 00 00 00 00 00 05 00  @   (
001F5910  10 00 00 00 18 00 00 00  21 40 CB 45 D0 59 E6 11          !@ËEÐYæ
001F5920  BC 70 3C 15 C2 D0 E7 BD  80 00 00 00 30 00 00 00  ¼p< ÂÐç½▮    0
001F5930  00 00 18 00 00 00 01 00  18 00 00 00 18 00 00 00
001F5940  46 69 6C 65 20 63 6F 6E  74 65 6E 74 20 66 72 6F  File content fro
001F5950  6D 20 41 2E 74 78 74 2E  80 00 00 00 48 00 00 00  m A.txt.▮   H
001F5960  00 0A 18 00 00 00 06 00  18 00 00 00 30 00 00 00              0
001F5970  73 00 65 00 63 00 72 00  65 00 74 00 2E 00 74 00  s e c r e t . t
001F5980  78 00 74 00 6D 00 65 00  46 69 6C 65 20 63 6F 6E  x t m e File con
001F5990  74 65 6E 74 20 66 72 6F  6D 20 42 2E 74 78 74 2E  tent from B.txt.
001F59A0  FF FF FF FF 82 79 47 11  00 00 00 00 18 00 00 00  ÿÿÿÿ▮yG
001F59B0  FF FF FF FF 82 79 47 11  00 00 00 00 00 00 00 00  ÿÿÿÿ▮yG
```

Unnamed stream data
Name of the ADS
Named stream data

Figure 5.14 Example of an alternate data stream.

INDX records contain filename attributes for associated files, as shown in Table 5.20. These, in turn, contain filenames, parent directory MFT references, and file sizes. See Hamm and Ballenthin (2012) for more in-depth examination of INDX records.

5.3.2.3 Orphan Files

Files whose parent directory has been deleted and whose MFT record is overwritten are known as *orphan files* or *lost files* (see Definition 5.7). The MFT record for a file in such a state therefore has no parent. To mitigate file system corruption by placing deleted files in the wrong directory, the MFT matches the parent directory MFT references with the data stored in the file's MFT record. Many forensic tools place these files in a virtual folder so that the examiner still maintains access – regardless of whether the file's content has been overwritten or not.

Table 5.20 NTFS INDX record content.

Offset	Size	Data
0x00	4 bytes	Signature (INDX)
0x04	2 bytes	Offset to fixup array
0x06	2 bytes	Number of entries in the fixup array
0x08	8 bytes	$LogFile sequence number (LSN)
0x10	8 bytes	The VCN of this child record
0x20	Varies	Node header

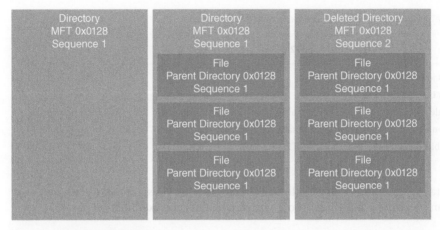

Figure 5.15 Orphan file, part 1.

Definition 5.7: Orphan File

A file whose parent directory has been deleted and whose MFT record is overwritten is known as an *orphan file* or *lost file*.

Figure 5.15 shows a directory with the record number 0x0128 being created. When the directory was created, the sequence number was set to "1." Files were then added and knew they belonged to the parent directory with the MFR record number of 0x0128 and the sequence number of "1." The directory was then deleted – and so were all the files in the directory.

When the MFT record 0x0128 was reused for a new directory (or file), the sequence number of the record was not incremented, but remained at "2." Therefore, the files that used to belong to the directory for record 0x0128 cannot be placed back into the new directory, as shown in Figure 5.16. If the files' records were not likewise overwritten, the

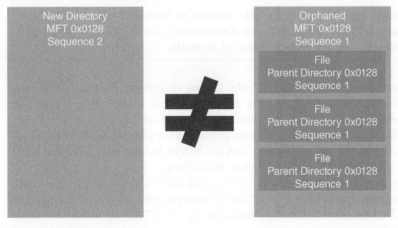

Figure 5.16 Orphan file, part 2.

Table 5.21 Significant feature differences in EXT file systems.

	EXT2	EXT3	EXT4
Supports journaling	No	Yes	Yes
Supports born (created time)	No	No	Yes
Time scale	Seconds	Seconds	Nanoseconds
Maximum date	January 18, 2038	January 18, 2038	April 25, 2514
Compatibility	EXT2	EXT2	EXT2 and EXT3

metadata for the files is recoverable and the file data may also be recovered. Forensic tools can therefore place them into a virtual container for examination.

5.3.2.4 EXT2/3/4 (Second, Third, and Fourth Extended Filesystems)

The EXT (extended) file system is the most common file system supported natively by Linux distributions. Linux is very flexible, however, so it can support many other file systems and can even boot to several different file systems such as XFS (X file system). The EXT file system has seen three major versions in commercial use: revisions 2, 3, and 4. Table 5.21 lists some of the feature differences between the EXT file systems that are significant for forensic examiners.

An inode (index node) is used in EXT file systems to track metadata for files and directories (see Definition 5.8). The metadata in an inode are: the file modified time-stamp, last accessed timestamp, inode changed timestamp, file deleted timestamp (in EXT3 and EXT4), file created timestamp (in EXT4 only), file size, user permissions and ownership, location of the direct blocks that contain the file data, and location of indirect blocks. Indirect blocks contain pointers to blocks that point data. There can be double indirect blocks or even triple indirect blocks if a large number of blocks is allocated to the file's data storage.

Definition 5.8: Inode

An *inode* (index node) is used in EXT file systems to track metadata for files and directories. Some tools refer to an MFT record as an inode as well, since the purpose of the MFT record is roughly equivalent to that of an inode.

Data for a file or directory is stored in blocks. During file system creation, the user can specify block size (1, 2, 4, or 8 KB), but the default block size is 1 KB (1024 bytes). The block is the smallest addressable allocation unit on an EXT file system. Blocks are organized into block groups. Each block group contains a copy of the superblock, a block bitmap, an inode bitmap, an inode table, and the blocks themselves. The superblock contains boot code and is backed up in every blockgroup.

Directory entries in EXT file systems contain the file name length, the file name itself, and the inode number of the file. In EXT2, the directory entries are sequential, while in EXT3 and EXT4, directory entries are managed by an HTree algorithm for faster searching capabilities.

5.3.2.4.1 *Deleted Files*

EXT2 files can, for example, be recovered by using the foremost or debugfs programs, and by searching for deleted files in the inode tables. EXT2 files do not zero out block pointers when a file is deleted.

EXT3 and EXT4 file systems zero out the direct block pointers in an inode when a file is deleted. EXT3 and EXT4 files may be possible to recover by using ext3grep and the EXT3 or EXT4 file system journal. Traditional carving techniques can also be employed, but this can be difficult at best, in part due to the block group descriptors' presence in the data area of the file system.

5.3.2.4.2 *Lost Files*

Inodes do not maintain a copy of a file's name or directory. If the file system becomes corrupt and a directory entry is deleted, but not the associated inode, the file still may be recoverable. During a FSCK (file system check) process, inodes may be recovered that no longer have an associated file name and directory name. In this case, the file system will place these into the *lost+found directory* with the inode number as the file name. This is similar to the NTFS orphan files operation. A lost+found directory is in the "/" directory of each volume.

5.3.2.4.3 *Journaling*

EXT3 and EXT4 are both journaling file systems. A file system that supports journaling acts much like database transaction fault tolerance with data integrity. It functions to store data in a journal until an act – such as writing a file – is completed. There are three levels of journaling in EXT file systems:

- *Writeback:* Only caches metadata in the journal. However, file data can be written to disk prior to journaling, making this the least reliable form of journaling.
- *Ordered:* Only caches metadata in the journal; however, the file data is not marked as committed to the disk until the data write process is completed.
- *Journaled:* Both metadata and data are cached in the journal until the write-to-disk process is complete. This ensures data integrity in the event of a failure, but it can impact performance due to the data being written twice.

Forensic examination of a system can be affected by journaling. If the system was set to full journaling, file data that no longer exists on the file system may be recovered from the journal. In the other two levels, metadata – such as a file name and file modified time – may be evidentiary even though the content was not recovered. Additionally, journaled file systems may try to roll back changes if the examiner tries to mount the file system. However, data can also appear incomplete or incorrect if the journal is not restored.

5.3.2.5 Operating System Artifacts

An OS is the interface between the user of a system and its hardware and software (Definition 5.9). OS artifacts are approached here as being native artifacts to the OS. For an introduction to analysis, two OSs are described here: Windows and Linux.[10] Common artifacts examined during an analysis are described from an investigation standpoint. This book, for example, does not intend to describe an engineering or programing level

---

10 Mac OSX artifacts of commonly examined forensic significance will be described in future editions.

of the Windows Registry, but knowledge of the Windows Registry and how it relates to an analysis is essential for even an entry-level examiner.

Definition 5.9: Operating System
A system that provides an interface between hardware, software, and a user. An OS is largely independent of a file system but may only support a limited number of file systems.

The OSs examined here can only be installed on Intel-based processors, and therefore memory operations are Little-Endian. Motorola-based OSs are Big-Endian and include OSs such as SunOS and BSD (Berkeley Software Distribution).

Various functions of an OS are designed to enhance the user experience. These operations typically leave behind artifacts to indicate what a user accessed, installed, typed, and even deleted. Again, this is not a comprehensive attempt to describe all forensic artifacts that an analyst should be aware of. This is a starting point for examining Windows OS artifacts and how they can tell a part of the story of what happened, and when, on a system.

Finally, many artifacts in an investigation may be add-on applications and do not vary across applications.

5.3.2.5.1 Windows

At the time this was written, Microsoft Windows had over 90% of the market share of desktop OSs as identified on NetMarketShare (2015). This includes the more than 10% that are still running Windows XP. The importance of understanding OS artifacts for the Windows OS cannot be overstated. Windows has versions from Windows 3.x through Windows 10. The various versions have introduced and changed the way artifacts interact with hardware, applications, store settings, preferences, and more. For a history of Windows, see Microsoft (2013).

Microsoft Windows is the intellectual property of Microsoft and as such is a closed source software. The documentation provided by Microsoft is enhanced by researchers and practitioners reverse engineering Windows artifacts with their causes and effects as they relate to digital forensics. As Microsoft continues to enhance or develop new versions of the OS, this reverse engineering, experimentation, and discovery of artifacts will continue to be important to the computer forensics field.

Additional resources for Windows forensics include *Incident Response and Computer Forensics* (Luttgens *et al.*, 2014) and *The Art of Memory Forensics* (Hale-Ligh *et al.*, 2014).

Registry The Windows Registry contains software and hardware settings and user preferences: "The *registry* is a system-defined database in which applications and system components store and retrieve configuration data. The data stored in the registry varies according to the version of Microsoft Windows. Applications use the registry API to retrieve, modify, or delete registry data" (Microsoft, 2015).

It is a hierarchical structure that at its base level begins four hives:

- HKEY_LOCAL_MACHINE
- HKEY_CLASSES_ROOT

- HKEY_CURRENT_USER
- HKEY_USERS.

The registry is loaded into memory during the OS boot process. The HARDWARE hive is only loaded while the system is running and is not a hive that can be examined if the system is shut down or an image of the volume is examined.

Files that store data for the registry that are most interesting for a digital forensic examiner are:

- NTUSER.DAT
- USERCLASS.DATA
- Software
- System
- SAM

The registry stores information in files in a proprietary database format. Each registry file begins with the header *regf*, and each entry starts with a header *hbin*. The hbin entries can be unallocated (or deleted) and recovered manually or with carving tools.

The following subsections describe specific information that can be derived from the files used to maintain the Windows Registry. For additional keys and techniques, see Carvey (2016).

NTUSER.DAT   The NTUSER.DAT file contains information specific to a user, including settings, most recently used (MRU) keys, startup scripts or applications, preferences, and more. Each user with a local profile on a system has an NTUSER.DAT file. The file is located by default in C:\Users\{profile_name}\for Windows Vista and later, and C:\Documents and Settings\{profile_name}.

Data contained in the NTUSER.DAT can indicate files the user accessed, URLs typed into a browser or Explorer bar, commands the user initiated, software the user installed, and file shares the user mapped.

USERCLASS.DAT   The USERCLASS.DAT file was added in Windows 7. It is located by default in C:\Users\{profile_name}\AppData\Local\Microsoft\Windows\. This file contains some information previously stored in the NTUSER.DAT. Specifically, the *Shell-Bag* information for a user profile is now stored here. ShellBags are registry artifacts that store user preferences for directories such as window size, sorting order, and placement on the screen. Of interest for the digital forensic examiner is that these artifacts can be used to show that a user account accessed and opened specific directories on a system. See also Tilbury (2011).

SOFTWARE   The software file exists on disk at %systemroot%\Windows\system32\config. The software file contains information on installed software, including the Windows OS and Microsoft applications. Any application can store configuration data in the software key.

With the addition of 64-bit OSs, Microsoft created a method to allow compatibility with 32-bit applications. These separate entries exist in the software key under HKey\LocalMachine\Software\WOW6432Node.

SYSTEM The system file exists on disk at %systemroot%\Windows\system32\config. When a system is running, a *current control set* is loaded into the software hive. The key itself contains two or more *control sets* – the last known good and the current control sets – in the event the registry becomes corrupted. If examining a dead image, both (or more) control sets should be looked at with the understanding that the current control set was in use the last time the system was booted.

SAM The SAM (security accounts manager) file exists on disk at %systemroot% \Windows\system32\config. This file contains account information for the local system. It includes local users, the user's encrypted password, and the location of the user's registry hive. Note that domain accounts will be stored in the active directory, and may not be stored locally in the SAM file.[11]

Prefetch The Prefetch folder is in the path C:\Windows\Prefetch. The files contain a .PF extension. The file name is represented as the name of an executable file followed by a hash of the original path. The contents of the Prefetch file include the date the executable was last run, the number of times an executable was run, the original path of the executable, and a list of dynamic link files required to run the executable.

For server versions of the Windows OS, the only file in Prefetch will be NTOSBOOT-*xxxxxxxx*.pf. This file will contain the full path of all DLLs, EXEs, and other files that are loaded at boot.

The analyst should examine the C:\Windows\Prefetch folder for entries. Ensure that the dates for the execution of suspicious files are checked. Ensure that common Windows binaries are being executed from the correct directories (rundll32, svchost, etc.). Also, consider carving for Prefetch entries.

For servers, the one Prefetch file (NTOSBOOT-*xxxxxxxx*.pf) will contain hundreds or even thousands of entries. It can be searched for malicious file names.

5.3.2.5.2 Volume Shadow Service (VSS)
The VSS, also called volume shadow copy, is a hybrid OS-level and file system–level data redundancy system. VSS tracks changes to user and system files and can contain previous versions of files and directories, including deleted data and files.

Example 5.9: Volume Shadow Service

The volume shadow service (VSS) maintains backup files. An examiner may be able to locate previous versions of files and re-create them from the various snapshots stored on a Windows system. This can be a valuable source of evidence even if a user deleted, wiped, or otherwise cleaned up files in an attempt to cover their tracks.

Additionally, don't consider the files as just a source of investigating previous files; also consider the fact that attackers have been observed to access VSS backups to extract system-protected files. Microsoft Active Directory servers maintain credential hashes for

---

11 If the user profiles are domain accounts only, the list of logins and associated security identifiers (SIDs) can be found in HKey_Local_Machine\SOFTWARE\Microsoft\Windows NT\CurrentVersion\ProfileList.

all domain users in the %systemroot%/NTDS/NTDS.dit databased file. This file is heavily protected by the system. Attackers can use a technique to leverage VSS to enable access to a backup of NTDS.dit, and thereby gain all credential hashes for the domain users in an environment.

5.3.2.5.3 Recycle Bin

The Windows Recycle Bin varies in name based on the OS version. Regardless of the name, the path is in the root of the volume. Each user that has logged into the system and accessed the volume will have a Recycle Bin subfolder with their security identifier (SID). The files the user sent to the Recycle Bin will be stored in their personal subfolder. Analysts have observed that attackers will frequently leave tools and utilities in the root of the recycle bin (e.g., C:\Recycler\ or C:\$Recycle.bin\).

5.3.2.5.4 Event Logs

The event logs AppData.evt, SecEvent.evt, and SysEvent.evt (or Application.evtx, Security.evtx, and System.evtx in Windows 7/Server 2008) contain logged information about the system. 540 and 528 events in SecEvent.evt and 4624 in Security.evtx record interactive logins. Application data can contain information including antivirus information and malicious services that have been launched. Table 5.22 lists the structure of Windows events in the EVT format.

Windows Vista and later introduced several new event log files that are focused on specific activities. The file format was changed from EVT to an XML-based EVTX. Some logs that require closer inspection and activation include:

- Scheduled Tasks logs,
- Powershell logs, and
- RDP logs.

5.3.2.5.5 Memory

Windows memory artifacts include the random-access memory (RAM) and a Windows page file. Windows uses a virtualized form of memory. The page file {system root}/pagefile.sys, by default, swaps memory to and from processes that are running in the background or foreground. Because the Windows virtual memory management is not completely understood by forensic tools, it's difficult to extract a running executable in memory in the same form it may have been stored on disk.

Forensically interesting artifacts that can be found in memory include:

- running processes,
- Windows event log records,
- plain-text passwords for various applications,
- Windows credentials, and
- strings.

Encrypted file systems can be difficult to decrypt without credentials. Fortunately, the Windows memory may maintain encrypted file system passwords in memory. Data collection should take into consideration the value of collecting memory before powering the system down or powering it off.

Table 5.22 Event log data.

Offset	Length	Field	Description
Header			
0x00	4 bytes	Length	The length of the entire entry
0x04	4 bytes	Reserved	The "LfLe" signature
0x08	4 bytes	RecordNumber	The event record number
0x0C	4 bytes	TimeGenerated	Time the entry was submitted
0x10	4 bytes	TimeWritten	Time the entry was written to the log
0x14	4 bytes	EventID	Packed bytes
0x18	2 bytes	EventType	Event type (error, failure, success, information, or warning)
0x1A	2 bytes	NumStrings	The number of strings in the log entry description
0x1C	2 bytes	EventCategory	Category of the event specific to the source
0x1E	2 bytes	ReservedFlags	Reserved
0x20	4 bytes	ClosingRecordNumber	Reserved
0x24	4 bytes	StringOffset	Offset to the description of the log entry
0x28	4 bytes	UserSidLength	The size of the UserSID (zero if no user identifier) ($E)
0x2C	4 bytes	UserSidOffset	(Variable length $B) Offset to the UserSID
0x30	4 bytes	DataLength	Size of the event specific data ($D)
0x34	4 bytes	DataOffset	(Variable length $C) Offset to the event specific data
Data			
	Variable string	SourceName	
	Variable string	Computername	
$B	$D	UserSid	
$A	Variable string	Strings	Pad with zeros to end the entry on a DWORD boundary
$C	$E	Data	
	CHAR	Pad	Pad with zeros to end the entry on a DWORD boundary
	4 bytes	Length	The length of the entire entry

Example 5.10: RAR Passwords

Attackers frequently use the Winlabs RAR compression application on the command line to encrypt and compress data they intend to steal. When the attacker encrypts the RAR file, the command switch "-hp" must be passed along with a password on the command line. Searching memory for the string "-hp" has resulted in successes in finding attackers' passwords in memory or on disk.

5.3.2.6 Linux Distributions

Linux is often referred to as an OS itself. The core of the system is the Linux kernel.[12] The original kernel was announced by Linus Torvalds in 1991 and was released under the GNU General Public License scheme, and it is actively developed by the open source community. Additional tools in a Linux distribution complete the OS by allowing interaction with the kernel, user interfaces, hardware, end-user applications, packaging systems, and more. Distributions[13] have been created by vendors, and support contracts for these distributions can be provided – thereby allowing the company to charge for the product.

Just like all things Linux, the distribution configurations can vary. This makes creating a single security tool, live response data collection, or even focused methodology document difficult at best. Some artifacts, however, are common among most distributions. Some standard places to investigate evidence on a Linux system are discussed in the remainder of this section.

5.3.2.6.1 /etc

The "/etc" directory on a Linux system generally contains system configuration. It can be thought of as roughly the equivalent of the Windows Registry. The files in the "/etc" directory, many in plain text, include information about the version of the distribution, services, runlevel, and time zone. The distribution will determine the exact structure of services, with RedHat and Debian having two different structures.

5.3.2.6.2 passwd/shadow

The passwd file contains a list of user and system accounts. Generally, the user hash will be marked with "X" if it is located in the shadow file. The shadow file contains the hash values of each user's password hash. The examiner can view the "passwd" and "shadow" files as text files. To search for accounts with login privileges, an analyst can use the "grep –v nologin" on the password file.

5.3.2.6.3 hosts

The hosts file maps hostnames to IP addresses and is given priority over DNS by default.

5.3.2.6.4 hostname

The hostname file keeps the host name of the current host.

5.3.2.6.5 *release* or *version*

Distributions such as Debian and RedHat styles of the OS keep their version in the/etc directory. This file can be found by doing an "ls *release*" or "ls *version*". It can then be viewed as plain text.

5.3.2.6.6 /var/log

The majority of log files on a Linux host will be contained in/var/log; on UNIX systems, some log files might be located in/var/adm. Also with the release of application packages

---

12 www.kernel.org.
13 See http://en.wikipedia.org/wiki/Comparison_of_Linux_distributions for a list of various Linux distributions.

such as XAMPP, the path to the related MySQL and Apache logs might be located in the/var/opt/lampp/subdirectories.

5.3.2.6.7 wtmp/utmp

The file wtmp is a binary log file that contains the historical login information for the system. The file utmp contains a list of currently logged-in users (more important when doing live response). The file can be viewed by using last –f {path to wtmp/utmp}, or a script that parses the data.

5.3.2.6.8 secure

Secure (or sometimes auth.log, depending on the Linux distribution) is a plain-text file that normally includes SSH logins and "su" (commands issued by the super user) events. Default settings roll the log over weekly, and historical copies are kept for four weeks. The historical logs may be gzipped. This file is a plain-text file if not compressed.

5.3.2.6.9 messages

Messages (or sometimes syslog, depending on the Linux distribution) is a plain-text file that includes system messages, software messages, and events that are not found in other logs. Default settings roll the log over weekly, and historical copies are kept for four weeks. The historical logs may be gzipped. This file is a plain-text file if not compressed.

5.3.2.6.10 dmesg

The dmesg file is a copy of the daily login events followed by hardware messages. This can include the most recently assigned DCHP address for a host. It also can contain USB information that may be valuable when an analyst is trying to export data to a USB device.

5.3.2.6.11 audit

If the auditd service is enabled on a system, it will maintain process accounting. These files can be read as plain text or can be processed using the "aureport –if {audit.log}" option (if the auditd package is installed on the analysis system).

5.3.2.6.12 Shell History

The shell history of a user is kept in their home directory. It is a hidden file in Linux and is prefaced with a dot (.). The version of shell determines the file name of the history file: BASH is stored in .bash_history or ksh, and zshell or cshell are typically stored in .history, for example. The most common, .bash_history, does not contain a timestamp, while other shells such as zshell maintain UNIX timestamps for every command. Shell histories do not contain a timestamp by default, but this can be enabled at the user level or globally. This file is a plain-text file if not compressed.

5.3.2.6.13 /home

Many applications maintain user settings in the user's home directory. They are frequently in a subdirectory that shows name beginning with a dot (.). Some application subdirectories are self-named, such as .mozilla (Mozilla Firefox). Some application subdirectory names are more obscure, such as .purple (pigeon chat client). The user's home directory is normally in the/home/{user name} path, but this can be specified during setup. To learn where a user's home directory is, the/etc/passwd file should be inspected.

5.3.2.6.14 /root

The directory/root is the default location of the root account's home directory. In early versions of UNIX, the "/" directory was used for root's home, but the number of files stored in "/" became unmanageable. Applications settings, the root account's history files, and configuration data are stored here in a manner similar to a user's/home directory.

5.3.2.6.15 Memory

Linux memory artifacts include the memory RAM and a Swap file. Linux also uses a virtualized form of memory. The swap file, called/*swap* by default, swaps memory to and from processes that are running in the background or foreground. Linux memory processes can be extracted from the virtualized/*proc* directory while the system is running.

Forensically interesting artifacts that can be found in memory include:

- running processes,
- plain-text passwords for various applications,
- log events, and
- strings.

LiME (Linux Memory Extractor) is a tool designed to retrieve memory from Linux systems. Prior to the kernel level 2.6, memory was unprotected and could be extracted using a "dd" command to copy/dev/mem to a file. Tools, such as Volatility, can be configured to analyze Linux memory images but must be fine-tuned based on kernel settings and configuration of the OS.

5.4 Analysis

Analysis methodology, to some extent, will depend upon the goals of the investigation. When investigating a system for malware, the focus is more likely to be on a timeline analysis, while investigating a system for proof of possession of contraband may focus on image collection and carving.

5.4.1 Analysis Tools

Tools for analysis may again depend upon the type of investigation being performed. Carving for contraband images will require different techniques than determining if malware was on a file system, for example.

There are several tools referred to as *digital forensic suites*. The idea of the suite is to attempt to perform as many analysis functions as possible inside the tool itself. These tools analyze file system data, Windows registry data, OS artifact data, and more. One of the drawbacks of having an all-in-one tool is that it becomes difficult to update the tool in a timely manner to address newly identified artifacts or techniques. To compensate for

Table 5.23   Examples of computer forensic suites.

Forensic Suite	Company
BlackLight	Blackbag Technologies
EnCase	Guidance Software
FTK	AccessData
Nuix Investigation and Response	Nuix
The SleuthKit and Autopsy	Basis Technology
X-Ways Forensics	X-Ways Software Technologies

this lack of flexibility, some of these tools allow users to script additional functionality. Table 5.23 lists an example of the available digital forensic suites.

Other tools used for analysis can be specialized to parse and analyze one artifact or a group of artifacts. These tools are often written to address a specific problem or newly identified technique. Table 5.24 lists examples of tools specialized on a single artifact or a group of artifacts.

5.4.2   Timeline Analysis

A common technique for analysis, particularly in an incident response investigation, is to perform a timeline analysis. In this technique, the analyst examines events chronologically. This can be used with any artifacts that maintain timestamps. There are tools, such as log2timeline, that are designed to poll various evidence sources and place the various timestamps and events in chronological order. This enables an analyst to identify artifacts touched by an attacker in a span of time. Figure 5.17 shows an example of a

Table 5.24   Examples of specialized computer forensic tools.

Analysis tool	Company	Artifacts analyzed
Event Log Explorer	FSPro Labs	Windows event logs
INDXParse.py	Willi Ballenthin	NTFS master file table
Net Analysis	Digital Detective	Internet browser history
Recon for Mac OSX	Sumuri LLC	Mac OSX forensics
RedLine	FireEye	Live response data collection
Registry Browser	Lock and Code	Windows Registry
SQLite Forensic Toolkit	Sanderson Forensics	SQLite database artifacts
Volatility	Volatile Systems	Memory
Windows Prefetch Parser	TZWorks	Windows Prefetch
dtSearch	dtSearch Corp.	Index searching
Scalpel	Golden G. Richard III	File carving
LiME	504ensics Labs	Linux memory acquisition

Time	Date/Time Description	Event	Notes
2015-07-01 03:26:33	Registry Key LM	HKEY_USERS\C._Documents_and_Settings_desktop.user_ntuser.dat\Software\Microsoft\Windows\ShellNoRoam\Bags\30\Shel	desktop.user user session indication
2015-07-01 03:29:23	Last Written	C:\Documents and Settings\desktop.user\Application Data	Likely last time user was logged in
2015-07-01 03:29:26	Created	C:\Windows\svch0st.exe	Backdoor
2015-07-01 16:12:22	Event Log	50	Error	The RDP protocol component X.224 detected an error in the protocol stream and has disconnected the client.	Backdoor
2015-07-01 20:45:59	Last Written	C:\Documents and Settings\desktop.user\Start Menu\Programs\Accessories\Command Prompt.lnk	Command prompt used
2015-07-01 20:46:12	URL History	http://fileserver.home.net	
2015-07-01 20:47:11	Registry Key LM	HKEY_USERS\C._Documents_and_Settings_desktop.user_ntuser.dat\Software\Microsoft\Windows\Shell\Bags\1\Desktop		desktop.user user session indication
2015-07-02 03:09:45	Event Log	50	Error	The RDP protocol component X.224 detected an error in the protocol stream and has disconnected the client.	RDP activity indicator
2015-07-02 05:15:35	Event Log	50	Error	The RDP protocol component X.224 detected an error in the protocol stream and has disconnected the client.	RDP activity indicator
2015-07-02 12:59:04	Event Log	50	Error	The RDP protocol component X.224 detected an error in the protocol stream and has disconnected the client.	RDP activity indicator

Figure 5.17 Example of a timeline for a single system.

timeline for a single system. The timestamp was derived from the artifact listed in the date/time description field. The event is the actual data the artifact created. The notes field comprises user interpretations of the data.

5.4.3 File Hashing

File hashing is the act of attempting to uniquely identify a file. Different hash algorithms can be used for this purpose, but some are weaker than others and are more likely to have collisions. Some common algorithms are provided in Table 5.25.

Once a file has been hashed, it can be compared with other file hashes. A common technique in incident response is to search for a file's hash value on Google and determine if the file's been seen before, and if so what its purpose is. Another technique used in contraband cases is to match a file's hash value with that of known contraband images to determine if the file had been seen before. In the case of trying to determine if a file is child sexually abusive material, identifying a file by hash value can help law enforcement prove the images are of a known victim.

File hashing can also be used to whitelist files based on their signature. The whitelisting process can result in data reduction in a case by removing legitimate files from a timeline. Doing so runs the risk of removing data from the analyst's view because attackers may use legitimate Windows files to perform their tasks.

5.4.4 Filtering

One of the challenges in computer forensics is an overabundance of sources of evidence. Modern OSs require thousands of interrelated files to function. The analyst, therefore, must differentiate between noise and the evidence that requires focus. Filtering can be used as a form of data reduction and is frequently an option in forensic tools, databases, and spreadsheets. An analyst can filter out all files by using hash values for whitelisting, for example.

Table 5.25 Common hashing algorithms.

Hash algorithm	Key space
CRC32	32 bits
MD5SUM	128 bits
SHA128	160 bits
SHA256	256 bits

It doesn't stop at hash values, however. An analyst can filter by date and time, file name, or file path. The options are limited only by the tool's functionality and the analyst. The challenges, as mentioned, are that an analyst can filter out attacker activity.

5.4.5 Data Carving

Data carving is the act of searching for particular strings or bytes within a structure. A hex editor or other data-viewing tools can be used to carve for data. The analyst determines a string or binary pattern to search for, then initiates a search across a device or structure for that string or pattern. The target can be of whatever scope is appropriate for the task, such as a file, slack space, unallocated space, a full volume, a memory image, or a swap file.

The technique can be used to carve for full files – such as recovering deleted JPG image files; or for records – such as recovering portions of a deleted Windows event log.

5.4.5.1 Files

Full files can be carved by searching for particular file headers or signatures. File carving is typically limited to carving for contiguous – nonfragmented – files in unallocated space or in other files. Techniques exist to carve data that is fragmented using fuzzy hashing (e.g., DigitalNinja, 2007) and are beyond the scope of this book.

5.4.5.2 Records

Carving for records involves searching for data where the full file may not be essential to recovering information (Hamm, 2012). Examples would be to carve for a weblog entry that contains full context in a single event: date and time, webpage visited, IP address accessing the page, browser ID, and so on. While a weblog is typically maintained in plain text, other data may be contained in binary blobs (such as Windows event logs) or a database format. The technique can be used to carve for either if the examiner is able to parse the information.

Example 5.11: Carved Records

Carving for records can be a very effective method of finding evidence when it's been deleted either intentionally or through normal system processes. As an example, the author received a server from law enforcement for examination. The system was seized because it was running a SpyEye server. When the system was analyzed, the Apache logs had been deleted and very little other logical evidence remained. The author carved for Apache Combined Log Format records and successfully recovered over one million entries. These entries were key in helping law enforcement determine the number of victims in the case because they contained information about all SpyEye infections from the infections checking into the server. Information retrieved included:

- IP address,
- system host name, and
- date and time of the check-in.

5.4.5.3 Index Search

An index search can be used if the examiner can preprocess data by indexing the image or structure. This can be used to perform quick searches – typically of plain-text data. Many forensic and e-discovery tools, such as dtSearch, contain the ability to preprocess and index forensic images. See dtSearch (2015) for more in-depth comparisons of indexed versus unindexed searching.

5.4.6 Memory Analysis

Memory analysis consists of examining a live memory image and a page – or swap – file. The way a virtual memory manager works is that it caches memory to disk when the information is not needed for immediate processing. This swapping function makes acquiring the memory alone not enough to rebuild processes that have been set to low priority in favor of high-priority processes running in the foreground.

Using a tool like Volatility can provide the analyst with, among other things, a way to determine:

- running processes,
- content of process memory,
- commands executed,
- strings (including passwords) cached in plain text,
- malware hooking or injecting other processes, and
- nonpersistent malware running in memory.

5.5 Summary

In this chapter, we've discussed computer forensics in three focused areas: disk and file system forensics, operating system forensics, and OS artifact forensics. The chapter is on a high level and provides only an overview of the artifacts discussed, so that the analyst or researcher has a baseline understanding of the concepts of computer forensics and can communicate effectively with others. Analysts and researchers are encouraged to go beyond the scope of this chapter, to engage in a more detailed analysis of the artifacts that have been discussed.

What becomes difficult is that, in a sea of artifacts and data points, looking for an anomaly in a largely user-customizable environment is met with large amounts of datasets and sources of evidence. It's not practical to look at every byte, sector, or file on a system and come to a conclusion of causality of every event in the digital environment. Instead, the analyst must frequently focus on artifacts that yield the most results and require the least amount of effort.

Additional file systems, artifacts, and OSs exist. Each has its own challenges and tool sets for examination, and each patch or change in these systems requires additional research to determine what effect they have on the ability to correctly read and interpret the data presented to the analysis by the toolkit they're using.

5.6 Exercises

1   Explain the difference between acquiring live data or acquiring a forensic image of a powered-down system. What are the complications and impacts of collecting live data versus creating a forensic image of a powered-down system's data?

2   Imagine an NTFS file system that was formatted with the cluster size specified as 8 Kb (8192 bytes). If a single-byte file was created, how many null bytes would be written to the sector? What would happen to the additional seven sectors in the cluster, and what might they contain?

3   Explain what a partition is and where hidden data could be placed intentionally by a technically apt individual.

4   On an NTFS file system, there can be more than one attribute of a given type. Explain theoretically where someone can hide data for an executable file in a legitimate system configuration file using the behavior of the file system attributes.

5   NTFS maintains at least two attributes with MACE (modified, accessed, created, and entry modified) times for every file and directory on the system. Explain the two attributes, and describe the differences in how the timestamps on these attributes can be updated.

6   Can deleted files be recovered from EXT file systems? Explain some of the challenges for recovery.

7   Explain why an attacker may use applications, such as WinRAR, to stage data for theft. What artifacts could an examiner look for in memory and virtual memory in order to determine if an attacker used WinRAR and derive the attacker's password?

8   A single date or time on a system can be unreliable given the many ways that they can be manipulated or even updated through the normal course of the operating system's functions. What type of analysis can be used to corroborate the accuracy of an event's timestamp? What other evidence might be identified from this technique?

6

Mobile and Embedded Forensics

Jens-Petter Sandvik

National Criminal Investigation Service (Kripos), Oslo, Norway and Norwegian University of Science and Technology (NTNU), Gjøvik, Norway

Over the past few decades, we have witnessed a revolution when it comes to computing power and the sheer number of computers around us. Intel cofounder Gordon E. Moore observed in 1965 that the number of transistors in an integrated circuit had doubled every year, and made the prediction that this would continue for at least ten years.[1] Later, in 1975, this forecast was modified to doubling every second year, and Intel executive David House rephrased it to say that with Moore's numbers, computing power would double every 18 months. Moore's law, as it became known, has withstood the test of time,[2] and today we can find computer systems everywhere from the biggest super-computers to the smallest medical implants.

Directly or indirectly, and knowingly or unknowingly, we often interact with electronic devices around us. Just think about all the electronic traces we leave behind in one day. We open doors with an electronic access card, and our phone records illuminance changes and counts the steps we take. We're in countless surveillance videos. The GPS in a car records where we are driving and tells us where to go, and some watches keep track of the atmospheric pressure. If one has diabetes, they may use insulin pens with a memory function that displays when previous insulin doses have been injected. All this information might potentially be used as evidence in an investigation.

Generally, more traces will be found on more powerful and personal devices. This means that much of this chapter will focus on mobile phones, since these devices tend to have an abundance of functionality, easy accessibility, and many options for communicating with others. Many embedded systems tend to have less functionality than a modern smartphone, but much of what is said about mobile phones is directly applicable to other embedded systems as well.

Another category of embedded systems is ICS (industrial control systems), the systems that control industrial processes. A part of ICS, which has gained popularity among both security professionals and malware creators, is Supervisory Control and

---

1 Moore actually observed that the "complexity for minimum component cost had increased at a rate of roughly a factor of two every year." "Complexity for minimum component cost" means the most cost-effective number of transistors in an integrated circuit.

2 The end of Moore's law has been predicted several times for at least two decades. Proponents have likewise predicted the continuation of Moore's law years into the future.

Digital Forensics, First Edition. Edited by André Årnes.
© 2018 John Wiley & Sons Ltd. Published 2018 by John Wiley & Sons Ltd.

Data Acquisition (SCADA). SCADA is the software part of ICS that acquires data from instruments and sends control signals to the equipment.

Another notable trend is found in the proliferation of small, low-power systems that are connected to the Internet through various network protocols. This Internet of Things (IoT) is still not fully developed or explored, but it is just a question of time before information gathered by these systems will be used as evidence in court.

6.1 Introduction

In this chapter, we lay out a foundation for mobile and embedded forensics, showing by examples which types of information can be found in different devices. In doing so, we aim to make the student able to understand the background for different methods, processes, and guidelines that exist within the field, and also to be able to select the best method for collecting and analyzing the results for a given device. As mobile phones and embedded systems often change, so do the specific methods, guidelines, and best practices for investigation. The best practices and state-of-the-art today soon enough become historical examples.

As described in Section 2.1, the stages in the forensic process are the same for both mobile and embedded systems as for computer systems. What make mobile and embedded devices special with regard to other technologies and sources of evidence are the challenges that come when dealing with the hardware. There are many different standards for interfacing with the devices, some of which are open and some proprietary. Because of this, we emphasize the collection and examination stages of the forensic process in this chapter.[3]

Our goal is to provide an overview. Yet, because it is so important to understand the technology we are using to understand the information we may glean, we also present some examples on specific methods and go in-depth on a few examples. However, a comprehensive introduction to the individual tools and methods is outside the scope of this chapter.

6.1.1 Embedded Systems and Consumer Electronics

Definition 6.1: Embedded System

An embedded system is a computer system that is designed to a specific set of functions within a set of constraints, which is smaller and more limited than a general-purpose computer system. The embedded system consists of software, hardware, and possibly mechanical parts.

An embedded system is a computer system, but one that is in general not easily reprogrammable to do other functions that a general-purpose computer system can do (Definition 6.1). The border between an embedded system and a general-purpose

---

3 Of course, the identification, analysis, and reporting stages should not be forgotten, even though they are not the focus.

computer system can be hard to draw, and we can find systems that fit into both categories.

Definition 6.2: Consumer Electronics
Consumer electronics refers to electronic technology meant for everyday use either at home or at the office. In this category, we find mobile phones, TV sets, hi-fi systems, watches, and computers.

A general-purpose computer is also in the category of consumer electronics (Definition 6.2), so we can't view consumer electronics as a true subset of embedded systems. We can, however, say that a big part of what is considered consumer electronics also falls into the embedded systems category. In this chapter, we will use the term *embedded system* as a general term for devices that fall into this category, and *mobile devices* or *mobile phones* where the text refers to this subset of embedded systems.

Figure 6.1 shows some examples of embedded systems and consumer electronics often used in daily life, and Figure 6.2 shows the internals of two systems from actual cases.

An embedded system usually consists of one or more central processing units (CPUs), random-access memory (RAM), and nonvolatile storage and peripheral devices, just like an ordinary computer system. The embedded systems usually have stricter constraints, including lower power consumption, smaller form factor, greater ruggedness, and real-time capabilities. The input and output are often more limited, such as buttons instead of

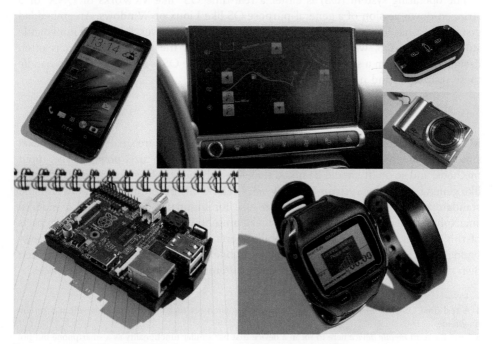

Figure 6.1 Embedded systems and consumer electronics from daily life.

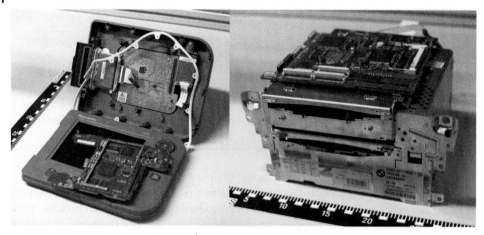

Figure 6.2 A map plotter for maritime use, and a car multimedia system with a GPS.

a keyboard, a small screen or even simple lights for status, and sensor inputs. An embedded system can also contain a system-on-a-chip (SoC). This is an electronic chip containing a CPU, memory, some nonvolatile memory for storing the boot code and operating system, and circuits for controlling peripherals.

Embedded systems often have many limitations, when it comes to both power consumption and sturdiness. The need for storage space is often limited, and we generally see flash memory instead of hard disk drives. Some systems have ROM for firmware and only volatile memory for dynamic data.

The operating system (OS) is either a real-time OS[4] like VxWorks or QNX, or a stripped-down version of a general-purpose OS like Linux or Windows. An embedded system often has limitations on processing power, electric power, RAM, and nonvolatile storage for the OS, which sets certain limitations for the OS. The system is often designed to perform a specific set of tasks; therefore, the OS is stripped down to handle these tasks well, and not necessarily much more.

6.1.2 Mobile Phones

Mobile phones are a special case of embedded systems. They are small, typically pocket sized, and they have some constraints with regard to screen size, power usage, input methods, and so on. It should be noted that smartphones are becoming more and more like general computer systems in many ways. The OS is becoming more powerful and standardized, and the interface easier to use for input and output. With a modern smartphone, we can browse web pages, make presentations, and write books. Even parts of this chapter were written on a mobile phone with a Bluetooth keyboard for easy typing. It is therefore natural to categorize mobile phones and mobile devices[5] in their own category, as the challenges are slightly different from other embedded devices.

---

4 A real-time OS (RTOS) is an operating system that guarantees that the OS responds within a certain timeframe.

5 I use the term *mobile device* here to mean a device that has similar functionality as a smartphone but not necessarily mobile phone functionality. Examples of this category are iPods, tablets, etc.

Table 6.1   The mobile network generations.

Generation	Description
1G (First-generation) networks	Analog networks, like NMT-450, and later NMT-900.
2G networks	The European GSM (Global System for Mobiles) or the CDMA (Code Division Multiple Access) used in USA. These were digital networks.
2G Transitional, or 2.5G	GPRS (General Packet Radio Service) and EDGE (Enhanced Data rates for GSM Evolution) networks. These technologies expanded the data transfer rates.
3G networks	UMTS (Universal Mobile Telecommunication Service) are the networks specified by 3GPP (3rd Generation Partnership Programme). The US equivalent is CDMA2000.
4G networks	LTE (Long-Term Evolution) is used both by traditional GSM and CDMA networks as the fourth-generation network.
5G networks	At the time of writing, this is still not standardized, but is planned to be ready in 2020.

Mobile phones are popular devices, and they are often considered even more personal than a computer. As mobile phones are used in most criminal cases, mobile phone forensics stands out as an important field and we put some extra focus on mobile phones in this chapter. The basic function of a mobile phone is the ability to connect to a mobile network, and make and receive calls. Later, functionality for sending messages and data has been standardized. Table 6.1 is a list showing the generations of mobile networks.

As discussed, a mobile phone is in many ways similar to a general-purpose computer. It can boot, can run an OS, contains both volatile and nonvolatile memory, and has a CPU for running the OS and applications. One of the differences is the system responsible for the radio transmissions, which runs on a second processor, called a *baseband processor*. This system contains its own RAM and firmware, so it runs separately from the rest of the OS on the phone.

There are several common OSs for mobile phones. Some are specially made for one particular type of phone; others are more general and can be found on several phones. We often see very simple OSs in the most low-cost phones, while more expensive phones tend to have more advanced OSs. Table 6.2 shows a few commonly found OSs on mobile phones.

On top of these OSs, there are applications that expand the functionality of the phones, such as the Messages app in Android that will send and receive SMS and MMS messages and the Camera app for taking pictures. Many of the OSs mentioned will let the user install new apps on the device in order to expand the functionality even further.

6.1.2.1   UICC (Formerly Known as a SIM Card)

Within the GSM (Global System for Mobiles) network, the subscriber information is in a module called the Subscriber Identity Module (SIM). This small smart card contains a microprocessor, some RAM, and some flash memory. It contains all the information about the subscriber that is needed in order to connect to the mobile network. In

Table 6.2 Operating systems (OSs) commonly found in mobile phones.

OS	Typical device
Various proprietary OSs	Inexpensive phones tend to have various proprietary OSs, like ISA for Nokia.
Android (Google)	Smartphones and other mobile devices from various manufacturers.
iOS (Apple)	Apple phones and tablets.
Windows Phone (Microsoft)	Smartphones from various manufacturers.
Blackberry 10/Blackberry OS	Phones from Blackberry Ltd.
Tizen (Samsung)	Samsung smart watches and some cameras, but also a few phones from Samsung.

addition, there is usually some storage space for saving call logs, contact lists, and SMS messages.

In the UMTS network, the SIM card is replaced by a Universal Integrated Circuit Card (UICC),[6] and this card runs SIM and USIM *applications* to connect to the network. The UICC looks identical to SIM cards, and is commonly just called a *SIM card*. This card can, in addition to the SIM and USIM applications, also contain other applications, such as authorization applications for banking services, and so on. The amount of storage on a SIM (or UICC) is limited, so phones often prefer to store call logs and text messages in their own internal memory instead of the SIM.

6.1.3 Telecommunication Networks

A mobile device connects to a mobile network, and necessarily leaves traces in the network infrastructure. First, we will take a closer look at a typical second-generation GSM network, then we will describe the third- and fourth-generation networks.

6.1.3.1 GSM Network

Figure 6.3 shows a simplified functional GSM network. It consists of three parts, namely the Radio Subsystem (RSS), the Network and Switching Subsystem (NSS), and the Operation Subsystem (OSS).

6.1.3.1.1 Radio Subsystem

The RSS (see Figure 6.3) consists of the parts of the system that are sending and receiving the radio signals. The Mobile Station (MS) is the mobile equipment like a mobile phone. This sends the signals to the Base Transceiver Station (BTS). One Base Station Controller (BSC) controls several BTSs. While the BTS handles the direct communication with the MS, the BSC allocates the frequency bands, handles the handover between the cells, and manages the BTS. One BSC with its BTSs are called a Base Station Subsystem (BSS).

---

6 The standard *ETSI TR 102 216* states, "UICC is neither an abbreviation nor an acronym," so we will only refer to it as UICC in the rest of the chapter.

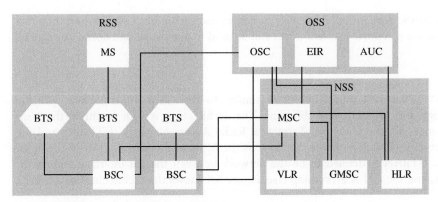

Figure 6.3 Structural architecture of a GSM network.

6.1.3.1.2 Network and Switching Subsystem

The NSS is where the setup and routing of calls and data happen. This subsystem consists of a Mobile Dervices Switching Center (MSC). The MSC controls several BSCs. The MSC will also talk to other MSCs and can hand over calls as an MS moves from a cell covered by one MSC to a cell covered by another. It also handles the setup of calls. Furthermore, a Gateway MSC (GMSC) connects the mobile network to an ISDN or PSTN network ("landline" telephone network).

The Home Location Register (HLR) stores the user information about a subscriber. This register contains the Mobile Subscriber ISDN number (MSISDN), the International Mobile Subscriber Identity (IMSI), the Location Area (LA) of the MS, the Visitor Location Register (VLR), and the MSC the MS is currently connected to. The location information is important in order to be able to route the calls to the MS.

The VLR is a register that keeps track of all MSs connected to the corresponding MSC. The VLR will contain a copy of the data from the HLR when an MS is connected to the corresponding MSC.

6.1.3.1.3 Operation Subsystem

The OSS takes care of the maintenance and operation of the network. This subsystem consists of an Operation and Maintenance Center (OMC), an Authentication Center (AuC), and an Equipment Identity Register (EIR).

The OMC takes care of high-level network management, such as administration of the network, user administration, billing information, security management, and logging.

The AuC works closely with the HLR in the NSS to authenticate users in the network. The AuC and the SIM are involved in the authentication and setting up of encryption of the radio interface. There are different algorithms involved. Algorithm 3 (A3) is used for authentication, A5 for encryption, and A8 for generating a cipher key. A3 and A8 are implemented in the SIM and AuC, while A5 is implemented in the MS and BTS.[7]

The EIR is a register of all International Mobile Equipment Identities (IMEIs). This register also contains a blacklist of reported stolen IMEIs, so these can be denied access

---

7 The A5 encryption only encrypts the data as it passes over the radio interface. From the BTS, the data continues unencrypted. The A5 algorithm has been shown to be cryptographically weak and can be broken with a limited amount of resources.

to the network. Not all mobile service providers use such a blacklist, so even though a mobile phone is reported stolen, it can still be used in a network that doesn't update its blacklist.

6.1.3.2 UMTS Networks

The UMTS network infrastructure is similar to the GSM infrastructure, but the technology and protocols are different. The architecture is split in three: the User Equipment (UE), the Universal Terrestrial Radio Access Network (UTRAN), and the Core Network (CN). The UE is the same as the MS and the SIM (USIM) in the GSM network, UTRAN is defined to be the network between the Uu interface and the Iu interface, and the CN is everything else. Figure 6.4 shows the architecture of a UMTS network.

The UE is connected via a Uu interface to a cell. This cell is managed by a Node B, which is connected to a Radio Network Controller (RNC). A system of one RNC, the connected Node Bs and the cells, are called a Radio Network System. The RNC talks to the CN through the Iu interface.

The UMTS CN has a mixed environment of packet switching (PS) and circuit switching (CS). Some of the systems are in the PS domain, some are in the CS domain, and some are in both domains.

6.1.3.3 Evolved Packet System (EPS)–Long-Term Evolution (LTE) Networks

In common speech, we often use the term *long-term evolution* for the 4th-generation mobile network. This is somewhat imprecise, as LTE covers only the radio access part of the network. LTE together with the System Architecture Evolution (SAE) form the EPS.

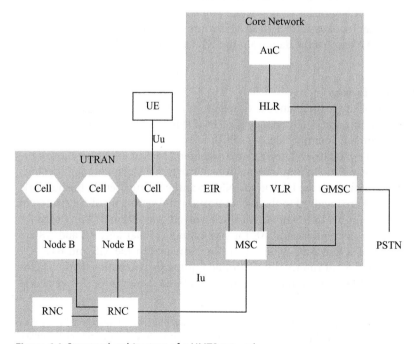

Figure 6.4 Structural architecture of a UMTS network.

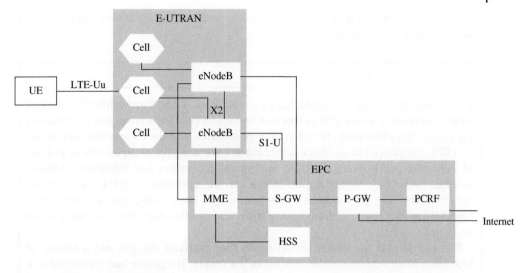

Figure 6.5 EPS structural architecture.

EPS is what most people refer to when they hear the term *LTE* or *4G*. As the name implies, this is not a complete redesign of the network architecture, but rather an evolution. The UTRAN element from UMTS is in LTE called Evolved UTRAN (E-UTRAN), and each cell is managed by an eNodeB (*evolved NodeB*). Figure 6.5 shows the parts of an EPS network, as described in this section.

In addition to the changes in the radio subsystem, there are also some changes to the core network, called Evolved Packet Core (EPC), which is a part of SAE. The Service Gateway (S-GW) is the gateway that handles all user data from the UE, and keeps statistics about the connection for billing. Lawful interception happens in this node. The Mobility Management Entity (MME) handles the signaling between the UE and EPC, and it is responsible for the security of signaling and user data. The Home Subscriber Server (HSS) contains subscription information and data about the whereabouts of the UE. The HSS might contain the UaC. The PDN Gateway (P-GW) is responsible for IP address allocation for the UE, and it handles Quality of Service demands. The Policy Control and Charging Rules Function (PCRF) handles policy control.

6.1.3.4 Evidence in the Mobile Network

With this overview of the GSM network in mind, which traces and evidence can be found in the network? The most common types of evidence found are call data records and data traffic logs. These are logs that show which calls have been made by or to a subscriber together with the duration, when SMS has been sent, and when and how much data has been sent and received. There is also information about the identity of the equipment that has been used together with a SIM card for connecting to the network.

Which BTS an MS has been connected to is also recorded, and can give valuable location data about where an MS has been, or where it is at the moment. The antenna of a BTS is often a directional sector antenna, where a sector is typically 120°. This means the data can contain information about which direction from the BTS a MS is located. We can also triangulate a device by using information about the signal strength between the MS and several base stations, or the time difference of the signals sent and received, if the information is available to us.

Example 6.1: Searching for a Mobile Phone

In February 2010, a girl was abducted by a man, bound, and thrown into the trunk of a car in Norway. She was able to free one hand, and called the emergency number to the police. The phone calls lasted in total 30 minutes, and the connection was traced to a BTS. The police set up check points around the area, checking all cars in and out of this area, and actively searched for the car the victim had described, without success. Based on the description of the car, the abductor, and the name of the person whom the girl suspected was behind the kidnapping, two suspects were found. After long interrogations, one of the suspects told where the dead body could be found.

The search area the police set up when they received the call was a couple of kilometers away from the actual location of the phone. The phone had connected to a BTS quite far away from the handset, and had not connected to any base stations closer to its location, even though several base stations had a better coverage where the phone was located. This shows that we have to be careful when looking at the coverage maps for the base stations, and keep in mind that the mobile equipment can connect to other base stations than the nearest ones.

6.1.4 Mobile Devices and Embedded Systems as Evidence

Data from mobile devices and embedded systems can be used as evidence just the same as data from computers. However, there is one major difference between evidence from an ordinary computer and from an embedded system: whereas the computer traditionally has a hard disk that stores the information with a standardized interface for low-level access, embedded systems tend to store information in flash memory with no direct, low-level access to the stored data.

This means that for evidence stored on a computer hard disk, there exist well-defined methods and best practices for acquiring and interpreting data, as discussed in Chapter 5. These methods and practices have been discussed and refined by a huge number of investigators, lawyers, and researchers, and are shown to be forensically sound as long as we follow the guidelines. For embedded systems, we do not have the luxury of these well-defined methods and practices. We need to be able to continuously assess the methods we use ourselves, and how we preserve evidence integrity and chain of custody throughout.

For a forensic investigator, this means that we have to know how the various methods we use can change the data, which data we can acquire with different methods, and also which data we won't be able to access with a particular method.

Two of the most important parts of the forensic process are to ensure the integrity of the evidence and the chain of custody. Not all the acquisition systems we use have built-in functionality for ensuring this, which means that we have to take certain steps to ensure the integrity ourselves. When acquiring data, we should make sure to calculate a digital fingerprint of the data, and to store the data and the fingerprint so it won't be deleted or modified in any way. The fingerprinting function is usually a cryptographic hash function (as discussed in Chapter 2), preferably SHA-2 or SHA-3.[8]

6.1.5 Malware and Security Considerations

No computer system can be guaranteed to be malware free. Smartphones and other embedded systems are no exception to this.

The malware SpyEye, described earlier in this book, also had a mobile component. This component is often called Spitmo, and it existed for Symbian, Blackberry, and Android. SpyEye was a malware that tried to perform bank transfers from the victim's account. Many banks have a two-factor authentication where an authentication number is sent as a SMS to a mobile phone. The functionality of the mobile component of SpyEye was to read the mobile Transaction Authentication Number (mTAN), as it was received from the bank, and to send it to a server so an unauthorized transfer could be done.[9] The installation of this component required somewhat cumbersome user interactions and downloading of an app from outside the official repositories, which was made to look like it was a necessary security update from the bank.[10]

We use point-of-sale (PoS) terminals whenever we pay for goods with a credit card. These systems can be exploited to gain access to payment card details. Modifications that have been seen for these systems range from physical modifications to malware infections. The physical modifications can be to add extra hardware inside the terminal to extract the credit card info together with a key logger for storing the typed PIN code. On the malware side, there exists a handful of malware designed to infect the PoS terminal and scan for payment card details in memory.

Not only financial services has been the target of malware. One of the most well-known malware campaigns directed toward industrial control systems is known as Stuxnet. This malware campaign targeted the centrifuges for enriching uranium, and would let them spin at excessive speeds while providing feedback that looked normal and concealed the actual speeds. Thus, the centrifuges would break, and the performance of the uranium enrichment facility decreased considerably. As most of this malware was found in Iran, the suspicion was that this specifically targeted the Iranian nuclear capabilities.

Hardware can also be infected with malware placed during the design or manufacturing process. Functionality that can be triggered during operations can be added to the hardware. A few possibilities to this functionality can be, for example, a kill switch that renders the hardware unusable at a crucial time, a slight modification to a random number generator (RNG) rendering a predictable output, or even functions that hide memory areas containing malware from accesses that look like a malware scan or forensic memory acquisition. Some research groups are looking at how to protect the

---

8 Even though the MD5 and SHA-1 algorithms have known weaknesses, they are still widely used. The reason for this is that the fingerprint is mainly protecting against undetected casual modifications or accidents. To protect against a targeted modification, we should rather use cryptographically strong digital signatures.

9 By unauthorized, we mean not authorized by the rightful owner or manager of the account.

10 More precisely, a certificate update.

design and manufacturing process against such attacks, and how to detect such threats after manufacture.

6.1.6 Ontologies for Mobile and Embedded Forensics

Definition 6.3: Ontology

A *conceptualization* is an abstract, simplified view of the world that we wish to represent for some purpose. An *ontology* is an explicit specification of such a conceptualization (Gruber, 1993).

Many have made overviews of the mobile and embedded forensics field, trying to find a good categorization for what we are doing and what we are examining. How we categorize the field depends on which insight we are trying to gain. A categorization made to help a first responder identify and prioritize digital evidence might look very different from the categorization made to help an advanced laboratory in identifying the embedded storage mediums and technologies used.

In this section, we will first establish one ontology (Definition 6.3) for mobile and embedded forensics that the authors find practical. After this, we will look at three other ontologies from the literature. The term *collection* is used for the phase in the forensic process, as described in Section 2.3, while the term *acquisition* is used for the methods applied as part of the collection phase.

6.1.6.1 An Acquisition Method Ontology

There are several ways of categorizing the assessments and methods we use. We therefore try to find a set of categories that will help our understanding of the collection process, and help us assess the risks and opportunities the methods hold.

We will define two views of the data collection process. The first view is the data view, where we describe the data in the system, including attributes of the information we want to collect. The other view is the method view, where we look at the method itself, and how it affects the system and the information we want to acquire. It is important to understand that both these views are a part of the collection process. The system view is in many ways the potential information we can get, while the method view is the realization of this potential. To select the best method, we should match the method with the information we want to collect.

6.1.6.1.1 Data View – Layers of Abstraction

If we start at the data view, we notice that the information exists at many of the levels of abstraction in the system we are investigating, as discussed in Section 1.3. Some information might be visible only at some of the abstraction layers, as the information is used at a specific level. We can, for example, think of a File Allocation Table that tells where each part of the file is located, but this information is not available if we look at the contents of the file. Some of the information will be easier to interpret at some of the layers, just like the contents of a file will be easier to interpret if we look at it from the top of the abstraction stack, instead of looking at each sector on a disk individually.

Note that encryption will make the information inaccessible on the lower layers of abstraction without the encryption key. We can gain access to the encrypted information, either by acquiring the data while, or where, it is unencrypted, or by decrypting the information after acquisition.

6.1.6.1.2 Data View – Trust

Another categorization that is useful within the data view, and closely connected with the layers of abstraction, is the trustworthiness of the system we collect the data from, or the reliability of the system. The correlation of the trustworthiness and the abstraction layers is easy to explain: the higher we are in the abstraction stack, the more of the underlying system we have to trust. This means that if we acquire at a physical level, the only part we can't control is the hardware of the acquired chip. If we do a logical acquisition, the running system can change the data before we are able to acquire it. An example of this is a root kit hiding a malicious process: to perform a logical acquisition, we have to trust the underlying system to give us all the data, but this trust is compromised. As the malware process is able to manipulate the data before we are able to read it, the acquired data can be misleading. Will this example of an acquisition give us all the information we need? Would the results be different if we could acquire the RAM directly without going through an infected OS?[11]

6.1.6.1.3 Data View – Volatility

The third aspect from the data view is the volatility of the data we want to collect. The order of volatility is defined in Section 2.3. The volatility is not only dependent on the storage medium, but also dependent on the necessity of the information to the system, and the allocation strategy of the system. Some information can be kept live in the system for the lifetime of the system, some might be kept while the system is running, and some might be cached just a moment. The discarded information might linger for a long time if memory (volatile or nonvolatile) doesn't get reallocated often, and might be quickly overwritten during aggressive reallocation strategies.

6.1.6.1.4 Method View – Layers of Abstraction

For the method view, the first and most notable category includes the abstraction layers we will acquire from. The scale is often defined as going from *physical acquisition*, where the data is read directly from the storage medium, to *logical acquisition*, where the data is read using application programming interface (APIs) on the running device, or even *manual acquisition*. There are many levels between the two; Coert Klaver calls the level right above physical acquisition "pseudo-physical acquisition" (Klaver, 2010).

6.1.6.1.5 Method View – Alterations

The next aspect of the method view identifies how much the method we use changes the system. There are two ways a system can be altered; physically and logically. We can also define a grading for the changes we do to a system. This list shows an example of a grading:

1) *"No alteration"*: This means that nothing will be changed. When we refer to "nothing," we also exclude miniscule changes that are hard to detect and won't have any implications for the interpretation of the evidence.

---

11 These were rhetorical questions; the correct answers are of course "not necessarily" and "probably," respectively.

2) *"Minor, detectable alteration"*: This includes changes to the system that make the method used for acquisition detectable after acquisition, either physically such as cleaning dirty connections or open seals, or logically such as entries in system logs and so on.

3) *"Alterations not affecting evidence data"*: Adding something, or changing the system, but without affecting traces. Physically this means to remove or change some parts of the system. Logically it might be to add software to the system, or change running software without changing user data.

4) *"Alterations affecting evidence data"*: This is to make changes such that user data or traces are changed. This doesn't necessarily make the evidence lose value, but we have to be careful when interpreting the traces and we probably have to show exactly how the traces have been changed. For example, metadata changes for a file when it is opened by the operating system.

5) *"Destructive alterations"*: This is where traces are destroyed. This approach should generally be avoided, but we might be in a position where acquiring one set of traces will destroy other traces.

6.1.6.1.6 Method View – Repeatability

Talking about changes to the system, it might be of interest to define a term *repeatability* of the acquisition method. This is to describe whether two acquisitions will render the exact same results. Two acquisitions of the flash memory of a running system will probably give different results, while a logical acquisition of a user's contact list can give the exact same results, even though the system has been running between the acquisitions.

A repeatable method does not imply that the data on the device is not changed. If we read the contact list from a phone using a high-level protocol, we are reading from a higher layer of abstraction, and the acquired information can be identical between two acquisitions. A physical acquisition of the device before and after the reading of the contact list will be different, as the alterations to the system happen on a lower layer of abstraction.

We can also look at the definition from experimental sciences, where a *repeatable* experiment can be done twice at the same lab and with the same lab setup with the same outcome, while a *reproducible* experiment can be done independently in another lab, with another lab setup, and give the same results.

6.1.6.1.7 Method View – Cost

The cost of a particular method is also a factor. The cost describes how much resources one needs in order to be able to do an acquisition, and it is not necessarily limited to monetary cost. A cost is better defined as a description of the resources needed to meet a set goal. We can split the cost into three periods of time, or stages: the first is the cost before the acquisition. This is the cost of the forensic readiness for this particular method, and is the topic of Chapter 4. The second period is the cost during the acquisition, which includes the resources that need to be available in order to use the method. This is an assessment that is especially important where the time is limited, for example if acquisition is done in an environment one can't control, we only have access to the device for a limited time, or the like. The third period is the cost of the resources one needs after the acquisition, which is the resources that will be used on examining the evidence and writing the reports. We can call these stages *forensic readiness, in-acquisition,* and *examination/reporting.* Other names for the first and last stages can be *pre-* and *post-acquisition,* to emphasize the focus on the acquisition methods.

The cost is the amount of resources we need to acquire, or use, in order to successfully utilize a method. The three types of resources are time, capital resources, and human resources.

Time is always a limited resource, and can be thought of as either clock time or person-hours. *Clock time* is the actual time something will take, as measured by the clock. *Person-hours* is how much time a task will take for one person to accomplish. If a task can be parallelized, more persons can do the task in a shorter amount of time. A task that doesn't need any human interaction can take quite an amount of clock time, but a minimal number of person-hours.

Capital resources is all the equipment we need. This is everything from the infra-structure to tools and software: all the physical "things" we need in order to successfully use a given method.

Human resources are the resources the persons doing the job possess. This includes knowledge, skills, number of persons, and so on. Different methods might require different skillsets and knowledge from the persons doing the acquisition and interpretation.

We can, of course, use the type of resources instead of the stages to assess the cost, or make a 3×3 cost matrix for the stages and types. This can work well for areas such as planning and administration of the resources for the laboratory.

6.1.6.1.8 Risks and Summary

When performing a forensic acquisition of a device, we seek to optimize the probability for acquiring all relevant traces that can be used as evidence. There is, however, a risk that the traces will be inaccessible or destroyed. We don't know in advance which traces we might find, and which will be most important, so we have to make qualified guesses for the data in the device.

The risk is determined in an assessment of the methods, together with the probability for the method to fail and the consequences. We don't need to do a quantitative risk analysis, as long as we have some thoughts about the methods and their corresponding failure probabilities and consequences. If we can acquire information with several methods, we should use the ones that are least destructive for the data we are interested in first.

Each of the acquisition methods we use can be categorized by assessing the informa-tion we can acquire by the particular method. We summarize the system view and the method view in Table 6.3.

When describing the methods in this chapter, we will only look at the method view. For the assessment, we give each of the categories a score from 1 to 5, putting it in a radar chart as shown in Figure 6.6.

- For the *abstraction layer,* the score 1 is as close to the raw data as we can get, while reading through the user interface or API on the device is 5.
- *Logical and physical alterations* follow the scale given earlier, with 1 as no alteration, and 5 as very destructive.
- *Repeatability* is scored as 5 if the results after two different acquisitions at different times are identical, while the device has been stored in accordance to the standard procedures, and 1 for very different results after two consecutive acquisitions. We can

Table 6.3   Overview of the system view and method view.

System view	Abstraction layer	At which level is the information we want most accessible?
	Trust/reliability	Can we trust the system at the various levels?
	Volatility	How volatile is the data at the various abstraction layers?
Method view	Abstraction layer	At which level can the method acquire data?
	Logical alterations	Which changes does the method inflict on the data?
	Physical alterations	Which changes does the method inflict on the physical device?
	Repeatability	Do two acquisitions give the exact same result?
	Cost; pre-, in-, and post-acquisition	What is the cost, and do we have available all resources we need?

say that 3 is a repeatable method, and 5 is a fully reproducible method, where *reproducible* means that the exact same result can be obtained by another independent lab on the same device. In the radar chart, we have marked this category with an asterisk ("*") to emphasize that a higher score is preferable, as opposed to alterations and cost.

- *Cost is a collective score*, where 1 is the least resources needed, while 5 is very resource demanding (*high cost*). We could have split the cost further into the individual resource types as described, but we only show one score for each of the stages for

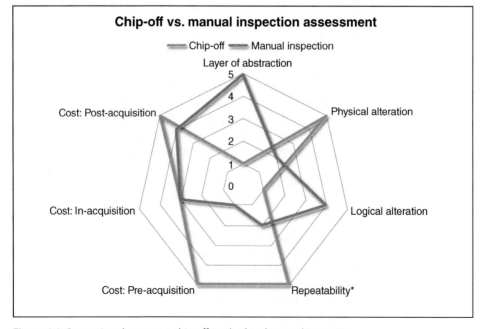

Figure 6.6 Comparison between a chip-off method and manual inspection.

simplicity. Note that different teams might weigh the cost of resource types differently, and therefore come up with different scores based on the same methods.

As there are many variables and conditions that can affect these categories, it is difficult to determine an objective score. Because this assessment model is a simplification, there will be uncertainties and probabilities one can't properly communicate through a simple score or radar chart. We should therefore use this as a tool to assess methods against each other and match them with the data from the data view, rather than use it as an objective measurement of how good each method is.

Furthermore, it is easy to think that the area of the radar chart correlates to how good or preferable a method is. This is not the case here, as for instance the abstraction layer doesn't say anything about how "good" the method is. The rationale behind the radar chart in this chapter is to give a visual cue of the differences between the methods based on the shape of the chart.

6.1.6.2 Technical Qualities

There are other ways to categorize the field, and the next three subsections will give an overview of other categorizations and models of mobile and embedded forensics.

One taxonomy[12] focuses on technical qualities. Harill and Mislan (2007) look at "small scale digital device forensics." Small-scale digital devices are understood as a subset of embedded systems where the form factor is smaller than that of an ordinary computer system. This ontology was made in order to identify small devices and the storage technology used, such that it would be easier to recognize at the scene of crime. The model they present categorizes the devices in four different categories:

1) Flash devices
2) Magnetic devices
3) Optical devices
4) PC extension devices.

The first three categories are based on the storage technology used, and the fourth, PC extension devices, is based on the functionality of the device. This latter category covers devices with processing power that are running some kind of firmware and are meant to plug into a PC, including mobile phones, gaming systems, GPS, and so on. An mp3 player in this model can fit into both PC extension devices, and flash devices or magnetic devices, depending on the technical storage solution.

6.1.6.3 Tools Used for Acquisition

Another way to categorize mobile and embedded forensics is to base the classification on the tools used for acquisition. Brothers (2008) has made a level hierarchy of the tools and techniques. The five levels described are:

1) Manual extraction
2) Logical extraction
3) Hex dumping/JTAG

---

12 A taxonomy is a categorization of the field.

4) Chip-off
5) Micro read.

With manual extraction, one reads the contents on the device manually by pushing buttons, writing down what is on the screen, taking photos, and so on. Logical extraction sends commands to the device and acquires the data sent from the device. Hex dumping/ JTAG uses debug interfaces or other methods to read raw data from the flash memory. Chip-off is done by removing the flash storage chip and reading this directly, and micro-read is the reading of the content of the individual gates on the silicon die itself. The further down the list one gets, the nearer they are to the raw data, and the costlier and more knowledge demanding an acquisition tends to become.

6.1.6.4 Data Acquisition Methods

Another taxonomy is described by Bommisety *et al*. (2014). They describe the data acquisition methods instead of tools or technologies. They split the main categorization into three categories:

1) Manual acquisition
2) Logical acquisition
3) Physical acquisition.

Physical acquisition here is defined as reading the contents of the flash memory chip directly, logical acquisition is to use the API for synchronizing the phone contents with a PC, and manual acquisition is to use the user interface for acquiring data.

6.2 Collection Phase

As described in Chapter 2, we can split the forensic process into multiple phases. In this chapter, we focus on the collection and examination phase, as these are the stages that are most significant to mobile and embedded forensics. The terms *acquisition* and *extraction* describe the methods used in the collection step of the forensic process.

There are several ways to acquire information from a device, dependent on which data one is interested in, the technical level of the laboratory, the availability of resources, and so on. Some of these methods might be described as destructive should the method permanently change the device or render it useless afterwards. We also have the choice between physical and logical acquisition, where logical acquisition uses ordinary interfaces in a live device in order to acquire data, while physical acquisition bypasses the control of the software running on the device.

As mentioned in the introduction, the acquisition itself can be a challenge when it comes to embedded systems. There are many different connection types, such as the communication protocols, the hardware, and the software running on the device. These variables change often, as new devices enter the market. Research on new methods of data acquisition is thus constantly in demand.

With all these methods for acquiring embedded devices, it also means that one often has more than one way to acquire the data. Investigators need to know about the strengths and weaknesses of the different available methods in order to ensure that they get the most valuable information from the process.

By the end of the section, you will have learned:

- the risks associated with the collection process step;
- to appraise different acquisition methods and assess their strengths and weaknesses;
- the difference between physical, logical, and pseudo-physical acquisitions; and
- the technology used in embedded devices.

6.2.1 Special Considerations for Embedded Systems and Mobile Devices

The forensic process as described in Chapter 2 is the basis for mobile and embedded forensics. One must use the most forensically sound method to collect the data from the device being examined, but in order to find the most forensically sound method, it is also necessary to know a few things about the system.

If it is a device or system that hasn't been examined before, one needs to find out how it works, how to get data out of it, and the risks faced when handling the device. This is best done by familiarizing oneself with an identical device. One can read the documentation of the device in order to get an impression of the functionality and interface. Keep in mind that the documentation doesn't necessarily cover the actual functionality of the device, as discussed in Example 6.2.

Example 6.2: Ring Buffers in Video Surveillance Equipment

One example of misleading product documentation was in a case where our lab acquired data from a video surveillance system in Norway around 2010. The documentation specified that the administrator of the system could set the retention time and the videos would be unavailable after this time. The user interface showed this setting; in this case, it was set to keep the video for 7 days. Unfortunately, the time we were interested in was 9 days previous, two days more than the retention time.

By examining the system, we found out that the ring buffers used for storing the video seemed to be a preset size, and the time setting only affected the playback user interface. The ring buffer didn't grow or shrink as the setting was adjusted, so the video would still record until the oldest part was overwritten by the newest. By adjusting the retention time to its maximum, we could access and acquire all the relevant data from the equipment by logical acquisition.

A forensic examination of an embedded device often falls in two different, albeit connected investigations. The most common form of examination is to reveal data stored on the device: written documents, communications between people, when the device was used, and so on. The other (and less common) form of examination is to reveal a device's functionality or capability as part of a reconstruction. Can the device be used in the way the hypothesis suggests, or should we make a new hypothesis based on what we know the device is capable of? Some questions one should try to answer when familiarizing oneself with a new device are described in the remainder of this section.

6.2.1.1 Functionality

What is the functionality of the device? The answer to this question tells the investigator what the device is and what it does.[13] This is important knowledge because it not only shows how it is meant to function, but also hints at what kind of data it might store.

6.2.1.2 Stored Data

What is stored in the device? This is closely tied to the first question about functionality. Two ways to get some initial answers are to check what it shows on the user interface, and to make some educated guesses about what we suspect it might store, given the functionality. We can make assumptions about not only the obvious data, but also the kind of data the device must store in order to have a given functionality.

6.2.1.3 Storage Media

What kind of storage media does the device contain? Is the storage media volatile, or is it nonvolatile? How much storage space is present? These questions make one consider how to handle the device. If there is only volatile storage in the device, one has to ensure that the device stays powered on. The size of the storage also gives some clues about how much data might be stored.

6.2.1.4 Security Measures

Are there any security measures that one should be aware of? This is a question that forces investigators to be aware of the risks regarding reading the data, as well as whether additional information is needed in order to acquire data. If not managed properly, they risk the loss of the data, or losing access to the information stored.

Some devices might encrypt the data, especially smartphones and other mobile devices. Other devices may contain tamper-resistant technology, which is often found in smart cards, military systems, and set-top media boxes. The inclusion of such technology is often used as a selling point for the device, so it is usually easy to find out which devices contain it. Details of their implementations, however, are often considered trade secrets, and many companies will not easily give access to detailed information about their security measures.

6.2.1.5 Communication Ports and Protocols

Which communication ports and protocols does the device use? This is an important question, as it will often point to different ports and protocols one can use to acquire data, each with its own advantages and drawbacks. In order to find the most forensically sound method for data acquisition, it is necessary to know the implications of using the different ports and protocols.

6.2.2 Handling Electronics – ESD

It is important to be careful when handling evidence so that one doesn't break it or impair its value. One significant danger to electronic equipment is electrostatic discharge (ESD) (Definition 6.4).

---

13 Or at least what it is supposed to do.

> **Definition 6.4: Electrostatic discharge (ESD)**
>
> An ESD is a discharge of electricity between two electrically charged objects when the objects are in close enough proximity for the charge to flow freely.

Figure 6.7 shows a warning sign that is often found in laboratories that handle exposed electronics. It shows that the devices are susceptible to ESD, and should be handled as such.

We have all experienced a flow of electric charges, received as a small electric shock, such as when gripping a metal handle. The most common way to build up an electrostatic charge is by *triboelectric charging*. The word comes from Greek, *tribo* meaning "to rub" and *elektros* meaning "amber," and it means the charge that builds up when two materials are in contact and then separated. The difference in electrical potential between the human hand and the environment can reach up to 35 kV in dry air, and the discharge current might reach several amperes for the duration of a few nanoseconds. For a person, this might feel somewhat uncomfortable; for a small chip, it can be devastating.

Electronic devices are usually made with ESD in mind. For most devices, it is not a problem to handle a modest amount of ESDs. I/O-pins typically have ESD protection circuits, and for the most part one only ever touches grounded areas.[14] For exposed

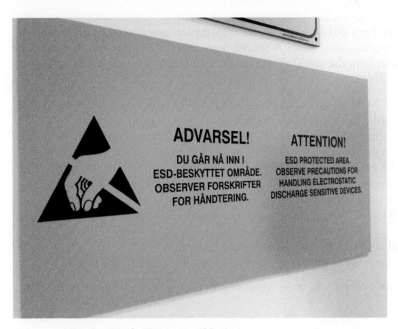

Figure 6.7 Warning sign for ESD-susceptible devices.

---

14 The reader might realize that the device isn't necessarily grounded directly to earth, but I use the term *ground* here to describe the electrical ground potential for the circuit, usually connected to the case or shielding.

electronics, the risk is much higher with the current flowing through the Integrated Circuits (ICs) instead of along the shielding. A discharge with an electric potential of only 30 V might be enough to destroy vulnerable circuits. ESD damage does not necessarily make an IC unusable or unreadable, but it can often result in vague errors that are hard to pin down. This affects the reading of data or the communication with the IC, and will lower the lifetime of the IC.

In order to minimize the risk of such ESD damage, one has to make sure that the triboelectric charges that build up are discharged before touching exposed electronics. The most basic precaution is to use a conductive mat on the desk and a conductive wristband connected to a common ground. The resistance between the mat and earth should be 1 MΩ to 1 GΩ, so that a static charge will dissipate safely to ground. It is also a good idea to remove sources that generate charges. Certain clothing material like wool and fleece have a tendency to build up a large amount of electrostatic charges. It is therefore necessary to avoid such fabrics while working on exposed electronics.

For the same reason, one should avoid storing exposed electronics in direct contact with paper. Use an ESD-protected box or bag when storing the disassembled device or moving it between locations in the lab. More advanced labs might have ESD flooring to use in conjunction with conductive shoes, as well as conductive materials for the inventory in order to make sure static charges are dissipated safely.

6.2.3 First Contact

In this chapter, we have discussed the initial information one should try to find about how the device works, which data is stored, and how to acquire the data. In this subsection, we start with the actual examination. Let's first look at a list of questions to consider:

1) Are there any hazards with handling the device? Blood or other bodily fluids? Chemical hazards? Sharp edges or broken glass?
2) Are there any physical traces that should be preserved, like fingerprints or biological material? If the device is at the scene of crime, be careful with touching or moving anything in the environment, as these things also may contain fragile traces.
3) Is the device broken in any way: scratches, broken interfaces, and so on?
4) State of the device? On, off, sleeping, or another state? Is power connected?
5) If the device is on, what is on the screen? Lock screen? Messages? Is it connected to a network?
6) Is the internal clock on the device correct?
7) Is there any information on the device that is in urgent need of acquisition?

We will look more into each of these questions in the remainder of this section.

6.2.3.1 Hazards

The first thing one must consider is health hazards. Blood or other bodily fluids might be contaminated with bloodborne diseases. One should therefore handle all material that might be blood or other bodily fluids as if it was contaminated. Use disposable gloves when handling devices of unknown origin, and if there is any suspicion of bodily fluids, use a mask, protective eyewear, and a lab coat. If the blood is dry, moving a device might whirl contaminated dry dust in the air (Ballou et al., 2013). Irritants or other chemicals that are on or around the device may also be hazardous.

In the same way that investigators treat bodily fluids as contaminated, they must also treat unknown chemicals as hazardous. Keep in mind that an unknown chemical might be toxic, corrosive, or irritant. Broken glass with sharp edges is also something one needs to pay special attention to. Please don't swipe an unprotected finger over a display where the glass is broken. Use thin gloves or a stylus for this instead.

6.2.3.2 Preservation of Other Traces

If there are fingerprints or other traces on the device that should be preserved, a forensic scientist in the specific field should be consulted. For preserving fingerprints, use gloves and touch the device in areas where it is unlikely to find good fingerprints, like corners or thin edges. It might be of interest to look for fingerprints on peripheral devices like SIM cards, memory cards, or batteries, so be careful when handling these devices also. Consider whether the parts containing other traces might be removed and handled independently.

Finger marks might also reveal the access codes for the device. In case of Android's unlock pattern, we can sometimes see traces from the finger on the display. This method is often called a *smudge attack* (Aviv *et al.*, 2010).

6.2.3.3 Damages and Unique Characteristics

Take notes or pictures of any scratches, bruises, or other special characteristics on the device, as complaints may come over the handling of the device. Pictures of these specific characteristics might also help to identify the device later. This is a part of the *chain of custody*, as defined in Section 1.2.

6.2.3.4 State and Information

The next step is to check the state of the device. Is it powered off? Then keep it off. If it's powered on, a decision should be made whether the device should be turned off, kept on, stored in a radiofrequency (RF)-blocking bag, flight mode turned on, or manually inspected on the site. Section 6.2.10.3 will give more details after the technical foundation has been laid out. Keep in mind that devices that are connected to a network might also be *controlled from* or *send information to* a remote location, or even remotely wiped. Take notes or photos of what is displayed on the screen, which buttons are pressed, any messages on screen, and any cables connected.

6.2.3.5 Clock Setting

A ground rule of digital forensics is to log the difference between the device's internal clock and a known clock. Some devices will reset the time if the battery is removed or is completely discharged. Most clocks drift, some more than others. Some devices adjust the internal clock from a remote source, and the clock will start drifting when the network connection is lost, thereby giving a more inaccurate reading when taken later.

6.2.3.6 Investigative Value of Information

There are usually many tactical investigative considerations in any case. Some information might be of more value early in the case than other information will be at a later stage, or vice versa. Be certain that the persons doing the tactical investigative choices know about the risks and possibilities for acquiring data from the device and the time frame they are discussing.

6.2.4 Physical Acquisition

In many ways, the physical acquisition of an embedded system can be seen as the equivalent procedure to the imaging of a hard drive. Just as one removes the hard drive, connects it to a write blocker, and reads the raw data, physical acquisitions remove the flash memory chip, put it into a device for reading the chip, and read the raw data. The procedure sounds simple, but there are a few challenges that don't come when imaging hard drives.

One of the big differences between removing a hard disk drive from a computer system and removing the flash memory from an embedded system, is that flash memory is often soldered on a printed circuit board (PCB), or even inside a SoC package. This makes physically removing the storage part much more demanding. Furthermore, the software running on the system will usually restrict access to raw data. The system is locked down more tightly than a PC system, which creates challenges in acquiring raw data through the OS. Investigators often have to handle the device in a way that will increase the risk of permanent changes to it, possibly affecting evidence. Keep in mind that it is not only the digital information in the device that might be evidence, but also fingerprints, tool marks, physical wear, and DNA.

Figure 6.8 shows a schematic figure of a generic embedded device, with the storage medium at the bottom, the OS in the middle, and the services and programs running on top in the box called "Processor." We can acquire data from several places. The lower down we acquire data, the more exact we will preserve raw data, low-level system data, and deleted data.

When acquiring data from the memory chip, we don't have a running OS or a flash translation layer (FTL) accessing and writing data. This is intuitively a more forensically sound method than acquiring data while the OS is running. The memory chip might, however, contain an embedded multimedia card (eMMC) controller or other protocol controller (UFS, SATA, or USB) that restructures the raw data before we can access it. This means that even though we read directly from the memory chip, the data is already interpreted, and some traces might be hidden. An introduction to FTLs can be found in Section 6.3.1.

If we do the acquisition from the top of the figure, we can use apps or services running on the device to access the data. The data is often well structured, but the interface is not always well documented. We can connect the device to a PC, and it can present itself as a mass storage device (MSD) or a Media Transfer Protocol (MTP) device. The problem at this level is that the programs or services themselves have limited access to the raw data on the phone, and the OS is running in the background. We generally won't be able to get deleted information from this approach.

We can also acquire data directly through the OS. However, this does require higher access rights than the OS offers ordinary processes. JTAG is a test/debugging system that we can use to debug the system, as described in Section 6.2.4.3, "JTAG/In-System Acquisition."

Finally, the box named Interface IC is an integrated circuit between the flash memory chip and the processor. This is typically a chip that is found together with the flash

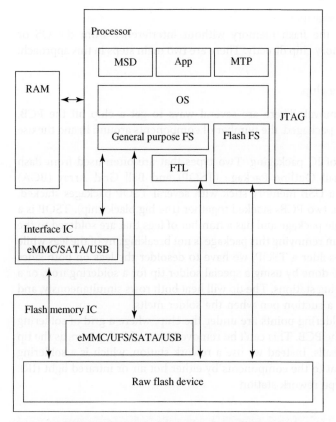

Figure 6.8 Main components of a generic embedded system.

memory. We can either go through the module interface or try to acquire the raw flash directly, something that might involve prying, desoldering, and/or use of other tools. As most of the embedded systems contain a flash device, we will concentrate on acquisition of data from this technology rather than magnetic disk drives.

6.2.4.1 Two Approaches to Physical Acquisition

As described in Section 6.1.6.1, there are two approaches to physical acquisition; one is to remove the memory from the device and read the contents through auxiliary hardware, and the other is to let the memory stay in the device and use the system itself to acquire the information. The former often tends to be a more destructive method, as one can alter the device physically by this approach.

We can name these two approaches *in vivo* and *in vitro*, respectively. The author borrowed the terms from biology: *in vivo* means that something is done or observed in a living organism, while *in vitro* means that something is done or observed outside a living organism (e.g., in a petri dish). To compare these two approaches with computer forensics, we can look at *in vitro* as removing the hard drive, and *in vivo* as booting a system with a live USB stick or CD and acquiring the disk with acquisition software running directly on the examined computer.

6.2.4.2 Chip-Off/In Vitro Acquisition

The intuitive way to read the flash memory without interference from the OS or firmware is to read the memory chip directly. There are two main steps in this approach:

1) remove the chip, and
2) read the contents on the chip.

Let us first look at the removal. There are several ways to get a chip off the PCB, depending on how the IC is packaged, the number of components around it, and the use of underfill.

There are several types of IC packaging. Two types that are often used from flash memory are the Thin Small Outline Package (TSOP) and Ball Grid Array (BGA) package. Figure 6.9 shows a USB memory stick with several TSOP packages stacked, one chip on each side of the two PCBs stacked together (the big black chip). TSOP is a surface-mounted, low-profile package and has a number of legs that are soldered to the PCB. One of the challenges in removing this package is not breaking any of the legs while removing it. In order to desolder a TSOP, we have to desolder the legs on both sides simultaneously. This can be done by using a special solder tip for a soldering iron, or a special tip for hot-air soldering stations. The tip will heat both rows simultaneously, and the chip can be lifted with a suction pen when the solder melts.

In a BGA package, all soldering points are under the chip, where a grid of soldering balls connects the chip to the PCB. This can't be removed by a soldering iron, as the tip won't reach the soldering balls. Instead we use a rework station, which is a soldering station that can transfer heat to the components by either hot air or infrared light (IR). Figure 6.10 shows an IR-type rework station.

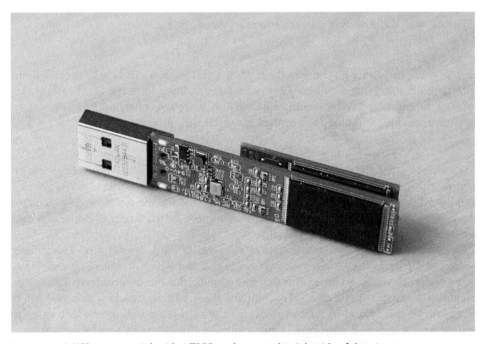

Figure 6.9 A USB memory stick with 4 TSOP packages at the right side of the picture.

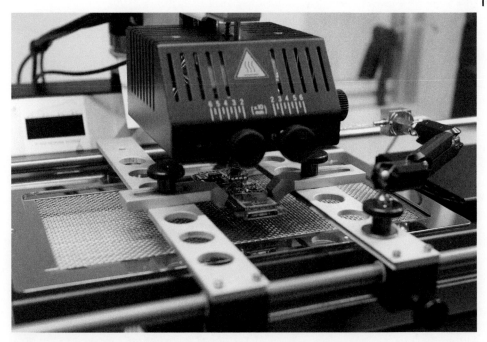

Figure 6.10 An IR rework station with a phone PCB mounted for desoldering.

Materials tend to expand when heated. Different materials will expand at different rates, something that can lead to the layers cracking and destroying the chip. A rule of thumb is that the core of the components should not be heated by more than 3 °C/s. The chip itself can withstand quite high temperatures as long as it is heated slowly, but the hotter the component becomes, the shorter the time it is safe to stay at that temperature. A heater at the bed of the rework station will preheat the PCB before the IR or hot air is applied. The station usually has temperature sensors to ensure it stays within the process window.[15]

Be aware that some components, especially phase-change memory (PCM), will lose the stored data when heated. PCM is a different storage technology than NAND. This technology uses chalcogenide glass that can switch between an amorphous and a crystalline state by applying heat, thereby changing the electric properties. These chips can therefore not be removed by desoldering, as they will be erased by heat. Instead, they have to be removed by other means that don't produce excessive heat.

Sometimes, producers will use underfill to keep the package in place during manufacturing or to make the solder joints more resistant to external forces. Underfill is epoxy-based "glue" used under (or on top of) the chip, between the solder balls on a BGA package. While underfill can improve the reliability of the device, as there is less probability of solder joint damage, it increases the challenges of desoldering the

---

15 A process window is a range of the parameters that yields a certain result in a process. For a soldering process this typically include maximum and minimum temperature, maximum time at maximum temperature, and temperature rise rate.

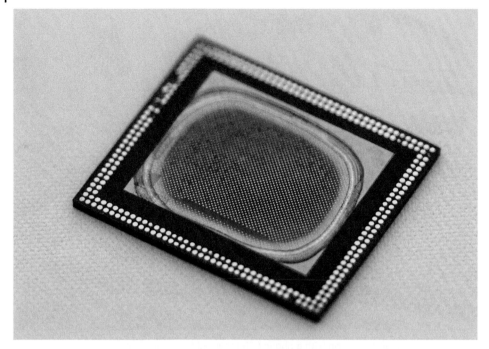

Figure 6.11 A chip that has been grinded using a lapping machine.

chip. Some products exist that can dissolve the epoxy, but these work only for the special underfill compound that they are designed for.

Another way to get the chip off, preferably undamaged, is to cut the PCB around the chip and grind away the PCB under the chip until the soldering balls are exposed. This method is called *lapping*, and one can use a machine to grind layers with high precision. Figure 6.12 shows a lapping machine, where the work piece is placed under the circular metal block, and the black base is revolving with an abrasive on top. The lower black, circular area revolves, and the work piece (in our case, a memory chip) is fastened on the metallic block that is lowered onto the revolving surface. Figure 6.11 shows a chip where the PCB has been removed by this process.

The next step in the process is to read the flash memory. There are a few options for this. One method is to use a universal programmer. This is equipment made for programming (or writing) to chips such as flash memory, electrically erasable programmable read-only memory (EEPROM), and field-programmable gate array (FPGA). These programmers also have the ability to read out the contents on the chip. One disadvantage of using this type of programmer is that they aren't made for forensics, and will typically skip bad blocks while reading. It is also possible to overwrite the contents on the chip by mistake if one doesn't understand all the options and configurations of the programmer. In order to read the contents of a chip, the manufacturer has to have the algorithms for that particular chip. If the chip is exclusively made for a company making a particular device, the programmer might not have the algorithms for reading that chip.

In order to fit a BGA chip in the programmer's socket, one needs to "reball" the BGA package. This means cleaning the solder pads on the BGA and soldering new soldering balls on the BGA package. See Figure 6.13 for a reballed BGA chip. As the ball grid and

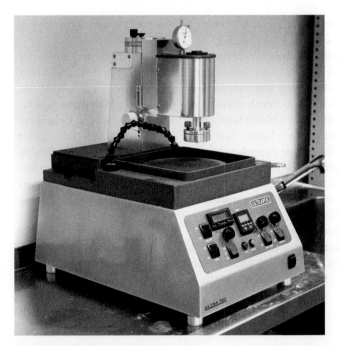

Figure 6.12 A lapping machine.

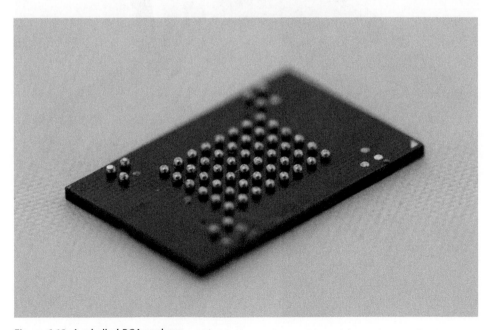

Figure 6.13 A reballed BGA package.

pinout are different on different packages, different physical sockets are necessary for reading the contents of the chip.

Instead of using a universal programmer, we can use equipment made exclusively for forensic use, like the Memory Toolkit from Netherlands Forensic Institute (Knijff, 2010). It reads the chip contents in the same way as a universal programmer, but in addition, reads bad blocks and allows users to tweak existing algorithms or write their own for unknown devices. Since the Memory Toolkit is designed for forensic use, the sockets are also optimized for this by using an adapter that doesn't need a reballed package for getting a good connection. This *pogo pin adapter* is an adapter that has spring-loaded pins as connectors. See Figure 6.14 for an example of a pogo pin adapter from the Memory Toolkit. Figure 6.15 shows a close-up of pogo pins, which are in the center area of the adapter. The central cylinder contains a spring that pushes on the pins protruding from the edges of the cylinder.

There exist many different manufactures of NAND flash, and some of these have joined forces in order to standardize a NAND flash interface. The Open Nand Flash Interface (ONFI) workgroup have made a standard for NAND interface that makes it easier for manufacturers of electronics to change the memory module without needing

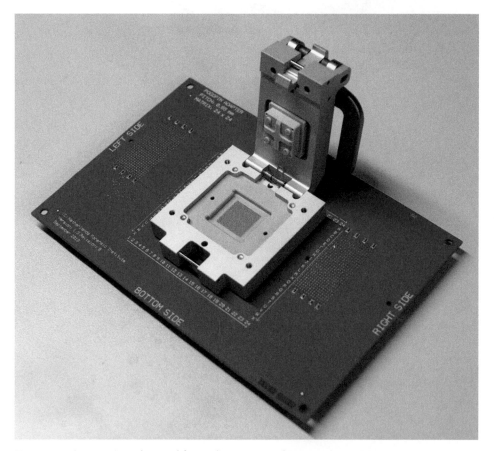

Figure 6.14 A pogo pin socket used for reading memory chips.

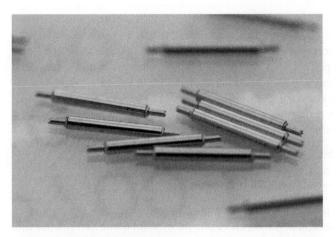

Figure 6.15 Close-up of pogo pins.

to redesign the memory interface. It also makes it easier to design electronics without deciding the memory chip before the end of the design process. Fortunately, it also makes it easier for investigators to read the NAND flash modules. ONFI also tried to future-proof the standard such that new innovations won't necessitate a new standard, which can be promising from a forensic perspective.

Figure 6.16 shows a radar chart of the assessment of this method. We can see that it gets data from a low layer of abstraction and that it alters the physical device. On the other hand, it doesn't affect the logical information in the device, and the method gives reproducible results. The cost is rather high, so one has to invest in advance when it comes to both capital and human resources. During the acquisition, a skilled person must do the chip-off manually, and the cost after the acquisition includes mainly the efforts of data interpretation.

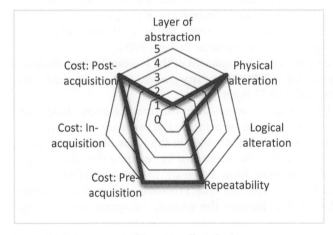

Figure 6.16 Assessment of the chip-off method.

6.2.4.3 JTAG/In-System Acquisition

Device manufacturers test their devices before shipping them, and it is necessary to debug the devices on a physical device rather than an emulator. The first standard from the Joint Test Action Group (JTAG) standardized boundary scans, so manufacturers could easily scan the electronics for nonworking parts and bad soldering joints. IEEE standardized this in 1990 in standard 1149.1–1990, entitled *Standard Test Access Port and Boundary-Scan Architecture*.

The standard describes three test levels during the production of a system:

1) *IC level*: IC testing and built-in self-tests
2) *PCB level*: board testing and production testing
3) *Module or system level*: testing of higher level systems.

The standard describes two modes of operation; a noninvasive mode that is guaranteed to be independent of the core logic in the IC, and a pin-permission mode that can use the I/O pins of the IC and isolate the core logic from the outside world. When the IC is powered up, it will always start in the noninvasive mode, so the IC will be working normally on all other I/O pins. Commands to the JTAG interface can later set the circuit in a pin-permission mode. In addition to these two standardized test modes, JTAG can also be used to put a processor in debug mode, and the JTAG interface can be used to debug the processor.

The boundary scan logic can be used to identify defects on the board, in the core logic of the ICs, and in the programmable logic. It can also send signals to other peripheral devices and debug firmware or software running on a processor or microcontroller. It is these two last points that are of most interest to investigators, as they can access the memory either by contacting the flash memory through the I/O ports while the core is disconnected, or by using the debugging system of the processor. The former is called *extest*[16] *mode*, and the latter *debug mode* (Breeuwsma, 2006).

A model of the JTAG architecture is shown in Figure 6.17. The heart of the system is the TAP controller, or the Test Access Port. This is a finite-state machine that will keep track of the instructions sent to the JTAG port. The registers around the core in the figure are the boundary registers. The communication to the JTAG interface is through five pins, where one is optional. These pins are not shared with any other functionality on the chip. Table 6.4 shows the JTAG pins and a description of the pins.

It is out of our scope to describe the state machine in the TAP here, but for the interested reader, more information can be found in Parker (2003).

In order to test a whole board, the JTAG component of the ICs can be daisy chained. Figure 6.18 show a setup where TDI and TDO are daisy chained into a scan chain, and have a common TCLK, TMS, and TRST* input.

Unfortunately for us, the JTAG test ports on consumer electronics are often hidden on the PCB, the JTAG connections are covered by paint, or the paths are even physically broken from the factory. JTAG might also be disabled in the IC by blowing a fuse, or setting a protection register that can only be re-enabled by resetting the whole chip.

Let us look at an example processor from Freescale to see how JTAG access restrictions are implemented by this producer. The Freescale multimedia processor has an IC Identification Module that handles the security subsystem on the chip,

---

16 External test.

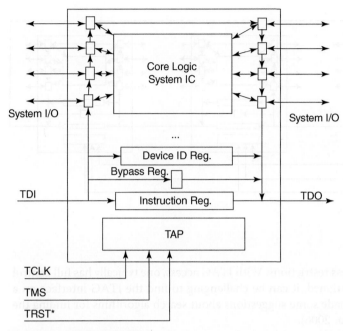

Figure 6.17 JTAG architecture.

including setting the operating mode for the Secure JTAG interface. These operating modes are Debug Enabled, Secure Debug, and No Debug, and they are set by blowing one-time programmable eFuses. These can't be reset after they are blown. No Debug will deny access to the JTAG port altogether, and Debug Enabled will be an open debug interface. Secure Debug can be enabled in order to facilitate field-testing or debugging of malfunctioning systems while in use, without giving access to the debug features for everyone else. Secure Debug is a protocol that will hand out a challenge, and if the response is right, access to the JTAG interface is granted. This means that one needs to know the key for enabling JTAG debug access.

When the JTAG port is found, and one is connected, we can use, for example, a JTAG-to-USB interface and communicate with the TAP on the processor. From here, we can read out memory directly, debug the chip using a debugger, or even change the running

Table 6.4 JTAG signals.

PIN	Name	Description
TDI	Test Data In	Serially shifted input. Float high.
TDO	Test Data Out	Serially shifted output
TCLK	Test Clock	Clock signal for JTAG logic
TMS	Test Module Select	Control signal for the TAP state machine. Float high.
TRST*	Test Reset	(Optional) Reset the TAP state machine. Active low. Float high.

TDO

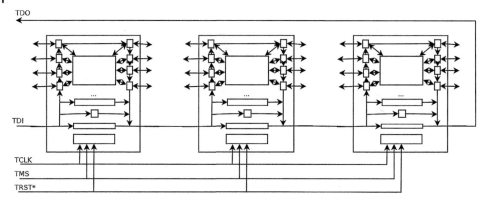

TDI

TCLK

TMS

TRST*

Figure 6.18 JTAG daisy chain.

system to get around access restrictions. With JTAG access, one typically has full control of the processor. As mentioned, it can be challenging to find the JTAG interface on a PCB. M. F. Breeuwsma made some suggestions about search algorithms for finding the JTAG points (Breeuwsma, 2006).

The assessment for JTAG acquisition is shown in Figure 6.19. We can see that this method usually collects data at a little higher layer of abstraction than chip-off; it can affect the device physically, as we might need to open it and alter it a bit to get access to the JTAG points. The method doesn't affect the data much, but since it does run through the processor of the device, one has to power on the device, which can affect the raw data. The method is repeatable, and cheaper than chip-off. To use it, however, one does need some equipment and training. After extraction, we have to interpret the data in the same way as the chip-off, rebuild the FTL, and so on. The post-acquisition cost is consequently similar to the post-acquisition cost of chip-off.

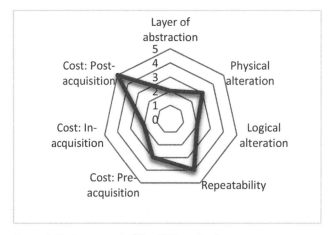

Figure 6.19 Assessment of the JTAG method.

The acquisition of data on embedded systems is traditionally split into two types: logical and physical. As we will see, this is not necessarily a model that fits reality, but it is close enough at least to give an idea about what we are doing and what we can expect. In Section 6.2.4, we looked at the physical acquisition, and in this section, we will look at logical acquisition: using the device's "ordinary" interfaces and data exchange protocols while it is powered on.

How this works is that the OS interprets the raw data on the device before it is sent to the external endpoint. In most cases, with a logical acquisition, we will not get access to deleted data. On the other hand, we will get information interpreted and easily accessible to the investigator. In many ways, a logical acquisition is similar to a "live acquisition" as we do with a computer system described in Section 5.2.1.1.

6.2.5.1   Manual Inspection

The simplest form of logical extraction is to use the main interface for accessing the device. For a phone, this will typically be done by entering data through the keyboard or touchscreen, and viewing information on the screen. The advantage of this type of examination is its speed. It can be done instantly as a triage at the scene of crime, to quickly acquire needed information at the start of an investigation. Sometimes, it can be the only practical option for acquiring information.

The drawback to this method is that it is more challenging to document the information. Either the information has to be written down while examining the device, or it has to be documented with photos. Both options generate manual, repeating, and error-prone work. This method also changes the data on the phone, so it is important to document as much as we can about what we do with the device, as well as any negative findings.

Manual inspection gives access to the parts of the phone that are accessible by the user through the user interface. Keep in mind, though, that this does not only mean text messages, call logs, and contacts, but also information from apps, emails, and other logged-in services.

Figure 6.21 shows a setup from ZRT with a camera to document a manual inspection of devices. The camera can take both still pictures and video, and an optional microphone can record audio from the device.

The assessment radar chart in Figure 6.20 shows that the data extraction is from a high layer of abstraction. One extensively handles the device while doing this, so the probability for something happening physically is higher, and of course the logical data will be altered by using the device. The repeatability is quite low, as information might be marked as read and timestamps will be updated. Next time one looks at the same data, we will get different results. The cost is actually close to zero pre-acquisition. In-acquisition cost is higher due to the person-hours used for documenting everything on the device, and the post-acquisition cost is high due to the person-hours used for facilitation of the information for further use and presentation.

6.2.5.2   SIM Acquisition

As mentioned in the introduction, a UICC (SIM card) is in itself an embedded system with its own microcontroller, RAM, and flash storage. The only exposed interfaces are

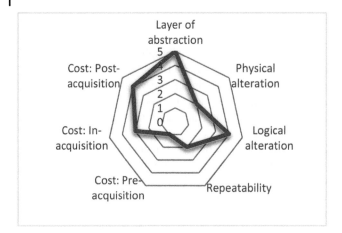

Figure 6.20 Assessment of the manual inspection method.

the pads on the card. This means that one will often be able to acquire data from the card logically, unless we can find a flaw in the software or firmware on the UICC, or have a lab that can expose the ICs and get direct access to the embedded flash.[17]

The UICC contains SIM and USIM applications that handle telephony-specific functions. Each UICC will contain an ICCID (Integrated Circuit Card ID). This number identifies the physical card and is sometimes referred to as a SIM Card Number. This is the number that is printed physically on the UICC. The number consists of three parts, as shown in Table 6.5. The SIM and USIM also contain an IMSI. This is the number that will identify the subscriber on the mobile network.

Apart from these two identification numbers, the UICC contains a list of networks it is not allowed to join. This list is updated when the phone sees a network that the subscriber's mobile network provider doesn't have any roaming deals with. This list might therefore tell us in which countries the UICC has been used.

Furthermore, the UICC also contains storage for a limited number of SMS, contacts, and a call log. Some phone models don't use this functionality as default and will only store messages in the UICC if the user explicitly specifies that preference. Other models store the first messages in the UICC, and continue to write to the phone memory only when this storage is full. In addition to the SIM/USIM functionality, the UICC can contain other apps that will store other types of information, like DRM (Digital Rights Management) apps, payment apps, and so on.

In order to communicate with the UICC, we often need to enter a personal identification number (PIN) before the SIM/USIM application accepts commands for reading stored data or connecting to the network. The user can disable PIN authentication. If the UICC is locked with a PIN, we will have three unsuccessful attempts before the PIN itself is locked. The PIN can be unlocked with a PIN Unlock Key (PUK). After 10 unsuccessful authentication attempts, the UICC will be

---

17 Smart cards in general implement many tamper-resistant technologies to make direct access to the IC difficult.

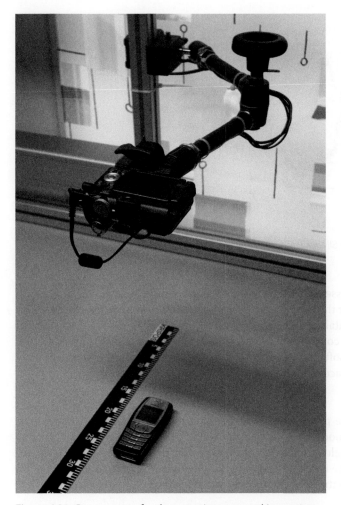

Figure 6.21 Camera setup for documenting a manual inspection.

completely locked without the possibility to unlock it. The PUK can usually be found on the letter accompanying the UICC from the mobile network provider together with the original PIN. The mobile network provider also stores the PUK in their subscriber database.

Table 6.5 Layout of ICCID.

Issuer Identification Number (IIN)	Major Industry Identifier (MII) (2 digits, always 89 for telecommunication)
	Country code (1–3 digits)
	Issuer identifier (1–4 digits)
Individual account identification	Variable length
Check digit	Using Luhn algorithm

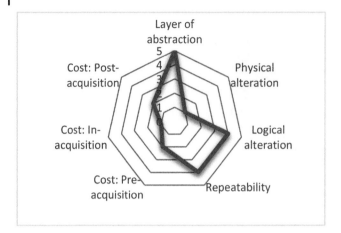

Figure 6.22 Assessment of the SIM logical acquisition method.

Figure 6.22 shows the assessment of this method. It collects data at a high layer of abstraction, so it won't alter the card physically, but it alters the information stored in the card. The method is repeatable, and we can read SMS without marking it as read. It would, however, reset the counter for failed PIN attempts. The cost is quite low; one needs a card reader and software to read the UICC, and the data might need some interpretation in the post-acquisition stage.

6.2.5.3 SIM Replacement
In order to ensure that the phone won't connect to a mobile network, we can either ensure that it is in flight mode by removing the UICC (SIM card), or we can put the phone in an RF-shielded enclosure. There is a risk when turning the phone on in order to turn on flight mode, as there is a short time where the phone might be connected to the network, where it can be controlled remotely. By removing the UICC, we will reduce this risk.

Some phones, however, won't start properly if they don't have a UICC present, and some will even delete data, like call logs or messages, if it detects a new UICC inserted. This behavior doesn't apply for all phones, but it is common with simpler phones, whereas smartphones are designed to be used also without a UICC.

To mitigate the risk of losing data, we can replace the UICC with one that won't connect to the mobile network. This means that the ICCID and IMSI are read from the original UICC and copied to another UICC that doesn't contain the keys needed for connecting to a mobile network. This is often referred to as *SIM cloning* or just *cloning*. With a cloned UICC inserted into the phone, it assumes it is still the same UICC as before it was powered down, while it will also be isolated from the network. Finally, we need to ensure before powering up the phone that it doesn't connect to other networks (such as Wi-Fi networks or Bluetooth).

6.2.5.4 Device Backup
One can find information from a device in other places than on the device itself. Some devices, especially phones and other smart devices, can have backups stored on a

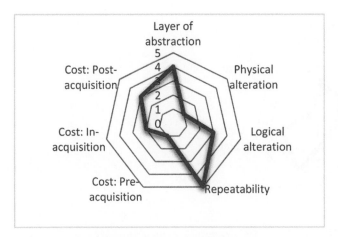

Figure 6.23 Assessment of the device backup method.

computer or "in the cloud." These backups can be encrypted. One can use the backup functionality to acquire a fresh backup from the device. An authentication token might be necessary to present to the phone, or type the password/pin on the phone for the computer to be allowed to connect and receive the backups.

For an Apple iPhone that is synced with a computer with iTunes, the phone and computer need to be "paired." After the phone is paired with the computer, the phone can be backed up, even when it is locked. If the iPhone backup is encrypted, the backup also includes Wi-Fi passwords, keychain, and other "secure" data. Be aware that, especially for cloud-syncing services, we might find traces from all the devices associated with one account on all other devices associated with the same account. A message sent from an Apple computer might be synced with the messaging application on the iPhone, and even show up on the phone.

Figure 6.23 shows the assessment of this method. Even though the data on the device is changed, the backup can still be identical. As the backup is taken from a higher layer of abstraction than the changed data, the process might be repeated with nearly identical results. The cost is quite low, as one won't need much equipment for this. Post-acquisition, we need to interpret the contents of the backup and report on the findings.

6.2.5.5 USB Mass Storage

The USB Mass Storage Device Class (MSC) is a part of the USB standard describing an interface to a mass storage block device over USB. This protocol is used when connecting a disk drive, a USB memory stick, or a SD card reader to a computer. For the computer or host, mass storage devices will look like locally connected disks, and one can access the file systems through the host's file system drivers. As the host will see the block device and interpret the file system, one might recover deleted files from an MSC device by using ordinary forensic hard disk imaging software. Note that an embedded device might present only one of its internal partitions as an MSC device when connected to the USB port of a computer. This means that system files and many user files won't be visible for the connected computer at all.

Many USB MSDs use the SCSI protocol for communication between the computer and the MSD. Commands for reading and writing are specified in the SCSI standard.

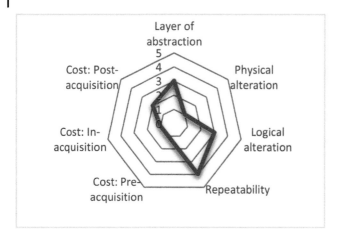

Figure 6.24 Assessment of the USB mass storage method.

This standard allows for proprietary SCSI commands, which are different from vendor to vendor, and these commands are often undocumented. These commands can, for example, implement functionality for flashing firmware and unlock access restrictions on a device. This can make for interesting functionality from a forensic perspective, as investigators can find ways to unlock devices without the password.

The assessment of this method is shown in Figure 6.24. We can see that the layer of abstraction has gotten a score of 3. This is because the OS will decide which data to show, so it is a layer of interpretation underneath the file system one is looking at. There are small if any physical alterations, but the data can be altered since the system is running. The cost is negligible, apart from the reporting and eventual interpretation.

6.2.5.6 Media Transfer Protocol

The MTP was introduced by Microsoft as a part of their Media Framework, and it was designed to transfer multimedia files and metadata between a computer and a multimedia device. Originally, it used USB as a transport; later, it was also used on top of TCP/IP and Bluetooth.

The difference between an MTP connection and a USB mass storage connection is that while MSDs have direct access to the block device, an MTP device will only have access at the file level. As the device interprets the file system, and transfers individual objects (or files) back to the investigator, one is not able to acquire deleted files through this protocol. As the protocol doesn't give direct access to the files on the device, a file cannot be changed directly. In order to change a file, it has to be transferred to the computer, changed, and pushed back to the device.

Figure 6.25 show the assessment of this method. We can see that the method will operate on a high layer of abstraction; it won't affect the device physically. The method will alter the data on the device, but it will still be repeatable. Also, the cost is low.

6.2.5.7 OBEX

The OBEX (OBject EXchange) protocol is in many ways a communication protocol similar to HTTP. While HTTP is a text-based protocol that serves web pages, the OBEX protocol is a binary protocol meant to transfer objects over an IR connection. The

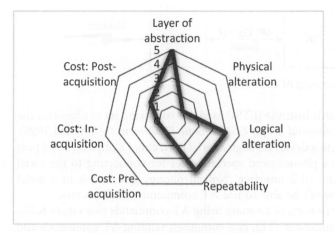

Figure 6.25 Assessment of the MTP protocol method.

objects can be pictures, contact cards, messages, or other types of information. Even though OBEX originally was made for infrared protocols, it can also be used with other transport protocols like Bluetooth, USB, or TCP/IP. Since this protocol is commonly implemented in many mobile devices, it can be used to acquire common telephony and multimedia files from a mobile device. These typically include contact lists, MMS messages, and calendars.

Figure 6.26 shows the assessment of the OBEX method. It collects the data at a high layer of abstraction, but as the amount of data is quite limited, one isn't able to read the changed data, so the repeatability is high. The cost is quite low for this method too.

6.2.5.8 AT Commands

AT commands, also called Hayes AT command set or Hayes commands, were developed by Dennis Hayes in 1981. They were originally used for communicating with modems that would modulate digital signals from the computer into electric waves in the audible specter, and send this through the telephone network. Later, the European

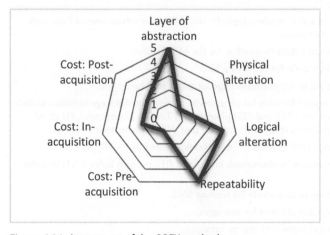

Figure 6.26 Assessment of the OBEX method.

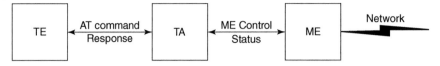

Figure 6.27 The parts of a system using AT commands.

Telecommunications Standards Institute (ETSI) used this command set as a basis for the standard GSM 07.07, *AT Command Set for GSM Mobile Equipment (ME)* (ETSI 1996). The AT commands are sent to a device through a serial port, either a physical serial port or a virtual serial port. Some phones need special cables for connecting to the serial interface, and others use the USB interface. Not all phones give access to a serial interface, which means we won't be able to use AT commands on all phones.

The standard specifies three parts of a system using AT commands (see Figure 6.27). One part is the Terminal Equipment (TE), or a computer, sending AT commands and reading the response from a Terminal Adapter (TA). The TA will itself send control messages and receive status responses from the Mobile Equipment (ME), which is responsible for the network communication. In most mobile phones, TA and ME are in the phone, while TE is, for example, a computer sending AT commands over USB, Bluetooth, IR, or another connection.

The AT commands can be divided into four command sets: a basic command set, an extended command set, a proprietary command set, and a register command set. The basic command set does not have any prefixes, the extended commands are prefixed with "+," and the proprietary commands are prefixed with "%." The register command set is used to set or read register status, which all have the name S<n> where <n> is a number for the register to be set or read.

The commands for a GSM phone are found in the extended command set. A few of the commands for reading information from a phone are described in Table 6.6. Please

Table 6.6 Some common AT commands for GSM.

AT command	Description
+CGSN	Returns a serial number, typically the IMEI. Can return several lines with more information.
+CNUM	Returns the MSISDN number for the ME if stored.
+CPIN=<pin>	Enters PIN code for unlocking SIM.
+CPBS=?	Returns list of supported storage locations for phonebook.
+CPBS=<storage>	Selects storage location for phonebook. Some defined storage locations include MT (combined ME and SIM phonebook), TA (TA phonebook), FD (fixed dialing numbers from SIM), and LD (last dialing phonebook from SIM).
+CPBR=?	Lists supported indexes for phonebook selected by +CPBS.
+CPBR=<i1>[,<i2>]	Returns entries in phonebook on index 1 (i1), or from index 1 (i1) to index 2 (i2).
+CMGF=1	Puts phone in text mode for reading SMS.
+CMGL=?	Lists available statuses for messages.
+CMGL="<status>"	Lists all messages with status <status>.

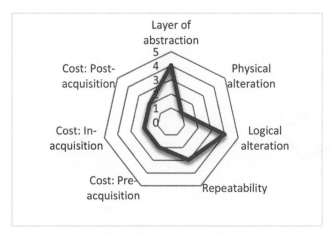

Figure 6.28 Assessment of the AT command method.

note that all AT commands are prefixed with *AT* (for *attention*) before sending it to the TA. The command *Z*, or *reset*, is therefore sent as *ATZ*.

Figure 6.28 shows the assessment for this method. We can see that the method alters data on the device. Reading unread SMS messages will mark them as read, but other types of data will be identical when repeating the method. Cost is not high, but investigators need some knowledge and time to perform the acquisition, and some resources for reporting afterwards.

6.2.5.9   Vendor-Specific Protocols

Many vendors use their own proprietary protocols to communicate with the devices. These protocols can be used to read content from the phone that is not accessible from other logical acquisition methods. One such vendor-specific protocol is FBUS, which is used in Nokia phones. This protocol is used to read the file system, or primary memory (PM). The PM file system doesn't contain folder or file names; they are numbered. The numbers tend to change between phone models, so the folder containing, for example, the IMEI might be "51" in one model and "23" in the next.

For some historical models (before BB5), we can also read a dump of the flash memory directly through the FBUS protocol. In order to get the flash dump, investigators need to know the address of where the flash is loaded. Some tools can guess where it is, but they are often wrong. In this case, one needs to manually try addresses until the start point for the flash memory is found.

6.2.5.10   Android Debug Bridge (ADB)

The Android OS and development kit (Android SDK) has an ADB, which is a command interpreter used for developers. It is turned off by default in Android phones, but it can be turned on by going to the Settings menu, selecting Developer Options, and enabling USB debugging. This will allow a PC to connect to the phone and have some access to the file system. Files can be browsed by the *ADB shell* command, and files or directories can be copied by the *ADB pull* command. In a nonrooted device, one won't get access to all files, just a subset of the file system. One can often get user data from some applications

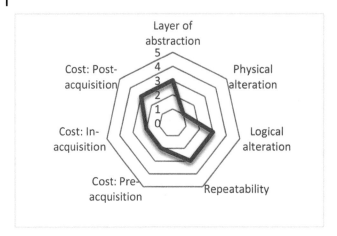

Figure 6.29 Assessment of the ADB method.

and other stored files on the device. Be aware that in newer versions of the OS, the computer has to be authenticated by the device. This means that even though USB debugging is turned on, the device has to be unlocked in order to gain access.

Figure 6.29 shows our assessment of the ADB method. We don't get access to much of the file system, and metadata in the file system will be altered. This reduces the repeatability. We don't need much resources, apart from knowledge for the staff doing the acquisition and some time for the reporting.

6.2.6 Somewhere between Physical and Logical

The terms *logical* and *physical acquisition* are just models of what one is actually doing. If we define a "physical" acquisition to read the data on the lowest possible level without the system interpreting the data, there is a quite huge and diverse amount of methods that can be classified as a "logical" acquisition. If we, on the other hand, define a logical acquisition to be an acquisition of data where we use the public interface of running services or applications on the device to acquire data, then we will leave a diverse field in between these two extremes.

If one acquired the data from a device from one level below the file system, but above the FTL, one would get data that seems to be from a physical acquisition, with deleted data, but still missing data that are in pages hidden by the FTL. This can be called a "pseudo-physical" acquisition (Klaver, 2010). We use this term to describe an acquisition that looks like a physical acquisition, but where there is a layer that interprets and changes the layout of the data before handing it over to us. Even though investigators use the system itself to read raw data from the flash device, the system is still a layer between the raw data and the interface from which we can read.

Before one can extract data from a device, one will often have to gain access to the data. In order to gain this access, we might have to manipulate the system, thereby increasing the risk of changing the data. The extraction will often be the same between the various methods, but the steps leading toward the extraction will be different. We can call these methods by the collective name of *access-enabling acquisition methods*, as one will need to gain access to the data by circumventing encryption or other restrictions.

These two methods are often interconnected, as it is often necessary to gain access in order to do a pseudo-physical acquisition, or a physical in vivo acquisition (see Section 6.2.4).

6.2.6.1 Root Access

When the OS is locked down, apps and services won't have direct access to the memory. Different OSs have different security measures. Some of the more common security measures are sandboxing, secure boot process, and encrypted storage. Sandboxing is where each process is given their own address space where they can't access other processes' memory or storage. Communication between processes is possible through an Inter-Process Communication (IPC) subsystem provided for this. Each app is therefore operating in its own sandbox. Android, with its Unix roots, also lets each application run as its own user, without root privileges.[18]

One method (referred to as *rooting*) to get access to flash memory is to trick the OS into giving one the access rights one needs, typically root access. With root access, one may read the raw block devices or the unencrypted file system. In order to get this access in a forensically sound way, an investigator often has to rely on local privilege escalation exploits in apps or the system running on the phone. The drawback with this method is that it is usually dependent on vulnerabilities in the software versions, the OS patch level, and hardware. An exploit for one version on one device won't necessarily work on another, updated device. Overzealous investigators might also crash the system by exploiting vulnerabilities that they don't understand well enough. The OS's own API can also be used for reading the block devices, and might therefore not get all the underlying data.

Figure 6.30 shows the assessment for the rooting method. We see that this is quite similar to the ADB method described earlier in this chapter, and many of the same assessments are also valid for this method. One difference that is not obvious from Figure 6.30 is that the rooting will affect the system on a deeper level than just by reading the data with ADB. Reading the data affects the user data to a greater degree than the rooting process, but the rooting process affects the OS itself. The root access might be permanent until a system upgrade or factory reset is performed.

6.2.6.2 Boot Access

Another way to access the flash memory is to boot another system and read the contents of the flash from this other system, just like booting a Live CD/USB and acquiring data from an OS. Many systems support writing to one of the recovery partitions with custom firmware, and this will give access to reading the contents of the flash memory without mounting the partitions. Some devices have a strict checking of signatures, and these might not allow booting custom firmware, or ROM (read-only memory). The typical method to bypass this is to boot the device into Device Firmware Upgrade mode (DFU-mode), or recovery mode. The names tend to change with the makers, and the functionality might be spread over several modes, so don't get confused with different

---

18 *Root privileges* is a term from Unix, where the user "root" (user id 0) has full privileges in the system. To have root access, or to be root, is therefore to have full access to all parts of the system.

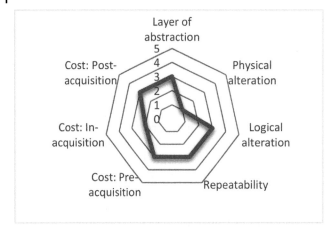

Figure 6.30 Assessment of the root method.

naming schemes. The most important thing is that from this mode, you will be able to flash a custom boot image.

In many of the devices, the boot code will check the signature of the rest of the boot chain, so unsigned code won't boot. Some devices have an option to turn this feature off, like HTC's S-OFF setting (Security-OFF). In many cases, this is not a good idea for forensic investigations as the switch to an unlocked boot loader will result in a factory reset of the device and loss of user data. Other devices don't have strict checking of signatures during the boot process, which makes the process easier.

Figure 6.31 shows our assessment of the boot code method. This method bypasses the running OS so one can get to a lower abstraction layer. It will access the system data, but not the user data. The process can be reproducible, with the exception of the boot code that can differ between acquisitions. The cost is a bit higher pre-acquisition because one

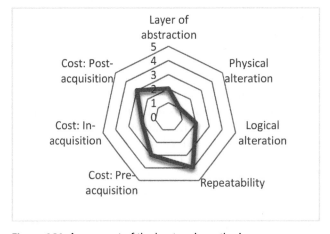

Figure 6.31 Assessment of the boot code method.

needs to find a way to get the boot code running, and it is necessary that the people doing this have the appropriate skills.

6.2.6.3 Encryption Keys

Many devices offer encrypted storage. This is often implemented in a co-processor so that the main processor won't use its own processing power on encryption and decryption. In a co-processor setup, the keys are stored in a secure, non-accessible memory on the co-processor itself. The keys can therefore not be acquired by commands from the processor. In such systems, a reset will wipe the keys from the co-processor and render the encrypted data inaccessible. The boot loader trick won't work either, as one needs the authentication method to decrypt the data on the device. A chip-off process won't yield anything but encrypted data, so in this case we need to use the device's own crypto engine to get access to the data. For systems that are designed to provide a secure environment, getting access represents a challenge that could take more time and resources than are at hand during an investigation.

iPhones from 3GS and up use encrypted storage, even if no password is set. The encryption used is a file encryption and not a full-disk encryption. It is therefore possible to acquire the file system and file metadata without decrypting the device. The content of the files will be encrypted, though.

As with all other encryption, even though the encryption algorithms are well designed and hard to break, we can often find vulnerabilities such as insecure handling of keys, nonoptimal implementation of the Pseudo-Random Number Generator (PRNG), and bugs in screen locks.

6.2.6.4 Flasher Tools

When searching the Internet for ways to read or write memory from a mobile device, we can find many commercial devices that will flash a certain family of mobile devices. These are typically designed for phone repair shops that are not considered official service centers. A *flasher tool* is considered low-cost equipment that seldom has good documentation or intuitive user interfaces.

Some of these flasher tools, however, offer the functionality we need for forensic examination. For reading the flash memory directly or flashing a new boot loader on the system, some even offer the functionality of brute-forcing access codes. It is important to know that forensic use is not the main intended usage of this equipment. Figure 6.32 shows a flasher box together with a rig for connecting a Nokia Lumia 800.

If it is the only practical option we have, we will still use flasher tools for forensics, but we have to be careful to ensure the integrity of the acquired data. In order to use these tools, it is important to test their functionality on test devices thoroughly before using them on seized devices. One click on the wrong button might overwrite traces on the phone, or even do a factory reset.

Figure 6.33 shows the flasher box method. The assessment is similar to that of the boot code method, but it will often alter the hardware to a higher degree than the plain boot code method, as one may have to physically open the device.

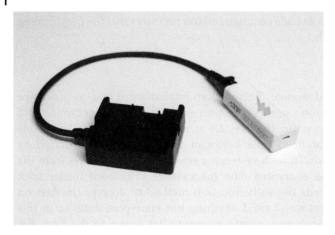

Figure 6.32 An ATF box (white) used both for flashing a device and for connecting to JTAG.

6.2.6.5 Chip-Off Continued

In the past few years, this has become more popular with eMMC ICs. These ICs have an MMC interface instead of a NAND interface. eMMC ICs contain an on-chip microcontroller that will do all the flash management internally, so that the OS doesn't need to implement FTL functionality. It might be unnecessary to point out, but this makes it easier for the developers as they don't need to think about wear-leveling and error-correcting codes in their product. These devices are also called *managed flash devices*, as the on-chip controller manages the flash peculiarities.

For Android devices, we currently see fewer NAND flash devices with YAFFS2, and more devices with an eMMC chip and an ordinary file system like ext4 without an FTL. The same is true for other smartphones.[19]

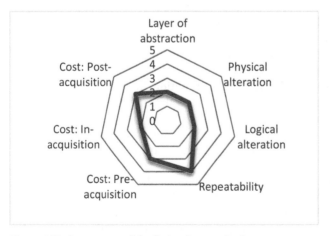

Figure 6.33 Assessment of the flasher box method.

---

19 Other operating systems use other file systems, though.

Table 6.7 eMMC signals.

eMMC signal	Direction	Description
CLK	I	Clock
DS	O	Data strobe
DAT0 - DAT7	I/O	Data
CMD	I/O	Command/response
RST_n	I	Hardware reset
V_{CC}	–	Supply voltage for core
V_{CCQ}	–	Supply voltage for I/O
V_{SS}	–	Supply voltage ground for core
V_{SSQ}	–	Supply voltage ground for I/O

The Multi Media Card (MMC) interface was originally a 7-pin standard with a 1-bit serial data bus. It was made public in 1997 and was one of the earlier standards designed for NAND flash instead of NOR flash. Later, MMCplus with an 8-bit data bus was standardized, and after this eMMC came into being. Table 6.7 shows the electric signals for eMMC.

The eMMC chips are electrically compatible with MMC readers, so if one desolders the chip, it can be read by connecting the corresponding signals to a MMC card reader. The default configuration of eMMC contains one user data block, two boot blocks, and (in version 4.4 of the eMMC standard) a *Replay Protected Memory Block* (RPMB). These additional storage areas are used for boot code and to establish a secure boot chain.

A newer standard, called Universal Flash Storage (UFS), has become more popular. This standard promises greater speeds than eMMC can deliver. Functionally, UFS devices are similar to eMMC devices, and the standard offers a similar management system, including protected memory blocks. The difference is in the interface: a UFS device doesn't have a dedicated clock line. The clock is encoded together with the data signal in something called 8b10b encoding.[20] UFS also implements a simplified SCSI command set.[21]

The eMMC or UFS controller simplifies the work for phone developers, but it also means that we don't get direct access to the flash, even after a chip-off. The interface controller will be between the I/O-pins on the chip package and the raw NAND storage. Deleted data might still linger in the NAND cells, but won't necessarily be visible or accessible from the standard interface. We can therefore call chip-off and acquisition of these chips *pseudo-physical*. One will get something that looks like a physical dump, but it is in fact already interpreted by a flash controller.

---

20 An 8b10b coding is a way to code 8-bit symbols into 10-bit symbols such that it is a balance between "1" and "0" (DC balance), there are no consecutive runs of more than five bits of the same value, and the clock can be recovered from the data stream.

21 SCSI stands for *small computer system interface*, and it is an old standard, originally used for hard disks, printers, etc. Even though we don't see many "SCSI"-labeled products today, the protocol itself is still widely used.

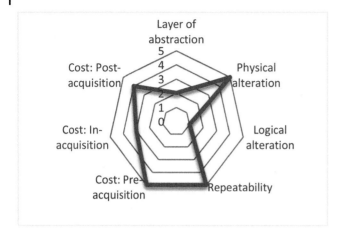

Figure 6.34 Assessment of the eMMC chip-off method.

Figure 6.34 shows the visual representation of this method. It is similar to the chip-off method, but with a slightly higher layer of abstraction. The post-acquisition cost is also somewhat less than the chip-off described earlier, as one won't need to rebuild the FTL.

6.2.7 Commercial Forensic Products

There exist many commercial forensic products for acquisition and interpretation of data from mobile devices. These commercial products are using many of the described methods for acquiring data. The forensic products also tend to use checksums of the acquired data to ensure the integrity of the stored data. They are tested for *forensic soundness*, and the products facilitate selecting and presenting information in reports.

Many commercial forensic products offer both logical and physical acquisition of data. Logical acquisition in these products will use the standard communication protocols for accessing the device, while the physical acquisition will use the methods we have described in this chapter as *pseudo-physical*, or "somewhere in between physical and logical."

While these products claim to support a wide range of mobile devices, this doesn't mean that the products can actually acquire all the data from the list of supported devices. For logical acquisition, only a few of the implemented protocols might be supported, or there might be proprietary extensions to protocols that are not implemented in the forensic product. For physical or pseudo-physical acquisition, we can extract the data, but the commercial products might not be able to interpret all relevant data.

No software is without errors, and this remains a valid statement for commercial forensic software. If the software can find deleted messages, it might not be able to find all traces of deleted messages. Other types of information might also be misinterpreted, so keep in mind that the information could be erroneous. In order to detect errors described here, it is preferable to use dual-tool verification as described in Section 2.3.

Figure 6.35 shows an assessment of an example forensic product. One of the strengths with a forensic product is that it will ease the post-acquisition work considerably, as it

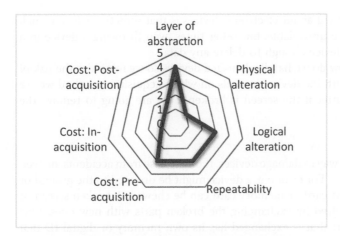

Figure 6.35 Assessment of a commercial forensic product.

often has a good report functionality. The products also often minimize their footprint on the system, especially when it comes to user data alterations.

6.2.8 What about RAM?

There has been much talk about flash memory so far, but what about the RAM? In the past few years, there has been an increasing focus on dumping memory, reconstructing memory, carving out memory, and reconstruct running process memory from computer systems. Why don't we do this on embedded devices too? One reason there has not been too much research into this is that the RAM is more inaccessible in embedded devices than in PCs. The interfaces to the system are often limited, and in more advanced systems, the OS itself gives strict limitations for running programs to access the RAM. The RAM is more volatile than a solid-state disk, so one must ensure that the system is in a powered state. To acquire the RAM, one can use the running OS (possibly bypassing security restrictions), use JTAG, or boot the system with alternative firmware without resetting the RAM.

In advanced systems with nonvolatile memory, data tends to be written to flash memory more often than on a computer. Therefore, more information from running processes is in nonvolatile storage. This is because a device often will operate on battery power, and there is a real probability for the battery to fall out or run out of power. The device should be able to recover from such incidents, so there is more focus on data integrity and writing to disk (or flash) in embedded systems.

Having said this, there can still be much valuable information in RAM, and it is likely that we will see more focus on memory forensics for embedded devices and mobile phones in the future.

6.2.9 Damaged Devices

Devices that are easy to move around are easier to accidentally damage than stationary systems. Mobile phones kept in a pocket can be damaged by humidity, fall on the ground and break, or be dropped into water. Furthermore, some might try to willfully destroy evidence. The interesting thing about electronic devices is that sometimes just a small ESD will make the evidence unreadable, but other times even throwing a device in a bonfire won't destroy the device enough to delete any data.

The question is often: how do we handle damaged devices so we minimize the risk of losing data? What we do with the device depends on which acquisition method we are going to use. It doesn't matter if the screen is broken if we are going to remove the memory chip anyway.

6.2.9.1 External Force

External force is a common way to damage devices. It might arise from accidents, or even attempts to destroy evidence. For example, a device might be dropped to the ground or thrown at a wall, or the SIM card or memory card can be chewed. A broken screen or input device might be repaired by exchanging the broken parts with new ones. One should be careful if the part that is exchanged has its own memory or digital ID that might interfere with the data stored on the device.

If the PCB is broken and for some reason one can't read the memory chip, one can try to remove the memory chip, reball[22] it, and solder it on a new PCB. This should be tested on a similar device before attempting to do it with potential evidence. When a suspect tries to destroy a device, he or she will often try to damage it by force. The PCB will be damaged, but the memory chip is often still intact.

Furthermore, if the memory chip is damaged, there are some possibilities to repair the chip, depending on the type of equipment the laboratory has. If the soldering pads are broken, one can try different techniques to get a good enough electrical connection. If the bonding threads are damaged but the die itself is undamaged, it may be possible to bond new threads to the die.

Figure 6.36 shows a mobile phone that has been subject to external force. In this case, a bullet from a pistol has passed through the phone and the PCB. The memory chip was, however, still intact, and could be read by a chip-off procedure.

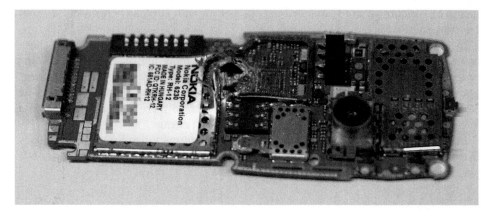

Figure 6.36 A mobile phone with damage from a bullet.

---

22 To resolder tiny balls to the soldering pads of the IC package.

With sufficient temperature, any electronic device will be destroyed. Luckily, the temperature that electronics is exposed to is typically not high enough. Even if the equipment is left in a fire, the cover can melt and protect the ICs on the inside. In the field, we have seen both memory chips in mobile phones and hard disks in video surveillance equipment that have survived fires. On the other hand, we have also seen equipment that has been thrown into a fireplace and been completely disintegrated by the fire.

In order to repair equipment damaged in a fire, one can first remove the damaged parts and clean the parts that look intact. If he proves lucky, most of the inside will still be working, and possibly only a few parts need to be changed, such as keyboards or displays. As said previously, if the PCB is damaged, one can do a chip-off, as the memory chip might still be intact.

6.2.9.2 Water, Liquids, and Blood

After a broken enclosure, perhaps the most common damage to an embedded device is water damage. There are many ways moisture can end up in a device. One can drop it into the water or store the device in a moist place (like a pocket during physical activity), or it can be soaked in bodily fluids in a number of ways. Bringing a device from a cold to a warm place will create condensation.

The most common damage for electronic circuits that have been in water is oxidation of the electrical conducting materials. This process happens much faster when we add water-soluble salts, electric potential, and oxygen in the mix. This means that if we find some electronic device submerged in saltwater with a battery connected and pull it out of the water, into the air, we have all the ingredients we need for damaging the device beyond repair in a short time. Blood also contains salts and makes a conducting liquid. It is not, however, only the oxidation process that makes an electric potential damaging; the device might short-circuit such that more current will pass through sensitive components than it can withstand.

The procedure for handling water (or moisture) damaged devices is, then: remove the battery or other electric power sources. Next, make sure that the oxidation process proceeds as slowly as possible before we can clean the device. For submerged devices, this means that one should not add oxygen by pulling the device out of the water.

When the device is in the lab, we can start cleaning. Disassemble the device as much as possible. Remove any salts from the device by cleaning it in isopropyl alcohol or deionized water. We can use a supersonic bath or a soft brush to remove debris on the board. At last, we have to dry the device. This can be done by packing it together with desiccants like silica gel bags; also, we can dry it in a vacuum chamber, or bake it in an oven at a low temperature.

6.2.10 Wrapping It Up

We have now seen many different techniques for acquiring data, and a few considerations before starting the acquisition. In this section, we set this into some context so it will be easier to remember the key points.

6.2.10.1 Matrix of Information Availability

As discussed in Chapter 2, there are many factors to keep in mind during the collection stage of the forensic process in order to ensure the availability of the information in a device.[23] All the factors that affect the availability of the information will often have interdependencies that one has to take into consideration during the planning of the collection step. These also cover mobile and embedded devices. It is important to remember that it is not just the data alone that is important, but also the information that is stored or encoded in the data.

Just as in a computer system, one needs to take into account the order of volatility. This will affect how fast the data can disappear, if it is possible to cut the power or not, and how quickly one must collect the information from the device.

For mobile and embedded systems, access restrictions and encryption are challenges that often arise. PIN codes block access to the available interfaces. In the last few years, encryption on mobile phones has become more common, which represents a challenge, especially for chip-off methods.

Then there is a catch-22 factor that arises from the state of the device; we can call it the *powered versus shutdown* factor. Automatic processes in the OS or firmware will overwrite data if one keeps the device on, and they will overwrite data if we shut it down. The processes in question can, for example, be garbage collection, automatic updating of logs, and updating of GPS track data. The question is this: which of these will overwrite the least amount of data, and the least important data? Pulling the battery will make sure the shutdown process won't run, but data held in RAM will not be synced to nonvolatile memory.

The next two factors deal with the interfaces and protocols that are actually available for us to use. Does the investigator have access to a physical dump, or only a logical copy of the data? If the only interface available is a numeric keyboard and a 7-segment display, the information one can acquire is often different than if one has a JTAG interface available. The communication protocols are also important – a USB interface can provide several protocols that each access data on different levels.

As related to the interface factor, we can look at the lab resources available. Does the lab have the equipment, staff, and training to do all the operations needed to get access to the data from a given interface? Even though the flash memory is a well-known chip, one might not have the resources available to do a chip-off acquisition.

At last, we can look at the interpretation factor. Is the investigator able, given some acquired data, to interpret the information stored or encoded in the data? This means that investigators should acquire data in a form they are able to understand. For example, a video surveillance system might store data internally in a proprietary format, but export it either in a known video format or together with player software. If one acquires the raw data, it may be necessary to reverse engineer[24] the format, and transcode it to a format that can be played using available software.

As an example of how these factors affect each other, we can think of a situation where an investigator has a mobile phone believed to contain a deleted text message and a video clip stored on the internal flash chip. If he does a logical acquisition, he will surely get the video file, but the automatic processes going while the phone is powered on might overwrite the deleted text message. On the other hand, if he does a chip-off and acquires the raw NAND data, he has a better probability of finding the deleted text message, as

---

23 The term *information* here means something like "meaning" or "data with meaning," not necessarily the same as the term *information* in Shannon's information theory.
24 *Reverse engineering* is to find the functionality or data formats a program used.

this data typically fits in one page on the flash, but he might have problems reassembling the video that is spread over several memory pages if the FTL or file system is unknown. It might not be possible to reverse engineer it within a reasonable amount of time.

6.2.10.2   Cheat Sheet
Table 6.8 gives an overview of the different methods together with a few advantages and disadvantages.

6.2.10.3   On or Off?
Now that we have more understanding of the technical details and the strength and weaknesses of the different methods to acquire data, we can also more easily consider what to do with a device when one is found.

Even if the power is cut, there might be a backup battery that keeps the system running, and it can even overwrite important data. Devices that seem to be off, with turned-off displays or lights, can still be running. Even when the device is apparently off and the OS seems to be shut down, the flash controller can still be reordering pages as long as it has power.

Example 6.3: Alarm Central

Our laboratory examined an alarm central in a Norwegian case, where all information stored in the flash were alarm messages for the missing main power every few seconds. These messages were generated after the crime scene investigator, who wasn't aware of the backup battery inside the device, cut the power in order to send the alarm central to the forensic laboratory.

First of all, see if the system contains any access restriction mechanisms, like passwords or PIN codes. It is important to be careful to verify that access codes actually work before turning the device off if one is going to acquire data by booting the OS. A passcode is usually a precondition for encryption, but newer iPhones (from 3GS and up) will encrypt the data even without a PIN code. If given a PIN code, verify that it is the right code before locking the device or turning it off; this can typically be done by trying to disable the access code.

The next question is whether to do a physical, logical, or pseudo-physical acquisition. If choosing a physical or pseudo-physical acquisition, it is best to power off the device, as more data will be intact. If one instead has to do a logical acquisition, turning the device on or off might trigger cleanup procedures that overwrite traces. Keeping a device on might also trigger garbage collection in the device. On the other hand, most logical acquisitions won't acquire deleted data, so this won't necessarily pose a big problem. The rule of thumb can therefore be: turn the device off, or remove the battery if it is not going to be acquired at once.

If we have to turn the device on before acquisition, it is a good idea to either remove the SIM card so it won't be able to communicate over a network when powered on, or enable flight mode before shutting the device off.

If the device can't be turned off and one can't acquire the data on-site, it is possible to transport the device isolated from any networks by storing it in a Faraday bag. This is an

Table 6.8   An overview of various acquisition methods.

Method	Advantage	Disadvantage
Chip-off	Acquire deleted data. Can bypass access codes.	Need advanced resources, equipment, time, and knowledge. Can't decrypt hardware-encrypted data during read process. Usually need datasheet for memory module. Destructive procedure. Can't acquire nonvolatile memory.
JTAG	Can read raw flash through processor. Can debug boot chain and OS. Can change behavior of running system. Don't need as much equipment as chip-off. Can acquire volatile memory.	Can be hard to find JTAG interface. Many devices have disabled JTAG or use security settings. Can be slow to read flash directly. Can be time-consuming.
Device backup	Accessible from a paired computer; contains much user data. Can trigger device to hand out a fresh backup. Can find backups in cloud storage.	Backup can be encrypted. Need a paired device. No deleted data, unless deleted between two backups.
OBEX	Standardized protocol. Supported by many phones.	Only a few object types can be transferred. No deleted data.
AT commands	Standardized protocol. Often easy to use on older or simple phones.	No deleted data. Some phones don't reveal a serial interface directly. Only some types of information are supported.
ADB	Easy connection. Have commands for acquiring files.	OS running, might have to change settings on the phone to turn on USB debugging. If no root, no deleted data. Only partial nondeleted data.
Manual inspection	Simple procedure, quick access.	Might take a considerable amount of time to report if many traces. Error prone; no deleted data; examination will change data.
Rooted dd	With root over ADB, can get access to block device and get deleted data.	Need to change the running software in order to get root. Different exploits for different phones. Not all devices have known exploits. OS has to be running.
Boot loader	The OS is not running; can acquire raw flash. Connection usually over USB.	In many devices, the device needs to be factory reset in order to unlock the secure boot chain. Might brick the device.
Flasher tools	Inexpensive, somewhat easy to connect. Often get a raw dump of the storage device. Uses various techniques.	Not the best-quality assurance process before shipped. Often bugs. Errors in manuals. "Get what you pay for." If not tested properly, can delete user data.
Commercial forensic products	Uses many techniques. Easy to use. Minimizes risk of overwriting data. Usually good documentation.	Implements the techniques they know, not necessarily most forensically sound. Can misinterpret data. Different products support different devices.

RF-shielded bag, such that the device won't be able to connect to wireless networks. Be aware that for a mobile phone, this will impact the battery time considerably, as the phone will try to connect to the network at maximum transmitting power. If we use cables to charge the phone while it is in the shielded container, be aware that the cable itself might act as an antenna.

6.3 Examination Phase

After extracting data from a device, the next step is to interpret the data. In this section, we look at the examination from two angles. One is the *top-down* approach. The "top" in this case is from the point of view of the embedded OS. This way will interpret the data as the OS sees it, or has seen it, building up the data structures and putting the data nicely into each structure as it fits. We can rebuild a file system and look at the data inside, or reverse engineer a specific protocol or file format such that one is able to interpret the acquired data. Sometimes, the protocols, file system, or format is completely unknown, and there isn't time to analyze and find out exactly the format. In these cases, one can quickly search for data that looks interesting, and instead figure out what we have found later.

Bottom-up in this chapter refers to the approach that first prioritizes interesting data or structures (on the bottom), and then tries to figure out what they mean (toward the top). Two methods are described here: looking for specific patterns that match known structures, and looking for specific known information and then interpreting the context of the information. The former method is called "*carving*, and the latter a *keyword search*.

When interpreting data, either from a commercial tool or from our own analysis, it is important to cross-reference the data with external sources or the investigative hypothesis. Sometimes the hypothesis is wrong; sometimes the external sources are wrong. Often, our own assumptions and interpretations are wrong and have to be corrected.

In this section, you will learn:

- How data is stored on the flash memory
- Flash translation layers and file systems
- Carving and keyword search.

6.3.1 Top-Down: Flash Translation Layer (FTL)

When acquiring data from a hard disk drive in a computer, it is important to remove the drive, connect it to another computer through a write blocker, and make a bit-by-bit exact copy of the hard disk drive. While making this copy, a hash of the copied data will be calculated and stored in order to ensure evidence integrity. After this procedure, one should employ other programs to interpret the partition table and file system(s) in the image file. In this way, one won't change the data while looking at it, and one will also be able to see deleted files and other data that might be hidden by, for instance, a root kit. A memory chip from a mobile phone can work similarly, but the data pass through another layer on the way from the raw flash to the file system driver. This layer is called a *flash translation layer*.

In order to understand the peculiarities of the data from a flash memory chip, we have to understand the inner workings of NAND flash memory.

In NAND flash, each bit can only be flipped from 1 to 0.[25] This is called *programming*. To change a bit from 0 to 1, one must flip a whole erase block to 1. This is called *erasing*.

---

25 1 is the default value in NAND flash. All bits in an unused page are therefore filled with 1 (or each byte is *FF* in hexadecimal).

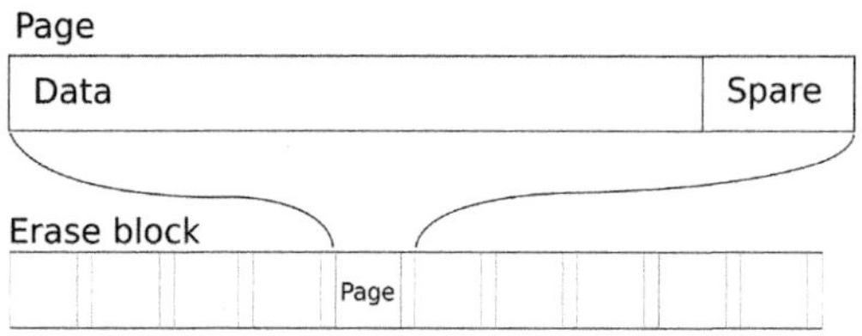

Page

Data	Spare

Erase block

Page

Figure 6.37 Erase block, pages, and spare area.

Flash memory is built by pages of data; these are typically 512 or 2048 bytes, and they also have some extra bytes per page. This extra data is often called *spare area* or *out-of-band* (OOB) area. A typical size for the spare area is 16 bytes per 512-byte page (or 64 bytes for a 2048-byte page). An erase block consists of several pages. One NAND flash chip from Spansion (S34ML04G1) has 2048 + 64 byte sectors, and an erase block is 64 pages, which are typical numbers for NAND flash memory. For the flash memory, the spare area is just a part of the addressable address space. It is the NAND flash driver that makes this area special, and uses it for an internal purpose. Just as a sector is the smallest writable area on a hard disk, a page is the smallest programmable area in a NAND flash memory. Figure 6.37 provides a schematic drawing of how the pages, spare area, and erase blocks fit together.

Flash memory is fragile. It can be programmed and erased just a number of times before it is expected to fail. For NAND type flash, this limit is typically 100,000 program–erase cycles (P/E cycles). To optimize the life expectancy for the memory, it is better to spread these cycles over all the blocks such that all blocks will wear out simultaneously. If one block is written and erased more often than other blocks, this block will be the limiting factor for the lifetime of the device. The FTL is a layer between the raw flash device and the file system that will spread the writes to the device, transparent to the file system above. Imagine a program writing one byte every minute to a file that spans an entire erase block in flash. Without wear leveling, the same erase block will be erased and written to every time. The lifetime of the memory will be:

$$\frac{100\,000\frac{PE\ Cycles}{fail}}{60\frac{PE\ Cycles}{hour}\times 24\frac{hours}{day}} = 69.4\frac{days}{fail}$$

There are several ways to optimize this number. For one, it is not necessary to write the whole file every time; one can write just the page that contains the change. If the block size is 64 pages, it isn't actually necessary to erase a block before it is filled up with 64 versions of the changed pages. Furthermore, one doesn't need to erase the same block every time, but can instead spread the P/E cycles to all available blocks. Let's assume we have 100 blocks available. The formula will be like this:

$$FR\times\frac{\frac{PB\times B_{availible}}{P_{used}}}{W_{freq}}$$

where FR is the failure rate (P/E cycles per fail), PB is the number of pages per block, P_{used} is the number of pages used in each programming operation, $B_{available}$ is the number of erase blocks available for wear leveling, and W_{freq} is the frequency of the programming operations. The example shows that:

$$\frac{100000 \frac{PE\ cycles}{fail} \times \frac{64 \frac{pages}{block} \times 100\ blocks}{1\ page}}{60 \frac{PE\ cycles}{hour} \times 24 \frac{hours}{day} \times 365.24 \frac{days}{year}} \approx 1217 \frac{years}{fail}$$

We see that it is a huge advantage to spread the writing over the whole memory chip.

In addition to wear leveling, the FTL often has other functions, like bad block management and error correction. A NAND flash device will have bad blocks already from the factory, and will continue to fail during the lifetime of the chip. The spare areas (OOB) for the pages are often used for managing the FTL, ordering the pages, marking pages dirty/ready for erasing, and so on.

Unfortunately, the flash management algorithms are often considered trade secrets, and companies making these algorithms will seldom reveal more of the inner workings of their intellectual property than they have to in order to ensure interoperability with other devices.

6.3.2 Top-Down: Flash File Systems

The advantage with using an FTL is that the file system doesn't need to know anything about the flash layout. There also exist file systems that are designed for use on a flash device, and include the functionality of the FTL. Figure 6.38 shows how the different file system models look schematically, showing an ordinary hard disk drive with a common hard disk drive file system at the left side. Examples of file systems that are made for flash memory are YAFFS, JFFS, JFFS2, and UBIFS.[26]

There are also other types of file systems found on embedded devices, like SquashFS, a compressed file system often used for static data like part of the OS or firmware. This doesn't store user data or logs, so it is just important to know about in case one wishes to reverse engineer parts of the OS or applications.

One of the differences between an ordinary file system and the flash file system is the integrated wear-leveling algorithms and bad block management. The OOB area will

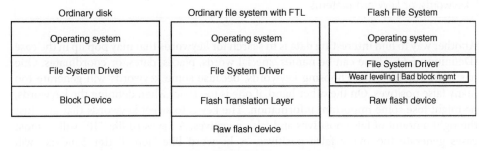

Figure 6.38 File systems on top of an FTL and a flash-aware file system.

___

26 UBIFS is the successor of JFFS2.

often be used for storing management data for these algorithms, as there is no FTL under the flash file system. As an example of a file system designed for flash, we take a closer look at YAFFS in Section 6.3.5.

6.3.3 Bottom-Up: Carving

Definition 6.5: Carving

Carving is a method that looks for data that fits into known file structures or other data structures, and interprets the data in light of these structures.

In order to find a file of a given file type, we can look for the known file header that includes the size of the file, and see if the rest of the file follows. How the file system actually stores the data will have an impact on the assumptions one can make about the layout of the data: a hard disk drive will try to store data sequentially because the read and write operations are faster at sequential access, and the OS wants to optimize the read and write time. For a flash drive, as we discussed, the optimization is focused on maximizing the lifetime of the device, and there is no added latency when accessing nonsequential pages. (See Definition 6.5.)

If the data we are looking for is stored in flash memory in a record that is smaller than the page size, the probability for finding data is better than if the data instead spanned several pages. A video will typically span several hundreds or thousands of pages, and for this reason has a large probability of fragmentation. A raw PDU for a text message will be less than 200 bytes, and will therefore have less probability of fragmentation.

As examples of structures that often are found in mobile and embedded devices, we look at SMS PDU in Section 6.3.7, and SQLite databases in Section 6.3.8.

6.3.4 Bottom-Up: Keyword Search

Definition 6.6: Keyword Search

A keyword search is a search for content that matches one or more keywords, parts of keywords, or keyword patterns.

Another way to find interesting data is to search for keywords that may pop up in the case (Definition 6.6). These can be names, special words, places, dates, or coordinates. One has to be careful when choosing keywords, because some keywords will generate too many false positives. On the other hand, if one is too strict when defining the keywords, he might lose some important information. The key is to select keywords that give just the right amount of false positives and false negatives. A keyword like "JP" will in most cases generate too many false positives. A keyword like "Jens-Petter Sandvik" will probably generate too many false negatives. A tip is to refine the search as one sees too many or too few search hits.

It is a fuzzy line between keyword search and carving. If one searches for regular expressions (regex), we often refer to this as *keyword search*, but as a regex is actually pattern matching, we see that we also can refer to this as *carving*. Often we use the term *keyword search* to mean finding data matching known data, and the term *carving* to mean finding structures matching known structures.

One thing to take into consideration is packed data. Some data is stored as Base64, ZIP, uuencoded, HTML-escaped, or other packed formats.[27] Depending on what one looks for, it might be necessary to unpack what one can find of packed data before searching for keywords.

An example of a program that does this is Bulk Extractor (Garfinkel, 2013). This program automates the process of scanning and unpacking data. As Bulk Extractor doesn't rebuild the file system, it will be susceptible to file fragmentation. Another caveat is that it splits the input into smaller blocks, and if the container is bigger than such a block, it won't be able to unpack the last part.

6.3.5 Technical Deep-Dive: FTL from Nokia 7610 Supernova

One example of an FTL we can look at is from a Nokia 7610 Supernova phone. This is a model from 2008, and the OS in this phone is Intelligent System Architecture (ISA), a Nokia proprietary OS. On top of this OS is the Series 40 platform and user interface.

The address space of the flash chip is split into two parts. First is a file system for static data such as boot loader, firmware, and OS. The partition we are interested in is the second partition. Each erase block is 0x20000 (131,072) bytes long, and each block has an 8-byte header. The first four bytes tell which partition this block belongs to. The one we are interested in has the value "F0 F0 01 00."

Within each erase block, there are pages that are 512+8 bytes. Each start with an 8-byte page header. The first 4 bytes tell if the sector is in use, is free, or is deleted. If the page is in use, the last 4 bytes in the header count as the index for this page. Figure 6.39 shows the erase block header and the page header for the first page in the file system. We see that the page index is "00 00 00 00," signifying the first page. Next, at location 0x22c0010, comes the page data; in this case, one can easily identify a FAT Boot Parameter Block in the boot sector.

By scanning the whole area for the erase blocks assigned to the right file system, scanning for the used pages within each erase block, and sorting the indexes, we can create a new binary file containing a FAT partition. Figure 6.40 shows this file system after it has been rebuilt.

Note that this FTL does not fit into the 512+16-byte scheme we said the flash usually has. It is important to remember that it is the driver that handles the layout of the FTL.

```
022C0000   F0 F0 01 00 00 FF 00 00   F0 FF FF FF 00 00 00 00   ðð    ÿ  ðÿÿÿ
022C0010   EB FE 90 66 73 69 6D 35   2E 36 30 00 02 01 01 00   ëþ fsim5.60
022C0020   02 00 02 40 E2 F8 E3 00   20 00 02 00 00 00 00 00     @âøã
022C0030   00 00 00 00 00 00 29 78   56 34 12 56 4F 4C 55 4D   )x V4 VOLUM
022C0040   45 4C 41 42 45 4C 46 41   54 31 36 20 20 20 00 00   ELABELFAT16
```

Figure 6.39 Erase block header for the first block in the file system.

---

27 Other containers might be virtual disks, compressed file systems, etc. This is not often seen in embedded systems, though.

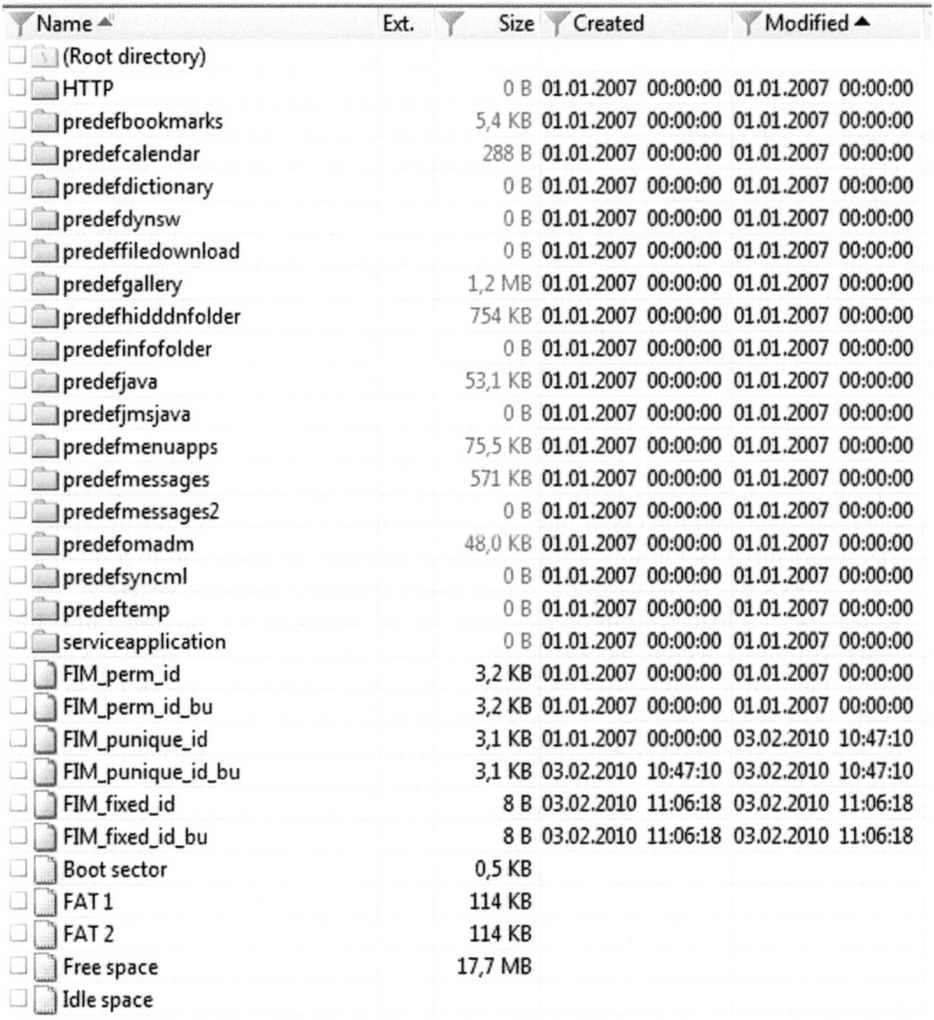

Name ▲	Ext.	Size	Created	Modified ▲
☐ ▣ (Root directory)				
☐ ▣ HTTP		0 B	01.01.2007 00:00:00	01.01.2007 00:00:00
☐ ▣ predefbookmarks		5,4 KB	01.01.2007 00:00:00	01.01.2007 00:00:00
☐ ▣ predefcalendar		288 B	01.01.2007 00:00:00	01.01.2007 00:00:00
☐ ▣ predefdictionary		0 B	01.01.2007 00:00:00	01.01.2007 00:00:00
☐ ▣ predefdynsw		0 B	01.01.2007 00:00:00	01.01.2007 00:00:00
☐ ▣ predeffiledownload		0 B	01.01.2007 00:00:00	01.01.2007 00:00:00
☐ ▣ predefgallery		1,2 MB	01.01.2007 00:00:00	01.01.2007 00:00:00
☐ ▣ predefhidddnfolder		754 KB	01.01.2007 00:00:00	01.01.2007 00:00:00
☐ ▣ predefinfofolder		0 B	01.01.2007 00:00:00	01.01.2007 00:00:00
☐ ▣ predefjava		53,1 KB	01.01.2007 00:00:00	01.01.2007 00:00:00
☐ ▣ predefjmsjava		0 B	01.01.2007 00:00:00	01.01.2007 00:00:00
☐ ▣ predefmenuapps		75,5 KB	01.01.2007 00:00:00	01.01.2007 00:00:00
☐ ▣ predefmessages		571 KB	01.01.2007 00:00:00	01.01.2007 00:00:00
☐ ▣ predefmessages2		0 B	01.01.2007 00:00:00	01.01.2007 00:00:00
☐ ▣ predefomadm		48,0 KB	01.01.2007 00:00:00	01.01.2007 00:00:00
☐ ▣ predefsyncml		0 B	01.01.2007 00:00:00	01.01.2007 00:00:00
☐ ▣ predeftemp		0 B	01.01.2007 00:00:00	01.01.2007 00:00:00
☐ ▣ serviceapplication		0 B	01.01.2007 00:00:00	01.01.2007 00:00:00
☐ ▢ FIM_perm_id		3,2 KB	01.01.2007 00:00:00	01.01.2007 00:00:00
☐ ▢ FIM_perm_id_bu		3,2 KB	01.01.2007 00:00:00	01.01.2007 00:00:00
☐ ▢ FIM_punique_id		3,1 KB	01.01.2007 00:00:00	03.02.2010 10:47:10
☐ ▢ FIM_punique_id_bu		3,1 KB	03.02.2010 10:47:10	03.02.2010 10:47:10
☐ ▢ FIM_fixed_id		8 B	03.02.2010 11:06:18	03.02.2010 11:06:18
☐ ▢ FIM_fixed_id_bu		8 B	03.02.2010 11:06:18	03.02.2010 11:06:18
☐ ▢ Boot sector		0,5 KB		
☐ ▢ FAT 1		114 KB		
☐ ▢ FAT 2		114 KB		
☐ ▢ Free space		17,7 MB		
☐ ▢ Idle space				

Figure 6.40 Rebuilt FAT file system.

The 528-byte page is just the smallest programmable entity in the flash. How it is used is up to the driver.

6.3.6 Technical Deep-Dive: Flash File System – YAFFS

The name YAFFS is an acronym for Yet Another Flash File System. The first specification came to light in 2002, and was designed for NAND flash with 512-byte page sizes. Later, YAFFS2 was designed for larger and more heterogeneous devices. YAFFS is a log-structured file system. This means that the file system data and metadata are written sequentially in a ring buffer, called a *log*. There is little metadata about the file system stored on flash. The beauty of log-structured file systems is that one can re-create the state of the file system just by scanning the stored data, and without the use of FATs or similar structures. This makes the file system more robust, or, as it is said in the documentation, "you can't corrupt something you don't store" (Manning, 2012). By scanning the file system at mount time, the file system driver builds the structures it needs to effectively manage the file system in RAM. As YAFFS2 is more widely used today, we look more specifically into YAFFS2 here.

In YAFFS, everything in the file system is an object. An object can, for example, be a file, a directory, a link (both hard and soft), a pipe, or a device. Each object has its own unique object ID. An allocation unit in YAFFS is called a *chunk*, and it can span one or more pages in the flash memory. A block is the same as an erase block in NAND flash. Chunks are written sequentially in each block.

When a new block is allocated, the file system increases the file system sequence number. This sequence number is used for keeping a chronological order of the chunks, and one is assigned to each block. Each chunk written to the page will include the file system sequence number, the object ID of the object written, the chunk ID, and ECC data. How this data is stored in the spare area is determined by the NAND driver.

The first chunk of a file (Chunk ID 0) is always an object header. This can be compared to an MFT entry in NTFS, and it contains metadata about the file such as object type, timestamps, filename, size, and so on. Table 6.9 shows the object header structure as it is defined in the YAFFS2 source code.[28] Two of the entries can be of variable size. The type field and the sum_no_longer_used field are defined as an "enum" and an "unsigned short" in the C source code. The enum doesn't need to be longer than 1 byte, and the unsigned int is only guaranteed to be at least 2 bytes long. In some implementations, we see that the unsigned short is in fact 2 bytes, but the compiler stores an additional 2-byte padding somewhere in the structure in order to align the next 4-byte integer to a 4-byte boundary.

We see that there are two sets of timestamps in the object header structure: one set of 32-bit values (yst_atime, yst_ctime, and yst_mtime), and one set of 64-bit values (win_ctime, win_atime, and win_mtime). There is only one set of timestamps in use in any OS. Windows will use the 64-bit values, and various Linux versions will use the 32-bit set of timestamps.

Figure 6.41 shows the start of an object header from a Huawei Android phone. The file name is at offset 0x0593064a, and says "nandread." Incidentally, this is the program used for acquiring the flash memory on this phone. We see the padding ("FF FF") after the 256-byte string buffer, at offset 0x0593074a. Note that offsets in the raw NAND dump are shown on the left side.

To understand the file system better, let us see what happens when doing a couple of hypothetical file operations, as shown in Table 6.10 Note that this is a simplified look at the process, where a block only contains four chunks: we create a file, write a couple of chunks, update the data in the second data chunk, and then delete the file. The background color in the table shows which chunks are written at each step (darker means older), and the last row is the current, valid chunk.

From a forensic perspective, we can see a couple of interesting things here. First, there exist two versions of this file, and both versions can be restored, with all metadata information intact for all versions. As each chunk is written sequentially in each block, and the order of the blocks can be identified based on the file system sequence number, we can re-create all changes in the right order.

---

28 From yaffs_guts.h, by yaffs.org.

Table 6.9 Objects as they are stored in flash (two of the values are compiler specific).

Offset	Size (bytes)	Name
0x0000	4 (can be 1 or 2)	Type
0x0004	4	parent_obj_id
0x0008	2 (can be 4)	sum_no_longer_used
0x000a	256	Name
0x010a	2	Padding (compiler dependent)
0x010c	4	yst_mode
0x0110	4	yst_uid
0x0114	4	yst_gid
0x0118	4	yst_atime
0x011c	4	yst_mtime
0x0120	4	yst_ctime
0x0124	4	file_size_low
0x0128	4	equiv_id
0x012c	160	alias
0x01cc	4	yst_rdev
0x01d0	8	win_ctime
0x01d8	8	win_atime
0x01e0	8	win_mtime
0x01e8	4	inband_shadowed_obj_id
0x01ec	4	inband_is_shrink
0x01f0	4	file_size_high
0x01f4	4	reserved
0x01f8	4	shadows_obj
0x01fc	4	is_shrink

```
05930640  01 00 00 00 0E 01 00 00 FF FF 6E 61 6E 64 72 65   ........ÿÿnandre
05930650  61 64 00 00 00 00 00 00 00 00 00 00 00 00 00 00   ad..............
05930660  00 00 00 00 00 00 00 00 00 00 00 00 00 00 00 00   ................
05930670  00 00 00 00 00 00 00 00 00 00 00 00 00 00 00 00   ................
05930680  00 00 00 00 00 00 00 00 00 00 00 00 00 00 00 00   ................
05930690  00 00 00 00 00 00 00 00 00 00 00 00 00 00 00 00   ................
059306A0  00 00 00 00 00 00 00 00 00 00 00 00 00 00 00 00   ................
059306B0  00 00 00 00 00 00 00 00 00 00 00 00 00 00 00 00   ................
059306C0  00 00 00 00 00 00 00 00 00 00 00 00 00 00 00 00   ................
059306D0  00 00 00 00 00 00 00 00 00 00 00 00 00 00 00 00   ................
059306E0  00 00 00 00 00 00 00 00 00 00 00 00 00 00 00 00   ................
059306F0  00 00 00 00 00 00 00 00 00 00 00 00 00 00 00 00   ................
05930700  00 00 00 00 00 00 00 00 00 00 00 00 00 00 00 00   ................
05930710  00 00 00 00 00 00 00 00 00 00 00 00 00 00 00 00   ................
05930720  00 00 00 00 00 00 00 00 00 00 00 00 00 00 00 00   ................
05930730  00 00 00 00 00 00 00 00 00 00 00 00 00 00 00 00   ................
05930740  00 00 00 00 00 00 00 00 00 00 FF FF ED 81 00 00   ..........ÿÿí...
05930750  D0 07 00 00 D0 07 00 00 D5 45 17 52 D5 45 17 52   Ð...Ð...ÕE.RÕE.R
05930760  93 40 D5 12 F3 B6 00 00 FF FF FF FF FF FF FF FF   "@Õ.ó¶..ÿÿÿÿÿÿÿÿ
```

Figure 6.41 YAFFS2 object header from an Android phone.

Table 6.10 Example of a file being created, written to, edited, and deleted in YAFFS2.

FS Seq. no.	Chunk no.	Object ID	Chunk ID	Description
1	0	100	0	Object header (file created, size = 0)
1	1	100	1	First data chunk
1	2	100	2	Second data chunk
1	3	100	0	Object header (file written)
2	0	100	2	Second data chunk updated
2	1	100	0	Object header (file written)
2	2	100	0	Object header (file truncated and unlinked)

This brings us to the second interesting finding, which unfortunately doesn't make things any easier for us. We see that none of the chunks in block 1 are valid anymore. This means that this block is marked as dirty and can be erased by the garbage collector when it needs a new block. If there are many blocks with only a few valid chunks, and the system is running low on free blocks, the garbage collector can start moving valid data to new blocks in order to free more blocks.

In order to re-create the deleted or changed files, we can do almost the same as the driver will do when scanning the file system during mount time. We make a list of the blocks in the order of the file system sequence, and then start scanning backward. The object headers and file data chunks we find first are the valid ones. The ones we find after this, with the same object ID and chunk ID, are deleted data. The file system driver will discard these, but we can use them to re-create the changed and deleted files instead.

6.3.7 Technical Deep-Dive: Structure – SMS PDU

SMS messages are often found in their raw format on devices. This format is also called a SMS PDU (Short Messaging Service Protocol Data Unit). Even though the SMS messaging program on the phone stores the data in various internal formats, we can also often find the raw PDU as it is sent from or received by the phone. With the rising popularity of smartphones, we see that more of the written communication is sent using other applications over the Internet instead of traditional SMS. Regardless of this, there is still a huge amount of communication over SMS.

When a SMS is sent, it is first sent to a SMSC (Short Messaging Service Center), where it is stored and sent to the recipient. If the recipient can't get the SMS (because the phone is turned off or out of coverage, or for some other reason), the SMSC will store the message for a predefined time and try to deliver it within this time. If the message still can't be delivered, it will be discarded. The format in which the SMS is sent is called a TPDU (Transport PDU). The standard uses the term *octet* to mean an 8-bit value, and *septet* to mean a 7-bit value. We will adapt the terminology here when discussing SMS.

An SMS-DELIVER message is a message that has been received on the phone, while a SMS_SUBMIT message is sent from the phone (or Mobile Station, as it is called in the specification). There are also four more formats defined in the standard: three report types (SMS-DELIVER-REPORT, SMS-SUBMIT-REPORT, and SMS-STATUS-

Table 6.11 SMS_DELIVER PDU fields.

Type	Name	Description	Size	M/O
TP-MTI	TP-Message-Type-Indicator	Message type (00 for SMS-DELIVER)	2 bit	M
TP-MMS	TP-More-Messages-to-Send	Indicates more messages	1 bit	M
TP-LP	TP-Loop-Prevention	Doesn't forward or inhibit automatic message generation	1 bit	O
TP-RP	TP-Reply-Path	Reply path exists	1 bit	M
TP-UDHI	TP-User-Data-Header-Indicator	TP-UD-field contains a header	1 bit	O
TP-SRI	TP-Status-Report-Indication	Sender has requested status report	1 bit	O
TP-OA	TP-Originating-Address	Address of the originating sender	2–12 oct	M
TP-PID	TP-Protocol-Identifier	The above layer protocol	Octet	M
TP-DCS	TP-Data-Coding-Scheme	Coding scheme of TP-UD	Octet	M
TP-SCTS	TP-Service-Center-Time-Stamp	Time when the service center received the message	7 oct	M
TP-UDL	TP-User-Data-Length	Length of the user data	Integer	M
TP-UD	TP-User-Data	Payload	Variable	O

REPORT) and one for sending commands to the service center (SMS-COMMAND). We only look at the two PDUs that are used for the actual text messages here. The formats for these two types are slightly different. We can first have a look at the TPDU for SMS-DELIVER messages, or messages received on the phone. TP in all the fields means *Transport Layer Protocol*, and M/O stands for *mandatory or optional*, as shown in Table 6.11.

The SMS-SUBMIT are messages that are sent from the phone, and these contain the fields, as shown in Table 6.12.

The first field in the PDU is the TP-MTI field, as shown in Table 6.11 and Table 6.12. The values this field can have are outlined in Table 6.13. The abbreviation SC in the table is for *Service Center*.

The TP-VPF field, found in the SMS_SUBMIT PDU, describes the size of the TP-VP field. This value can have the four values, as shown in Table 6.14.

The TP-VP field does not contain a record of the time of when the message has been sent, but may still give some clues if it is in absolute format (the value 11). This is the only format that contains a timestamp; the other formats only give the time relative to when the service center receives the message. Depending on the device, this field might be a set delay offset from the sending time. If the field is used for examination, it should be tested on a similar device first.

The TP-Originating-Address and TP-Destination-Address are given as Address fields. These fields contain one Address-Length field (one octet), one Type-of-Address field (one octet), and one Address-Value (variable length).

The Address-Length contains the length in number of *semi-octets*, or *nibbles* (4-bit values). If the number is odd, it means it will be one 4-bit value that is padded with binary 1111.

Table 6.12   SMS_SUBMIT PDU fields.

Type	Name	Description	Size	M/O
TP-MTI	TP-Message-Type-Indicator	The message type (01 for SMS-SUBMT)	2 bit	M
TP-RD	TP-Reject-Duplicates	Flag to instruct the service center to reject messages with the same TP-MR and TP-DA as previously sent message	1 bit	M
TP-VPF	TP-Validity-Period-Format	Is TP-VP field present	2 bit	M
TP-RP	TP-Reply-Path	Request for reply path	1 bit	M
TP-UDHI	TP-User-Data-Header-Indicator	TP-UD-field contains a header	1 bit	O
TP-SRR	TP-Status-Report-Request	MS requests a status report	1 bit	O
TP-MR	TP-Message-Reference	A value that is incremented for each message sent, identifying the message	Integer	M
TP-DA	TP-Destination-Address	Address of the destination Short Message Entity (SME)	2–12 oct	M
TP-PID	TP-Protocol-Identifier	The above layer protocol	Octet	M
TP-DCS	TP-Data-Coding-Scheme	Coding scheme in the TP-UD	Octet	M
TP-VP	TP-Validity-Period	Time when the message is no longer valid	oct/7 oct	O
TP-UDL	TP-User-Data-Length	Length of TP-UD-field	Integer	M
TP-UD	TP-User-Data	User data	Variable	O

Table 6.13   TP_MTI fields (Transport Protocol Message Type Indicator).

TP-MTI bit1, bit2	From SC to MS	From MS to SC
00	SMS-DELIVER	SMS-DELIVER-REPORT
10	SMS-STATUS-REPORT	SMS-COMMAND
01	SMS-SUBMIT-REPORT	SMS-SUBMIT
11	Reserved	Reserved

Table 6.14   TP_VPF (Transport Protocol Validity Period Format).

TP-VPF bit4, bit3	Description	TP-VP size
00	TP-VP field not present	0
10	TP-VP field relative format	1 octet
01	TP-VP field enhanced format	7 octets
11	TP-VP field absolute format	7 octets

Table 6.15 Type-of-address octet, with one 3-bit type of number, and one 4-bit numbering plan.

Bit 6, 5, 4	Description	Bit 3, 2, 1, 0	Description
000	Unknown (user or network have no information about the numbering plan)	0000	Unknown
001	International number	0001	ISDN/telephone number
010	National number	0011	Data numbering plan
011	Network specific number	0100	Telex numbering plan
100	Subscriber number	0101	Service center specific plan
101	Alphanumeric (7-bit encoding)	0110	Service center specific plan
110	Abbreviated number	1000	National numbering plan
111	Reserved for extension	1001	Private numbering plan
		1010	ERMES (European Radio Messaging System) numbering plan
		1111	Reserved for extension
		All others	Reserved

The Type-of Address is actually three bit-fields. The most significant bit is always 1, the next three bits describe the type of number, and the lower four bits describe the numbering plan, as shown in Table 6.15. Note that the most significant bit is always set.

The TP-Service-Center-Timestamp is a valuable source of information. This value is set by an external clock: the service center's clock. For example, by looking at this timestamp with regard to timestamps from the phone and from the telephone providers' traffic data, investigators can see whether the phone has been turned off at some point in time (e.g., TP-SCTS is one value, but the traffic data shows that the phone has received the message later, which correlates to the file times found in the phone) or if the phone's clock has been incorrect (e.g., TP-SCTS is one value, and the same in the traffic data, but the phone's timestamp is incorrect).

The format of the TP-SCTS field is given in *semi-octet representation*. This means that each nibble (4-bit value) has a BCD (Binary Coded Digit) coding.[29] Please be aware that when viewed in a hex viewer, these values seem to be *nibble-swapped*,[30] that is, two and two digits seem to be swapped. So when seen in a hex viewer, the timestamp in ISO format "2015-05-09T23:21:34 + 02:00" is coded as: "51 50 90 32 12 43 80." The last byte is the time zone. The time zone is stored in a signed magnitude representation, where the high bit in the first semi-octet is the sign (1 = minus, 0 = plus). The three last bits in the

---

29 BCD means that each decimal digit is represented by one binary number with the same value. The number 34 will therefore be represented at 0x3 0x4 (or binary "0011" "0100"; we need 4 bits to represent 10 values).

30 A *nibble* often refers to a 4-bit value, or half a byte. *Nibble-swapped* therefore means that we have to swap the nibbles in a byte to get the original value. The value 27, or "1B" in hexadecimal, will be stored as "B1" in the flash memory.

Table 6.16 User Data Header.

Offset	Size	Description
0	1 octet	Length of User Data Header (UDHL)
1	1 octet	Information-Element-Identifier (IEI) "A"
2	1 octet	Length of Information-Element "A"
3	0–n octets	Information-Element "A"
3 + n	1 octet	Information-Element-Identifier "B"
4 + n	1 octet	Length of Information-Element "B"
5 + n	0–m octets	Information-Element "B"
5 + n + m	1 octet	Information-Element-Identifier "C"
. . .	. . .	. . .

first semi-octet and the last semi-octet are the time offset to the number of 15-minute increments; 8 is therefore +2 hours (8∗15 minutes = 2 hours).

We see that sent messages don't contain a timestamp. This can make it more challenging to place carved sent messages on a timeline. We also see that the SMS-SUBMIT contains fields that contain the message reference. This can be used for finding the order of sent messages, but as the field is only one byte, it will therefore only hold values up to 255.

For multipart messages, there is also a User Data Header (UDH) at the start of the user data. This header contains the information shown in Table 6.16.

The list of Information-Element-Identifiers (IEIs) is long, and won't be included here. The most common one for SMS messages is for concatenated SMS messages. The IEI for these messages is "00" or "08," and the length is three or four bytes, respectively. The Information Element contains the bytes shown in Table 6.17.

The last part of decoding the SMS format is the actual message. The message can be stored as 2-octet Unicode characters, but it is often stored as 7-bit encoded text. Each character in this encoding will span 7 bits, or one septet. The SMS message size is 140 octets; this means that a message can contain (140∗8)/7 = 160 characters.[31] Table 6.18 shows the 7-bit default SMS character set.

Table 6.17 Information Element used in UDH.

Size	Description
1 or 2 octets	Reference number (8 or 16 bit)
1 octet	Part number this PDU
1 octet	Total number of parts

---

31 For 2-octet Unicode characters, the limit is 140/2 = 70 characters.

Table 6.18 Default SMS character set.

	0-	1-	2-	3-	4-	5-	6-	7-
-0	@	Δ	SP	0	¡	P	¿	p
-1	£	_	!	1	A	Q	a	q
-2	$	Φ	"	2	B	R	b	r
-3	¥	Γ	#	3	C	S	c	s
-4	è	Λ	¤	4	D	T	d	t
-5	é	Ω	%	5	E	U	e	u
-6	ù	Π	&	6	F	V	f	v
-7	ì	Ψ	'	7	G	W	g	w
-8	ò	Σ	(	8	H	X	h	x
-9	Ç	Θ	)	9	I	Y	i	y
-A	LF	Ξ	*	:	J	Z	j	z
-B	Ø	ESC	+	;	K	Ä	k	ä
-C	ø	Æ	,	<	L	Ö	l	ö
-D	CR	æ	-	=	M	Ñ	m	ñ
-E	Å	ß	.	>	N	Ü	n	ü
-F	å	É	/	?	O	§	o	à

SP, space; CR, carriage return (return to beginning of line); LF, line feed (return to beginning of next line); ESC, escape character (if equipment can't interpret the escape, it should show a space instead).

The characters are stored aligned toward the lower bit number in each octet. The remainder is padded with zeroes. For a single character, it is stored as this table shows:

Bit 8	Bit 7	Bit 6	Bit 5	Bit 4	Bit 3	Bit 2	Bit 1
0	c7	c6	c5	c4	c3	c2	c1

$c7$ is the most significant bit in the 7-bit character, while $c1$ is the least significant. Two characters are stored like this, where c is the first character and d is the second character:

Bit 8	Bit 7	Bit 6	Bit 5	Bit 4	Bit 3	Bit 2	Bit 1
d1	c7	c6	c5	c4	c3	c2	c1
0	0	d7	d6	d5	d4	d3	d2

The string *Yes* ("59 65 73" in hex; see Table 6.18) will be stored like this (with the corresponding letter in parentheses):

Bit 8	Bit 7	Bit 6	Bit 5	Bit 4	Bit 3	Bit 2	Bit 1
1 (e)	1 (Y)	0 (Y)	1 (Y)	1 (Y)	0 (Y)	0 (Y)	1 (Y)
1 (s)	1 (s)	1 (e)	1 (e)	0 (e)	0 (e)	1 (e)	0 (e)
0	0	0	1 (s)	1 (s)	1 (s)	0 (s)	0 (s)

or in hexadecimal notation as "D9 F2 1C." The three leading zeroes in the last line are the padding.

The GSM standard can be somewhat hard to read as there are many abbreviations and references that can be hard to remember. We still try to give an overview of a small part of the SMS specification, however, as it is a format one will often see when examining mobile phones. For more information, please refer to the technical specifications [3rd Generation Partnership Program (3GPP), 2015].

6.3.8   Technical Deep-Dive: Structure – SQLite3 Database

In mobile devices, especially Android phones, one often finds user data in SQLite 3 databases. The API makes it easy for apps to store both configuration and user data in SQLite. SQLite is a well-documented format, and details of all the data structures can be found in the sqlite.org webpage (SQLite, 2016).

An SQLite 3 database consist of pages that are of size 2^n bytes, where $9 \leq n \leq 16$ (i.e., the size is between 512 and 65536 bytes). All pages in a database are of equal size. SQLite supports either a legacy rollback journal (file name ending with "-journal"), or a write-ahead log (file name ending with ".WAL"). The rollback journal writes unmodified pages to a journal file before writing the changes, so the changes can always be rolled back. The write-ahead log does the opposite as the new data is written to a WAL file, and is only written back to the database during a checkpoint operation. We can see that in both scenarios, there might be valuable information in either type of file.

The header is located in the first page and is 100 bytes long. It is shown in Table 6.19.[32]

All numbers in SQLite are big-Endian. The page size at offset 16 will tell if each page will be fragmented over several flash pages, or if each page will fit nicely into one flash page. Figure 6.42 shows a hex dump of the header of a database from an Android phone. We can see that offset 0x10 contains the values "04 00" – that is, 0x400, or 1024 bytes per page. Furthermore, it is clear that the database has been changed and flushed eight times. This number won't tell us the exact number of changes, as several changes can happen before the file is closed or flushed. In WAL-mode, the counter might not be updated at all. Even though the number has some significant shortcomings, it can give an indication of how much the file has changed.

The in-header database size might be stored in the header; but if one isn't available, SQLite will use the file size instead, making this value optional. In the example, it is set to 0. The schema cookie is increased each time the schema changes; here, we see that it is set to 7. At offset 0x38, we can see the encoding used in the database; in the example, the value is 1, which means UTF-8. The header might tell us about the various settings for the database, but what about the data? What does it look like, and how can we search for it?

A b-tree is a data structure where each inner node has keys that separate and sort the nodes, or children, under it (Knuth, 1998). This is a common data structure found in many databases and file systems (Giampaolo, 1999). In SQLite, data is stored in two variants of such b-trees. In one variant, data is only stored in the leafs, and the inner nodes only store the keys for looking up the leafs. These are called *table b-trees* in SQLite terminology. In the other variant, trees only contain keys and don't have data. In SQLite

---

32 Based on the file format specification at sqlite.org.

Table 6.19 SQLite file header.

Offset	Size	Description
0	0x10	The header string: "SQLite format 3\NUL" (where\NUL is the null character, the value 0)
0x10	2	The database page size in bytes. 0x200 (512) to and including 0x8000 (32768). The value 1 means a page size of 0x10000 (65536).
0x12	1	File format write version. 1 for legacy; 2 for WAL.
0x13	1	File format read version. 1 for legacy; 2 for WAL.
0x14	1	Bytes of unused "reserved" space at the end of each page. Usually 0.
0x15	1	Maximum embedded payload fraction. Must be 0x40 (64).
0x16	1	Minimum embedded payload fraction. Must be 0x20 (32).
0x17	1	Leaf payload fraction. Must be 0x20 (32).
0x18	4	File change counter.
0x1c	4	Size of the database file in pages. The *in-header database size*.
0x20	4	Page number of the first freelist trunk page.
0x24	4	Total number of freelist pages.
0x28	4	The schema cookie.
0x2c	4	The schema format number. Supported schema formats are 1, 2, 3, and 4.
0x30	4	Default page cache size.
0x34	4	The page number of the largest root b-tree page when in auto-vacuum or incremental-vacuum modes, or zero otherwise.
0x38	4	The database text encoding. A value of 1 means UTF-8. A value of 2 means UTF-16le. A value of 3 means UTF-16be.
0x3c	4	The "user version" as read and set by the user version pragma.
0x40	4	True (nonzero) for incremental-vacuum mode. False (zero) otherwise.
0x44	4	The "Application ID" set by PRAGMA application_id.
0x48	0x14	Reserved for expansion. Must be zero.
0x5c	4	The version-valid-for number.
0x60	4	SQLITE_VERSION_NUMBER

terminology, these are called *index b-trees*. As investigators most often are interested in the data, the table b-tree leaf pages are typically what one looks for.

The page header will tell us which page we are looking at. Table 6.20 shows the table page header structure.

```
Offset(h)  00 01 02 03 04 05 06 07 08 09 0A 0B 0C 0D 0E 0F
00000000   53 51 4C 69 74 65 20 66 6F 72 6D 61 74 20 33 00   SQLite format 3.
00000010   04 00 01 01 00 40 20 20 00 00 00 08 00 00 00 00   .....@  ........
00000020   00 00 00 00 00 00 00 00 00 00 00 07 00 00 00 01   ................
00000030   00 00 07 D0 00 00 00 00 00 00 00 01 00 00 00 04   ...Ð............
00000040   00 00 00 00 00 00 00 00 00 00 00 00 00 00 00 00   ................
00000050   00 00 00 00 00 00 00 00 00 00 00 00 00 00 00 00   ................
00000060   00 00 00 00 0D 03 FC 00 06 01 5A 00 03 07 03 AA   ......ü...Z....ª
00000070   02 B5 02 5D 02 0E 01 5A 00 00 00 00 00 00 00 00   .µ.]...Z........
```

Figure 6.42 Hex dump of a SQLite header.

Table 6.20 Table page header structure in SQLite.

Offset	Size	Description
0	1	Page type: 2 = interior index, 5 = interior table, 0x0a = leaf index, 0x0d = leaf table.
1	2	Start offset of first free block in page.
3	2	Number of cells in the page.
5	2	Start offset of cell content area (0 = 0x10000).
7	1	Number of fragmented free bytes.
8	4	Only present in interior b-tree pages: page number for right-most pointer.

After the header, an array of 2-byte cell pointers follows immediately. The number of pointers are given in offset 3 of this page header. If this is the first page, the page header will follow the file header at offset 0x64. Figure 6.42 shows the page header starting at offset 0x64, after the SQLite file header. It is a leaf table page (value 0x0d) and contains six entries (offset 0x67 = 0x64 + 3). According to offset 0x69 (0x64 + 5), the cell data starts at page offset 0x15a. At offset 0x6c, we can see six 2-byte pointers: 0x307, 0x3aa, 0x2b5, 0x25d, 0x20e, and 0x15a.

Table 6.21 shows the leaf table cell structure. This is the structure the page header points to.

A *varint* is a special type of variable-length integer structure used for encoding 2's complement 64-bit integers. It will encode the integer in up to 9 bytes. There are 0 to 7 bytes where the high bit is set, and ends in one byte where the high bit is cleared; or 8 bytes where the high bit is set, followed by one byte where all 8 bits are part of the integer (which gives $7 * 8 + 8 = 64$ bit). Each of the bytes holds 7 bits of the integer, and is assembled as big-Endian.

Figure 6.43 is a hex dump of the leaf table cells as described in Table 6.21. If we look at offset 0x15a, we see that the bytes in the varint describing the length are 0x81 (high bit set) and 0x31 (high bit cleared). If we look at the bits, we see the first byte as "1000 0001," and the second as "0011 0001." We drop the most significant bit in both numbers and join them together: "000 0001" joined with "011 0001" becomes "00 0000 1011 0001" = "1011 0001" = 0xb1.

The next varint is the rowid, in this case 0x06, which is just one byte. Then the payload starts and continues for 0xb1 bytes. If we look at Figure 6.43, offset 0x15d (start of payload) + 0xb1 = 0x20e. At this offset it seems like another cell is starting, something we can confirm by looking at the pointer array at offset 0x74 in Figure 6.43, where we can find a pointer with this exact value.

The payload for a table b-tree leaf page is in a format called a *record format*. This format contains a header and a body. The header starts with a varint indicating the size of the whole header (including the size varint). Then follows one or more varints called *serial types*, describing the data in the body, which are shown in Table 6.22.

The body follows immediately after the header and contains the data without any delimiters, as we already know the sizes from the header.

If we look at Figure 6.43, we can see that the payload header of the first cell starts at offset 0x15d. The header is 7 bytes, and the varints that describe the payload body are

```
Offset(h)  00 01 02 03 04 05 06 07 08 09 0A 0B 0C 0D 0E 0F
00000150   00 00 00 00 00 00 00 00 00 00 81 31 06 07 17 1D   ...........1....
00000160   1D 01 82 35 74 61 62 6C 65 53 65 74 74 69 6E 67   ..,5tableSetting
00000170   73 53 65 74 74 69 6E 67 73 07 43 52 45 41 54 45   sSettings.CREATE
00000180   20 54 41 42 4C 45 20 5B 53 65 74 74 69 6E 67 73    TABLE [Settings
00000190   5D 20 28 5B 5F 69 64 5D 20 49 4E 54 45 47 45 52   ] ([_id] INTEGER
000001A0   20 20 4E 4F 54 20 4E 55 4C 4C 20 50 52 49 4D 41     NOT NULL PRIMA
000001B0   52 59 20 4B 45 59 2C 20 5B 41 70 70 49 44 5D 20   RY KEY, [AppID]
000001C0   54 45 58 54 20 20 4E 55 4C 4C 2C 20 5B 44 65 76   TEXT  NULL, [Dev
000001D0   69 63 65 49 44 5D 20 54 45 58 54 20 20 4E 55 4C   iceID] TEXT  NUL
000001E0   4C 2C 20 5B 51 75 65 72 79 54 79 70 65 5D 20 54   L, [QueryType] T
000001F0   45 58 54 20 20 4E 55 4C 4C 2C 20 5B 41 6C 74 49   EXT  NULL, [AltI
00000200   44 5D 20 54 45 58 54 20 20 4E 55 4C 4C 29 4D 05   D] TEXT  NULL)M.
00000210   06 17 2D 17 01 65 69 6E 64 65 78 4E 6F 74 65 73   ..-..eindexNotes
00000220   5F 4E 6F 74 65 5F 49 6E 64 65 78 4E 6F 74 65 73   _Note_IndexNotes
00000230   06 43 52 45 41 54 45 20 49 4E 44 45 58 20 4E 6F   .CREATE INDEX No
00000240   74 65 73 5F 4E 6F 74 65 5F 49 6E 64 65 78 20 4F   tes_Note_Index O
00000250   4E 20 4E 6F 74 65 73 28 4E 6F 74 65 29 56 04 06   N Notes(Note)V..
00000260   17 33 17 01 71 69 6E 64 65 78 4E 6F 74 65 73 5F   .3..qindexNotes_
00000270   43 72 65 61 74 65 64 5F 49 6E 64 65 78 4E 6F 74   Created_IndexNot
00000280   65 73 05 43 52 45 41 54 45 20 49 4E 44 45 58 20   es.CREATE INDEX
00000290   4E 6F 74 65 73 5F 43 72 65 61 74 65 64 5F 49 6E   Notes_Created_In
000002A0   64 65 78 20 4F 4E 20 4E 6F 74 65 73 28 43 72 65   dex ON Notes(Cre
000002B0   61 74 65 64 29 50 03 06 17 2F 17 01 69 69 6E 64   ated)P.../..iind
000002C0   65 78 4E 6F 74 65 73 5F 54 69 74 6C 65 5F 49 6E   exNotes_Title_In
000002D0   64 65 78 4E 6F 74 65 73 04 43 52 45 41 54 45 20   dexNotes.CREATE
000002E0   49 4E 44 45 58 20 4E 6F 74 65 73 5F 54 69 74 6C   INDEX Notes_Titl
000002F0   65 5F 49 6E 64 65 78 20 4F 4E 20 4E 6F 74 65 73   e_Index ON Notes
00000300   28 54 69 74 6C 65 29 81 20 01 07 17 17 17 01 82   (Title). ......,
00000310   1F 74 61 62 6C 65 4E 6F 74 65 73 4E 6F 74 65 73   .tableNotesNotes
00000320   02 43 52 45 41 54 45 20 54 41 42 4C 45 20 5B 4E   .CREATE TABLE [N
00000330   6F 74 65 73 5D 20 28 5B 5F 69 64 5D 20 49 4E 54   otes] ([_id] INT
00000340   45 47 45 52 20 20 4E 4F 54 20 4E 55 4C 4C 20 50   EGER  NOT NULL P
00000350   52 49 4D 41 52 59 20 4B 45 59 20 41 55 54 4F 49   RIMARY KEY AUTOI
00000360   4E 43 52 45 4D 45 4E 54 2C 20 5B 54 69 74 6C 65   NCREMENT, [Title
00000370   5D 20 54 45 58 54 20 20 4E 4F 54 20 4E 55 4C 4C   ] TEXT  NOT NULL
00000380   2C 20 5B 43 72 65 61 74 65 64 5D 20 54 45 58 54   , [Created] TEXT
00000390   20 20 4E 55 4C 4C 2C 20 5B 4E 6F 74 65 5D 20 54     NULL, [Note] T
000003A0   45 58 54 20 20 4E 55 4C 4C 29 50 02 06 17 2B 2B   EXT  NULL)P...++
000003B0   01 59 74 61 62 6C 65 73 71 6C 69 74 65 5F 73 65   .Ytablesqlite_se
000003C0   71 75 65 6E 63 65 73 71 6C 69 74 65 5F 73 65 71   quencesqlite_seq
000003D0   75 65 6E 63 65 03 43 52 45 41 54 45 20 54 41 42   uence.CREATE TAB
000003E0   4C 45 20 73 71 6C 69 74 65 5F 73 65 71 75 65 6E   LE sqlite_sequen
000003F0   63 65 28 6E 61 6D 65 2C 73 65 71 29 00 00 00 04   ce(name,seq)....
00000400   0D 00 00 00 01 03 04 00 03 04 00 00 00 00 00 00   ...............
```

Figure 6.43 Leaf table cells.

Table 6.21 Leaf table structure in SQLite.

Size	Description
varint	Size of payload.
varint	Rowid, also called integer key.
variable	Payload.
4	Page number of first overflow page if the payload won't fit into the b-tree page. Omitted if all payload fits into b-tree page.

Table 6.22 Serial types used in the record format.

Serial type	Size	Description
0	0	Value is NULL.
1	1	Value is an 8-bit integer.
2	2	Value is a 16-bit integer.
3	3	Value is a 24-bit integer.
4	4	Value is a 32-bit integer.
5	6	Value is a 48-bit integer.
6	8	Value is a 64-bit integer.
7	8	Value is a 64-bit float (IEEE 754–2008).
8	0	Value is 0.
9	0	Value is 1.
10, 11	0	Not used.
$N \geq 12$, even	$(N-12)/2$	Value is a BLOB with size $(N-12)/2$.
$N \geq 13$, odd	$(N-13)/2$	Value is a string with size $(N-13)/2$, without null terminator.

given in Table 6.23 together with the data in the body, which follow immediately after the header.

We know what both the header and data look like, and we can validate the data by looking at the sizes and the pointer structures in the page header and the record format header. Carving for schemas and mapping the data onto these schemas are left as an exercise for the reader.

6.3.9 Technical Deep-Dive: Timestamps

Time is often a challenge in digital forensics. One reason for this is that we tend to think about time as a strictly increasing number that is the same, globally, for all devices. The

Table 6.23 Payload header and body in the first cell at offset 0x15d in Figure 6.43.

Serial type	Type	Size	Value
0x17	String	(0x17-0x0d)/ 2 = 5 bytes	Table
0x1d	String	(0x1d-0x0d)/ 2 = 8 bytes	Settings
0x1d	String	(0x1d-0x0d)/ 2 = 8 bytes	Settings
0x01	8-bit int	1 byte	7
0x82 0x35	String	(0x135-0xd)/ 2 = 0x94 bytes	CREATE TABLE [Settings] ([_id] INTEGER NOT NULL PRIMARY KEY, [Aped] TEXT NULL, [DeviceID] TEXT NULL, [QueryType] TEXT NULL, [AltID] TEXT NULL)

sad truth is that the clocks that are used in devices are neither guaranteed to be strictly rising nor globally equal. Clock settings might be adjusted, and two clocks adjusted independently might not show the same value at the same time. When an investigator sees a timestamp, she needs to establish which clock this timestamp is related to. Is it from the device's internal clock, or is it set from an external server? She also has to know which time zone or time region the timestamp belongs to. A *time zone* is the term for how far a timestamp is offset from UTC,[33] while a *time region* refers to the logical region in which the timestamp is labeled. In addition to its being offset from UTC, a time region also contains information about daylight savings time (DST), both its offset from standard time and when DST starts and ends.

We also need to try to establish the difference between the various clocks that set the timestamps and an objective, precise clock. Most commonly one should assume that the clock on the device hasn't been adjusted more than to correct the drift, and comparing the clock with a known clock at the time of acquisition may glean a hypothesis about the actual time with regard to the timestamp. If this hypothesis doesn't seem to hold, one should investigate this further. (See Example 6.4.)

But how is time represented on devices? There are several timestamp formats, but fortunately only a handful are commonly used. Table 6.24 shows some of the different timestamps used in mobile devices, the size of the timestamps, and a description.

As mentioned in Section 6.3.8, SQLite has a special storage format called a *varint*. Java timestamps stored in an SQLite database will therefore often be stored as a 6-byte big-Endian number, not 8 bytes. As the timestamp will fit in 24 bits, there is no need to waste 2 extra bytes in the database.

Table 6.24 Various timestamp formats.

Timestamp	Size	Description
Unix epoch	4	Seconds since 1970-01-01T00:00:00Z
Java time	8	Milliseconds since 1970-01-01T00:00:00.000Z
Chrome	8	Microseconds since 1601-01-01T00:00:00.000000Z.
SQLite	19	Stored as text on the form "YYYY-MM-DD HH:mm:ss". The default is to store the values in UTC.
SMS PDU	7	Stored as BCD encoded swapped nibbles, "YYMMDDHHmmssZZ", where the timezone is the number of 15 minutes from UTC, stored in a signed magnitude representation. See Section 6.3.7.
Mac Absolute Time	4	Seconds since 2001-01-01T00:00:00Z.
Windows time	8	Number of 100 ns since 1601-01-01T00:00:00.0000000Z
Text representation	Var	Variable format.

---

33 UTC, or Coordinated Universal Time, is the correct term for the time at longitude 0°. Earlier, GMT (Greenwich Meridian Time) was used, but UTC has a more precise definition.

Example 6.4: Adjusting the Clock to Get an Alibi

When examining a smartphone in a Norwegian case in 2013, our lab incidentally found that one of the SQLite databases logged much of what was happening on the phone. The logged information itself included the phone connecting to wireless networks, and programs downloaded or deleted. The log was written sequentially, but in one instance, we saw that the next timestamp was 24 hours earlier than the previous one. This was evidence that the clock on the phone did not go correctly either before or after this instance. The probability that the suspect had thought about the possibility of getting an alibi by adjusting the time on the phone was suddenly higher. Our trust in the rest of the timestamps from the phone was also lower.

6.4 Reverse Engineering and Analysis of Applications

In many electronic devices, there is data stored by applications running on the device, and often we see that the commercial products can't interpret data stored by an application on a device. In these cases, we have to do the analysis of the data ourselves. (See Definition 6.7.)

Definition 6.7: Reverse Engineering

Methods for finding out how something works, how it is assembled, or what the functionality is.

The questions the reverse-engineering task tries to answer are often the same ones we ask ourselves during a forensic examination, and we should therefore be aware of the possibilities that are within the field(s) of reverse engineering. We won't be able to cover everything about reverse engineering here, but rather give an idea of what this is about.

In this section, you will learn:

- methods used for reverse engineering, and
- a few targets of reverse engineering.

6.4.1 Methods

We can typically split reverse engineering of digital information into three main methods: black box testing, static code analysis, and runtime analysis. The methods are often used in conjunction, as one uses insight gained from one method to help understanding or direct the focus for another method.

6.4.1.1 Black Box Testing

When examining an unknown device, one can use an identical test device, load it with known data, and make a journal of what is done. For an unknown phone, it might be to call known numbers, send and receive text messages, store contacts, and call the contacts. After acquiring the data using a forensic method, the investigator can start looking for the known data, and interpret the data structures from what he knows about the events recorded in his journal. If one doesn't have access to a test device, data from the seized device can be compared with known data from other sources (e.g., traffic data from the phone service provider, and known GPS locations).

This is a way to find the most changeable information, and it gives relatively quick results. The drawback to this method is that it requires many assumptions about the data and how it is stored, and it won't reveal all the information about the structures we are looking at. Flags in the protocols or storage formats might be difficult to interpret, and an investigator might misinterpret values.

One is dependent on building on prior knowledge when testing this way; for a call log, there must be a field for the caller or the recipient, information about whether it was an incoming or outgoing call (maybe a timestamp), and a field showing how long the call has lasted. With this knowledge, one can find these data in the vicinity, and interpret the structure.

Fuzzing is a special form of black box testing, where one feeds the buffers of the application under test with semirandom data, in order to provoke the application to enter an unexpected state. If this happens, it is often a symptom of a bug where the data fed to the application is interpreted. With some luck, this might be an exploitable bug.

6.4.1.2 Static Code Analysis

Static code analysis techniques use the binary machine code, or the source code,[34] to analyze the code without running it. This includes, for example, disassembling, decompiling, and reading the source code.

Disassembling translates the machine code that a processor can run, or byte code that a runtime environment can interpret, and makes it readable for humans. Typically, this means to use the machine code as the processor reads it, and translate it into assembly code.

Decompiling goes one step further, interpreting the patterns of the machine code and rebuilding this into a higher-level coding language pattern. Think of this as a reverse compilation process. The compilation process is a process that loses information on the way from source code to machine code: variable names disappear, and patterns that are easily understood by humans get translated to patterns that are optimized for computing speed. We can get something that is functionally the same by decompiling, but usually not identical to the original source code.

Static code analysis can also be done on the source code itself. One can look at the coding comments to give an impression of what the functions are meant to do, as well as for common programming errors, data structures, and so on.

6.4.1.3 Runtime Analysis

Runtime analysis is where a program is analyzed while it is executing on a processor or in an emulator. One of the most common ways to do this is by using a debugger. *Debugging* is a term originally used by programmers for finding errors in the running code, thereby removing "bugs" in the program. It is also used by security researchers and others to examine running programs in order to map functionality, weaknesses, and errors.

---

34 If the source code is available, that is. To paraphrase a blockbuster movie: "Use the source, Luke."

The debugger is often attached to a process in the OS, and we can set breakpoints in the program. A breakpoint can be an instruction in the machine code, the address of an executed instruction, an address for memory access, or other conditions. This will stop the execution of the program so the program state can be inspected, and interesting parts of the program can be stepped through one instruction at a time.

Debugging is not the only way to do runtime analysis. One can, for example, look for changes caused by the program, which files the program touches, which resources the program accesses during runtime, and network activity.

6.4.2 Targets

Just as we categorize the techniques for reverse engineering, we can also categorize the targets of reverse engineering. The targets listed in this section are not an exhaustive list, but rather a few that can help the understanding of data available in a forensic investigation.

6.4.2.1 Program Functionality
The first thing to do when starting the reverse-engineering process is to find out what the program actually does. What is the data it handles, does it communicate with other programs or over a network, and does it listen for incoming network connections?

6.4.2.2 Data Structures
One of the more common questions in digital forensics deals with the interpretation of data found stored in the flash memory of a device. We might find strings of interest in a file along with binary data, or data that looks like interesting timestamps, locations, or IP addresses without any other contextual data.

Reverse engineering the application that writes data can give the data context. Is it a coordinate that is written because the device has been at the location, or is it because someone has looked at that location on a map? Is the IP address another device's address, or is it just a node in a traffic-relaying network?

It is not only context to found data that can be discovered, but also additional information stored in the data structures, some that might be used in testing the investigation hypothesis. Unique attributes of the data structures can be used to carve data using carving techniques, as described in this chapter.

6.4.2.3 Protocols
The protocols that a program uses for communication can be as important as the data structures it stores. An investigator can use the knowledge of the protocols a program uses to communicate with the program itself, or its endpoints. For example, an investigator can reverse engineer a program reading data from an unknown device, and use the knowledge about the protocol the device uses in order to write software that might read data from the device and store it in a better way.

6.4.2.4 Encryption
One often encounters encryption when examining mobile and embedded devices. Even though the encryption algorithm itself is strong, the implementation of key handling routines can be nonoptimal, or PRNGs won't necessarily produce

exceptionally random numbers (Alendal *et al.*, 2015). By reverse engineering artifacts, bugs, and implementation errors, we can for example discover ways to access encrypted data. (See Example 6.5.)

Example 6.5: Encrypted Notes

In one case from Norway in 2014, our lab discovered a database on an Android phone that had been updated at an interesting point in time. The database belonged to an application that could be used for taking notes that would be encrypted before being stored on the phone. By reverse engineering the application, we found that the notes were indeed encrypted with AES-128 encryption, but the encryption key was hardcoded in plain text in the application. The password that the user had to enter did not protect the encryption key, and we were able to decrypt all the notes stored in the database.

6.5 Summary

In this chapter we have looked at the peculiarities of mobile and embedded forensics, but also at the common factors in the forensic process. Two of the most fundamental principles in the forensic process are the *evidence integrity* and *chain of custody*. These are important to always have in mind when working with evidence, as they are the assurance that the evidence is correct and has not been tampered with.

The part that differs most for mobile and embedded devices with regard to the forensic process is the collection and examination phase. As these systems tend to be specialized, they often have proprietary or limited interfaces. The systems also tend to have a limited functionality. The system one will investigate needs to be assessed in order to identify the type of evidence that can be found on it. Typical questions we can assess about the device are regarding its *functionality, stored data, storage media, security measures,* and *communication ports and protocols.* We often lack a predefined set of methods and tools that already have been assessed and verified to be *forensically sound.* We therefore often have to make this assessment ourselves. How do we optimize the probability to get the relevant evidence in the most reliable and trustworthy way possible?

Be careful when handling an unknown device. There might be health hazards present, such as contaminated bodily fluids, toxins, irritants, corrosive chemicals, sharp edges, or other hazards. Use protective clothing and eyewear, and wear gloves when handling devices. Electrostatic discharges can make electronic circuits fail. Use antistatic equipment to minimize this risk for ESD to damage exposed electronics. We also have to be careful to not destroy other evidence like fingerprints, DNA, or tool marks on the physical device.

Before we start working on a device, we need to record some information about it. This includes the *power state of the device, physical appearance, any digital information from the user interface,* and *clock settings.*

There are many ways to categorize the mobile and embedded forensics field. Previous work includes looking at the technical qualities, the tools used for acquisition, and the data acquisition methods. We have shown another ontology, which tries to assess the methods based on several factors. We split the factors into two "views"; the *data view*, which looks at the data, and the *method view*, which looks at the specific method. The method view consists of: *layer of abstraction, alterations, repeatability*, and *cost before, during and after acquisition*. The method should match up with the information one wants to acquire. The attributes of the information desired can be assessed by these factors from the data view: *layer of abstraction, trust*, and *volatility*.

There are several methods to acquire data from a device. *Logical* and *physical* acquisition are often mentioned, where logical acquisition implies the use of normal user interfaces and APIs to extract data. Physical acquisition resembles imaging of a hard disk drive, where one uses low-level access to the raw data. If the data resembles raw data, but is already interpreted by a layer, we refer to this as *pseudo-physical* acquisition. In order to gain access to the data, one might need to change the system by exploiting the system, entering passcodes, or other forms of handling the device.

After data has been collected, we need to examine the data. This interpretation of the data can be meticulous and time-consuming. Interpreting how data is stored and what the data means is a task that is riddled with assumptions and educated guesses. We have to make sure that we describe the assumptions we make that are important for the meaning of the information.

As flash memory has a limited lifetime, the system needs to spread the writing over the whole memory such that not a single memory address gets programmed more than others. To spread the writes is called *wear levelling*, and the *flash translation layer* will do this. Some file systems are made for flash memory and include flash management functionality. Memory chips that contain a microcontroller that handles the flash management are called *managed flash memory*.

Reverse engineering is an umbrella term for various ways to find out something unknown about a system, like *program functionality, data structures, protocols*, or *encryption*. We can do this by *black box testing, static analysis, runtime analysis*, or a combination of these methods.

6.6 Exercises

Here are a few exercises that touch into the topics in this chapter. They can be used for reviewing the chapter, or as a basis for discussion. The questions don't necessarily have one correct answer, as the answer might vary with the assumptions made. As an extra challenge to all the questions, it is interesting to identify these assumptions and to assess how changing the assumptions might influence the answer.

1   Which OSs exist for mobile and embedded systems?

2   What should we consider before picking up an electronic device at the scene of crime?

3   What is managed flash?

4   A text message has been received on an encrypted mobile phone. From the system view, in which layers of abstraction does the message exist, and where is it readable?

What can we say about the trust we have to place in the system for each case? What about the volatility of the data?

5   A nontechnical police officer calls in from a scene of crime during a search. The search team has found several phones, one is on, and they want to know how to handle these. What are your recommendations? How will your assumptions affect your advice, and can new information from the search team change or improve your advice?

6   In a drug case, you suspect there has been communication between two suspected ringleaders, as both know about the delivery and pickup. The lawful interception has not seen any direct communication between these suspects: no SMS, calls, or direct data streams. You suspect they have used their smartphones to communicate. What do you think you can find on their phones? How would you start looking for their communication? Anything you can do before the suspects are brought in? How would you acquire the data from the phones? And how would you search for traces?

7   The handling of evidence is an important consideration. The crime scene investigator has found a phone on the scene of crime, and suspects that there is crucial evidence in the phone. The phone seems to have some droplets inside the cracked screen. He hands you the phone, and says that due to the importance of the digital evidence, you should acquire the data first, and then the other forensic experts will look for fingerprints and biological traces after you are finished. How should you handle the device? What should you do in order to minimize the health hazards? And how to minimize the impact you leave on the other traces?

8   Continuing the case in question 4: you know you can read the eMMC contents with JTAG for this phone. What is the best way to handle the digital evidence from the acquisition in order to ensure the evidence integrity and the chain of custody for the acquired data? How should the checksums be computed, and how should they be stored? What about the storage solution?

9   What is a flash translation layer, why does NAND memory often include this, and which type of information does the FTL need in order to work? Why isn't an FTL always needed in addition to a file system for storing data on flash memory?

10   Compare two or more of the acquisition methods in light of the acquisition method ontology described in Section 6.1.6.1. What are the differences between the methods, and which type of data matches the methods?

11   What is the difference between rooting a device to acquire the flash memory and acquiring the flash memory with a boot loader? Discuss: which method is best to use if the device has storage encryption enabled, and which method is best for

acquiring evidence in RAM? Which method would you prefer if you suspect that malware is running on the device?

12 During an ordinary day, in which mobile or embedded systems do you think you leave traces? How can this information be collected? Can this information be used to strengthen or weaken an alibi? What else can this information tell?

7

Internet Forensics

Petter Christian Bjelland

Ernst & Young AS, Oslo, Norway

A digital forensics expert will sooner or later deal with evidence from network infrastructure and remote endpoints. In the literature, this is commonly referred to as *network forensics* and *Internet forensics*. Whereas network forensics relates to the examination of infrastructure to a large extent under the control of the investigator (e.g., an internal company network), Internet forensics relates to the examination of infrastructure out of one's control, such as servers in other countries. While many techniques are similar in both cases, this chapter focuses on forensic examination of artifacts found on and through the Internet.

Internet forensics applies to both investigations of crimes committed *on* the Internet and investigations of crimes committed *with* the Internet. The former includes crimes such as computer intrusion, denial-of-service attacks, and bank fraud. The latter includes crimes such as identity theft, extortion, and money laundering. Furthermore, because of the networked nature of the Internet, we essentially have three crime scenes to consider during our examinations: the adversary, the victim, and the infrastructure between them.

A forensic investigator will often have access to one environment, either that of the perpetrator or that of the victim. In the term 'environment', we include both endpoint computers, as well as the local network they are connected to. The investigator will also have some access to the infrastructure in that he can test how the infrastructure is configured. In addition, information found on open sources, such as the World Wide Web, may provide valuable leads and insights during an investigation. Different types of forensic artifacts may be found in different environments. In this chapter, we discuss what these artifacts are and how they can be acquired.

7.1 Introduction

The Internet evolves rapidly, and many of the specifics of Internet forensics quickly become outdated. You therefore need to acquire sufficient knowledge of how the Internet works, in order for you to come up with new solutions to existing and emerging

Digital Forensics, First Edition. Edited by André Årnes.
© 2018 John Wiley & Sons Ltd. Published 2018 by John Wiley & Sons Ltd.

challenges. We begin this chapter with a review of how the Internet is glued together. This is a vast topic to cover, ranging from the physical connectivity between computers to application protocols that allow you to play games with your friends overseas.

This chapter reviews artifacts that may be acquired in the realm of Internet forensics. These include those that may be found in the Internet infrastructure and in open sources, as well as those artifacts left behind on the endpoints (i.e., the clients and servers). The final section discusses how these artifacts may be examined and analyzed in a structured manner. Many types of Internet forensics artifacts are acquired from remote environments that one does not control, for example the lookup of domain name ownership. This chapter will also discuss how we can ensure evidence integrity and chain of custody under such circumstances.

By the end of this chapter, you should have:

- An understanding of how the Internet is glued together
- Insight into how Internet artifacts may be found and acquired
- Insight into the acquisition of artifacts left behind from the use of the Internet.

7.2 Computer Networking

Computer networks are what connect our devices, enabling a wide array of instant communication across large geographic distances. The artifacts we classify as part of Internet forensics are artifacts that either enable or are enabled by these networks. Throughout this chapter, we will discuss the various types of information that are part of either the infrastructure or the data being transferred. But before that, we'd like to show you a bird's-eye view of what we are working with.

When a computer connects to the Internet, it in fact connects to a single local or wide-area network. This network relays data between the computer and another Internet-connected computer. Both computers may not be connected to the same network, so data must be sent across one or more adjacent networks to reach both ends. To specify the recipient of some information, a network address is assigned to the information. This network address is most often referred to as an Internet Protocol (IP) address. The transmission of the information, or data, is handled by a set of devices called *routers* and *switches*. These devices have a number of network cables connected to them, called *legs*. When some data arrives at a router, the router looks at the recipient address to determine which leg is best suited to carry it further. This is referred to as a *hop*. This process is repeated on all switches and routers until the data either arrives at its destination or is dropped by a router for having used too many hops.

Put simply, the relationships between two computers are of one of these three forms: peer-to-peer, where all computers are both consumers and producers of services (i.e., they *both* send and receive information); client-to-server, where a server computer provides some service to a client computer (e.g., a web page); or server-to-server, where two servers share information, such as for load-balancing purposes in cloud deployments. For a computer to be able to receive data from another computer, it needs to have a *port* open from which it listens for data. This port is a numeric value from 0 to 65535. Some ports are more common than others (e.g., port 80 and 443 for accessing web pages). Thus, the port number may help identify the type of resource that is being accessed.

If we have access to the infrastructure transmitting the data, we can copy the data to disk for further inspection. Such copying is useful for debugging applications or services that rely on network communication, but also enables us to detect network intrusions and perform after-the-fact forensic analysis. It is not uncommon for organizations to maintain a cache of the data entering and leaving their networks for some period of time, e.g. one week. Among other things, the cache contains the IP addresses of the source and destination computers, as well as the source and destination ports. Depending on how the data copying is configured, the cache may also contain the actual data being transferred, such as a JPEG picture.

A computer can be connected to several distinct networks at the same time. This may be through multiple physical network interfaces that are part of the computer hardware, or virtual networks that are implemented on top of said hardware. Such virtual networking is common in virtual private networks (VPNs). The computer may thus have several IP addresses at a given time.

7.3 Layers of Network Abstraction

This chapter will review the technologies and protocols that support the Internet and what they may indicate for digital investigations. We use the layers of abstraction (see also Section 1.3.1) as defined in the Open Systems Interconnection (OSI) model as a reference for this review. These layers are: *physical, data link, network, transport, session, presentation,* and *application.*

7.3.1   The Physical Layer

The lowest level of computer intercommunication is the physical layer. This layer transmits the digital zeros and ones from one location to another through a physical medium, such as electricity over copper wires, optical light through fiber cables, or radio waves through the air. This layer is of interest when one wishes to do network traffic interception as part of their investigation.

7.3.2   The Data Link, Network, and Transport Layers

The layers above the physical layer ensure that the zeros and ones are correctly received, and they determine which physical medium a given piece of data should be transmitted through. Three important protocols operating at this layer are the IP, the User Datagram Protocol (UDP), and the Transmission Control Protocol (TCP). IP is an addressing scheme used to determine where a given piece of data is going, and there are currently two versions of the IP address being used on the Internet: version 4 (IPv4) and version 6 (IPv6). UDP and TCP are data transport protocols that manage how data is sent from one IP address to another. The major difference between the two protocols is that TCP ensures that every packet is correctly sent from end to end, in the appropriate order. Because of the extra verification steps, sending data with TCP is slower than with UDP. TCP is thus commonly used for transmitting information such as web pages and email, and UDP is a more popular choice for services such as Internet telephony and streaming, where a certain level of packet loss and corruption is accepted.

7.3.2.1   IP Addresses

RFC 791[1] describes three steps for sending a network packet from one endpoint to another using the IP. First, the identity of the recipient must be determined, then the location of the recipient, and finally a route from the sender to the recipient. IP addresses deal with the second part (i.e., indicating the recipient's location). As mentioned, there are two IP versions currently being used, IPv4 and IPv6. IPv4 has been used for decades and is still the most commonly used version of IP address by far. An IPv4 address is commonly represented as four bytes represented as four numbers between 0 and 255 each separated by a dot, or as a 32-bit integer between 0 and approximately 4.3 billion.

We can specify a range of IP addresses by writing the address as a prefix. A common syntax for such a prefix is an IP address, followed by a forward slash and a number between 0 and 32. Table 7.1 shows some example prefixes for IPv6 addresses. Both versions 4 and 6 specify network ranges on this format.

In the early days of the IP, large IP network prefixes were given to large organizations like IBM, meaning that a large part of these 4.3 billion IP addresses are reserved, though they may not be in use. This means that the rest of the Internet has far less IP addresses to share, and as more and more devices require addresses, available ones are running out. The IPv6 addressing scheme was extended – instead of using 32 bits to uniquely identify a network endpoint, it uses 128 bits, which gives us well over 340 trillion addresses to choose from.

7.3.3   The Session, Presentation, and Application Layers

The three upper layers of the OSI model provide further abstraction from how bits are physically transmitted between endpoints. The application layer enables protocols like

Table 7.1   IP networks and ranges.

Remainder	No. of addresses	Sample network	Low	High
0	1	192.168.0.1/32	192.168.0.1	192.168.0.1
1	2	192.168.0.0/31	192.168.0.0	192.168.0.1
2	4	192.168.0.0/30	192.168.0.0	192.168.0.3
3	8	192.168.0.0/29	192.168.0.0	192.168.0.7
4	16	192.168.0.0/28	192.168.0.0	192.168.0.15
. . .	. . .			
15	32768	192.168.0.0/17	192.168.0.0	192.168.127.255
16	65536	192.168.0.0/16	192.168.0.0	192.168.255.255
. . .				
30	1073741824	192.0.0.0/2	192.0.0.0	255.255.255.255
31	2147483648	128.0.0.0/1	128.0.0.0	255.255.255.255
32	4294967296	0.0.0.0/0	0.0.0.0	255.255.255.255

---

1 https://tools.ietf.org/html/rfc791.

the Hypertext Transfer Protocol (HTTP) and the File Transfer Protocol (FTP), two popular high-level protocols for requesting and transferring data.

7.4 The Internet

The topics we cover in this section reveal how computer networks are able to connect to each other, both directly and through other networks. Together they enable every pair of Internet-connected computers to reach one another. While this tangibly relies on technical specifications and implementations, the Internet is also highly dependent upon negotiations and agreements between large international corporations.

7.4.1 Internet Backbone

Beneath the applications we use every day are a set of core services that glue together networks around the world into what we call the Internet. These represent the backbone upon which all other Internet-connected protocols and applications rely. In this chapter, we discuss three of these services: the *autonomous system*, the *Border Gateway Protocol*, and *Internet service providers*.

7.4.1.1 Autonomous System (AS)

An AS is a set of IP prefixes under a single administrative control (e.g., a university network or the network of a corporation). Each AS is given a globally unique AS number (ASN) that identifies the network. These ASNs are managed by organizations called Regional Internet Registries (RIRs). There are five such RIRs, each responsible for a geographic area.

Each of these RIRs is given a range of ASNs by a global organization called the Internet Assigned Numbers Authority (IANA). In addition to assigning RIRs with ASN ranges, IANA is also a global manager of the IP address pool, as well as global root authority for the Domain Name System (DNS), which we will discuss later. Organizations obtain an ASN by filling out an application form and submitting it to its RIR. There are four types of ASs: multihomed, Internet exchange point, stub, and transit.

A multihomed AS is a network that is physically and directly connected to two or more other ASs. This provides the network with true Internet redundancy, so if one of the connections fails, the network will still be able to communicate with other endpoints on the Internet. An important difference between a multihomed AS and another type of AS is that network traffic is not allowed to flow through it. If for example network B is a multihomed AS, network A cannot communicate with network C through B.

An Internet exchange point is the infrastructure on which Internet service providers (ISPs) connect their networks to share traffic. One of the benefits of such an infrastructure is that ISPs do not have to build new infrastructure every time they establish new peering agreements with other ISPs.

Stub and transit ASs are similar to a multihomed AS; however, they allow network traffic to flow through their network. The difference between the two is that stubs are only connected with a single AS. Network traffic flowing through such networks is called peering, and there are three types of peering: *customer*, *transit*, and *peer*.

A customer is an individual or an organization paying an ISP to be connected to the Internet. In transit peering, an ISP pays another service provider for connection to the rest of the Internet. This type of peering is normal when a small ISP wants to connect to the Internet. Instead of having to build the physical infrastructure required to provide global Internet access for their customers, they pay a number of other ISPs that already have the infrastructure a settlement to connect to the Internet through them. As they often have their infrastructure located in various locations around the globe, it makes sense to cooperate with others to enable global reach for their customers and transits. If two ISPs see that they are mutually dependent upon each other for this global reach, they can agree on being peers, where they do not pay each other for the use of their networks.

Example 7.1: Verizon versus Cogent Peering Disputes

It is easy to imagine disputes between ISPs on whether or not they should have a peer or transit relationship. In 2013, the ISPs Verizon and Cogent disagreed on whether Cogent should have to pay Verizon for using their network. The dispute revolved around traffic going from the video streaming service Netflix. Netflix is paying Cogent for transit, and thus Cogent is responsible for delivering the content to Netflix customers. However, this traffic crosses the infrastructure of other ISPs, and they wanted to be paid for delivering the content as well.

7.4.1.2 Border Gateway Protocol (BGP)

ASs on the Internet connect with each other using a protocol called Border Gateway Protocol, as illustrated by Figure 7.1. Every router supporting BGP maintains a routing table that is used to determine the shortest route to the destination network. This table consists of network segments associated with a set of ASs that are between the router and the destination endpoint. These network addresses are defined as IP address prefixes, and the routers usually choose the path with the smallest number of ASs defined for the longest (i.e., most specific) prefix. BGP routers are manually configured, and special rules may thus be applied by the network administrator in deference to, for example, lower cost on a longer path. In addition to the manual configuration, BGP routers also

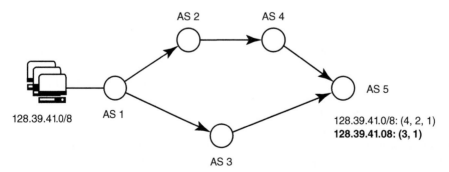

Figure 7.1 Connecting multiple autonomous systems and finding the shortest path (icons by Visual Pharm).

exchange route updates with one another so that changes made to one BGP router are propagated throughout the Internet.

Example 7.2: BGP Blackholing by Mistake

To see just how important it is for the Internet that BGP functions properly, we can look at an incident involving the Pakistani government and the video-streaming service YouTube in 2008. The government meant to block traffic from an AS in Pakistan going to YouTube. However, by what is assumed to be an accident, the configuration to send this traffic to nowhere was sent to a Pakistani ISP using BGP. Due to BGP's configuration propagation feature, this "blackholing" spread to the entire Internet, essentially taking down YouTube globally for a period of time.

7.4.1.3 Internet Service Providers (ISPs)

ISPs are organizations that provide access to the Internet to customers. Some ISPs are large, maintaining a global physical infrastructure, while others are small, providing Internet access to a relatively small number of customers in a small town or region. ISPs are organized into three tiers by their size: Tier 1, 2, and 3.

Tier 3 ISPs are the smallest, and they usually pay higher tier ISPs for transit on their infrastructure. Tier 2 ISPs are larger, maybe maintaining a national Internet infrastructure. These tier 2 ISPs may establish peering agreements with other tier 2 ISPs, sell transit to tier 3 ISPs, and buy transit from tier 1 ISPs. Tier 1 ISPs do not have to buy transit from any other ISP; they maintain large physical infrastructures, such as the subsea network cables connecting continents. Tier 1 ISPs establish peering agreements with other large ISPs to gain access to parts of the world where they do not have the infrastructure; they also sell transit to tier 2 and 3 ISPs.

7.4.2 Common Applications

There is no limit as to the types of applications that may run on the Internet. Indeed, it is infeasible to discuss every existing application within this chapter. However, some applications have manifested themselves over the years as so common that they are almost ubiquitous to the Internet itself. This chapter discusses three such applications: the *Domain Name System*, *Email* and the *World Wide Web*.

7.4.2.1 Domain Name System (DNS)

In our discussion about IP addresses, we discussed three steps required to transmit data from one Internet endpoint to another: naming, addressing, and routing. The DNS is responsible for naming. DNS is implemented by a set of hierarchically organized name servers that, through a series of requests, map a domain name to a set of valid IP addresses for that name. See Figure 7.2 for an illustration of a DNS lookup of the domain hig.no. At the top of the hierarchy are the global root name servers. This root is managed by IANA, the same organization managing the AS numbers for Internet networks.

A domain name consists of one or more alphanumeric strings separated by dots. The part at the far right is referred to as the top-level domain (TLD). Historically, the amount

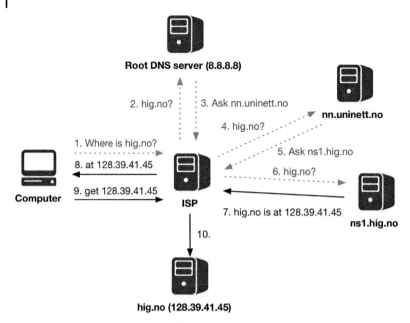

Figure 7.2 DNS lookup of the domain hig.no (icons by Visual Pharm).

of TLDs has been restricted to relatively few, containing only national identifiers, such as .no, .se, and .dk, and some generic names like .com, .net, .org, and .info. Recently, it has become possible to acquire complete TLDs, and we are now seeing TLDs like .google.

There are seven different types of DNS records; these are described in Table 7.2.

There are currently (as of April 2015) 13 root name servers on the Internet.[2] Due to the sheer number of domains in use on the Internet, it is not possible for these servers to keep track of all the domains. Therefore, requests are delegated to other name servers

Table 7.2 DNS record types.

Type	Description	Example
SOA	DNS zone's authority	ns1.hig.no hostmaster.hig.no 2015082800 43200 7200 2419200 3600
A	IPv4 address	128.39.41.45
AAAA	IPv6 address	2001:700:1d00:17::45
MX	SMTP mail exchangers	10 smtp.hig.no
NS	Name servers	ns1.hig.no
PTR	For reverse DNS	www.hig.no
CNAME	Domain name aliases	hig2.no

---

2 http://root-servers.org.

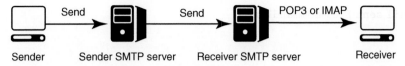

Sender   Sender SMTP server   Receiver SMTP server   Receiver

Figure 7.3 Email protocols (icons by Visual Pharm).

based on the TLD. These name servers may again refer to other name servers (i.e., respond with a NS record), before the name server holding the A, AAAA, MX, or CNAME record is found. These lookups are cached for some time determined by a value called time to live (TTL), saving network bandwidth, power, and time. Once the IP address of the domain we want to communicate with is determined, the lower layers of the OSI model make sure our data is transmitted to the destination endpoint.

7.4.2.2 Email

Electronic mail quickly gained widespread use on the Internet. Here we discuss three important protocols relating to the exchange of such data: the Simple Mail Transfer Protocol (SMTP), Internet Message Access Protocol (IMAP), and Post Office Protocol (POP). An overview of how these protocols interoperate to let you send and receive email is provided in Figure 7.3.

An email consists of a header and a body field, as shown here:

```
From: "Petter Christian Bjelland" <petter.bjelland@gmail.com>
To: "André Årnes" <andre.arnes@hig.no>
Subject: Mail sent from commandline

It works!
```

SMTP is a widespread delivery-only protocol that pushes email from one mail server to another. How an email may be sent from a SMTP server is illustrated below. And while webmail services such as Gmail and Hotmail are using their own custom protocols for transmitting emails within their own networks (i.e., sending email from one @gmail.com email address to another), they all use SMTP for sending emails outside their own network. When mail is pushed from one SMTP server to another, it does not consider the user recipient of the email, the value before the '@'. It only considers the domain name or IP address.

```
mpro:book pcbje$ openssl s_client -connect smtp.gmail.com:465 -crlf
-ign_eof
EHLO localhost
AUTH LOGIN <Base64 encoded Gmail username>
<Base64 encoded password>
MAIL FROM: <petter.bjelland@gmail.com>
RCPT TO: <andre.arnes@hig.no>
RCPT TO: <katrin.franke@hig.no>
DATA
From: "Petter Christian Bjelland" <petter.bjelland@gmail.com>
To: "André Årnes" <andre.arnes@hig.no>
```

```
Subject: Gmail sent from commandline

It works!
.

QUIT
```

Note that the actual recipients of an email and those stated in the email header may differ. The recipients not disclosed in the email header are often referred to as *BCC recipients* (BCC stands for "blind carbon copy"). The format supports attachments appended as Base64[3] encoded text added as part of the email header. Whereas SMTP is a delivery-only protocol, the IMAP and POP protocols are used for managing user mailboxes and transmitting emails to the end user. These are the protocols that allow users to download their email and manage their inboxes locally in applications like Microsoft Outlook. They also handle user authentication against the email server.

7.4.2.3 World Wide Web (WWW)

We conclude this section with a review of HTTP and Hypertext Markup Language (HTML), technologies central to the WWW. HTTP is at the application layer of the OSI model. It uses TCP for transferring requests and responses between servers. A HTTP request consists of a header field and a body field. The most commonly used version of HTTP, version 1.1, requires three elements to be present in a request header: a verb, a path, and a host.

Valid verbs are OPTIONS, GET, HEAD, POST, PUT, DELETE, TRACE, and CONNECT. However, GET and POST requests are by far the most common types of requests. Application developers are free to implement these verbs as they please, but IETF (1999) provides a detailed description of how they are supposed to operate. The request body can be any type of data, including binary data such as pictures and videos.

A HTTP response also consists of a header and a body field. The response header provides information about the status of the request (e.g., "200 OK," ""401 Forbidden," and "404 Not Found"). There are a large number of possible response codes, but in general, codes starting with 2 mean "OK," and requests starting with 4 or 5 mean "not OK." The response headers also contain information about what type of data is returned (e.g., pictures or text), as well as how long the information will be valid. This header field enables the requestor to cache the response and save time and bandwidth in the case of future requests for the same object. The response body consists of binary data, hopefully on the media type indicated in the header field.

On the WWW, the HTTP response type is often TEXT/HTML, meaning that the requester should parse the content as a web page. This is a text format that is a dialect of the eXtensible Markup Language (XML). Web browsers specialize in sending and parsing HTTP requests and responses. They will generate a view on the user's screen based on this text. Within the text, browsers can find elements that trigger new HTTP requests, such references to pictures, scripting files, or style sheets. How the response should be presented to the user is determined using these style sheets, and scripts can generate subsequent requests, potentially adding more content to the original request.

---

3 Base64 is a data-encoding scheme that allows binary data to be transferred as ASCII text.

7.4.2.4 Peer-to-Peer Networks

Previous sections of this chapter have described applications in a client–server model, where a number of clients access services like web pages or email accounts on a server. This section discusses some common applications that use another model called peer-to-peer. After some initial discovery process where peers figure out whom they may connect with, the peers (e.g., desktop computers) may communicate directly with one another without using any third server. This model allows for distributed computer communication and has been a vital part of many file-sharing networks over the years. Here, we discuss two applications that have made a significant impact in the field: BitTorrent and the Blockchain.

The BitTorrent protocol enables distributed sharing of files, where different pieces of a file may be downloaded from different peers. Once a peer has fully downloaded a piece of the file, that piece may be shared with other peers. When a peer has downloaded all pieces of the file, it becomes a *seeder.* To start sharing a file using BitTorrent, the sharer must create a torrent descriptor file and make this available to the downloaders (e.g., by email or on a website like thepiratebay.org). Among other things, the file contains a set of Uniform Resource Locators (URLs) that are *trackers* for that torrent, as well as information about which files the torrent contains. The torrent trackers store information about the *swarm* of peers sharing the given torrent. These trackers may be useful sources of artifacts, which we will discuss later in the chapter.

The blockchain is a vital part of the cryptographic currency Bitcoin. Whereas traditional online payments rely on central entities like Visa to ensure that money is not double-spent, bitcoin uses a distributed model of trust, where each transaction is verified by the other peers in the network. The way a transaction is verified is to check it against all other transactions. If a node determines that a transaction is valid, it adds it to a data structure called a block. As a block will contain references to previous blocks, each block provides a verification to the transactions in the previous ones. The block is later broadcasted to the network. The blocks of transactions and the network used to distribute them are called the Blockchain. When the transaction is present in a sufficient number of blocks, the receiving end of the transaction can feel confident that the transaction is valid and that the sender will not be able to retract or somehow undo it.

As all nodes in the network need to be aware of all transactions, it is possible to trace transactions. While anonymity is a key benefit of bitcoin, it only disconnects the involved public keys (called *addresses*) of a transaction from their identities. In criminal investigations, we might find these public keys on acquired computers and we may thus, to some extent, be able to trace its transactions. Such tracing is discussed later in the chapter.

7.4.2.5 Other Media

As more and more services are being embedded into the web browser, the technology has adapted to incorporate new types of applications, including video, storage, and rich media like 3D engines. This section describes some of the traditional as well as emerging technologies that may leave traces of web browsing.

One technology that was embedded early on in browsers was the *Java applet*. A Java applet enabled web applications to perform tasks that other client-side application logic like JavaScript couldn't, with its additional permissions to allow access to resources like reading files on the client computer. It has been heavily criticized for its many security vulnerabilities, which have caused many browsers to disable the applets by default. Another early rich media technology was Adobe Flash, which enabled streaming of videos, animations, and user interaction. It too proved to be a source of many vulnerabilities over the years and enabled attackers to execute arbitrary code on the client computer. Many of the features of the HTML5 standard have reduced or removed the need for these technologies.

When a user sees a web page, it is the result of multiple requests made by the browser and subsequent parsing of the responses. With the exception of objects like Java applets, Flash movies, and pictures, most of the responses are text that the browser must parse or execute. Browsers have different ways of doing this parsing, and unless there is a standard for how these texts should be handled, the visible result can vary.

The HTML5 specification is an attempt to standardize how the parsing is done, and with it comes a set of new technologies designed for modern web usage. Some of these technologies include: *WebSQL*, which allows a web application to create and maintain relational databases within a sandbox on the client computer; *Websockets*, which enables clients and servers to push messages to each other, in contrast to the traditional request-response; *EventStream*, which allows the web server to push messages to the client, but not the other way around; *WebGL*, which enables rich visualizations within the browser (e.g., 3D games); and *WebRTC*, which enables peer-to-peer real-time video and audio chat between two browsers.

Many of these technologies also relate to the recent HTTP/2 standard, which was released in May 2015 to replace the previous HTTP/1.1 standard from the 1990s. While HTTP/2 does not alter most of the topics covered here, it may be assumed that its performance is optimized by techniques such as bundling resources, and that multiplexing requests may affect the artifacts we acquire.

We will most likely continue to see a rapid development where more and more features are pushed into the browser. It is thus necessary to stay up to date with the various types of browsers and the artifacts they leave behind. We will discuss some of these artifacts later in the chapter.

7.4.3 Caveats

When you encounter an IP address that appears to be of interest in some digital evidence, there may be several reasons why that address may be misleading or inaccurate. Two common scenarios are that the discovered address may be shared among multiple endpoints (e.g., in a school) or that the address is a proxy for the real address. This section discusses two common caveats that you will certainly encounter as an Internet forensic investigator: *network address translation* and *onion routing*. We will, in addition, discuss web shells in this section.

7.4.3.1 Network Address Translation (NAT)

While surfing on the Internet, you may share an IP address with multiple other users. This is common on shared networks in workplaces and schools. Users connected to the same wireless network typically have the same public IP address. Within the shared networks, the endpoints are identified by local IP addresses. This means that endpoints connecting to different networks may have the same local IP address, but different public

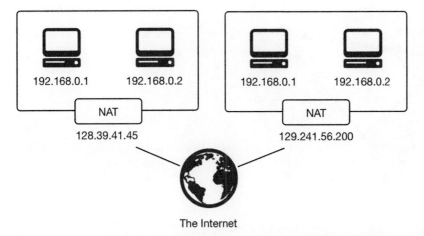

192.168.0.1   192.168.0.2   192.168.0.1   192.168.0.2

NAT   NAT

128.39.41.45   129.241.56.200

The Internet

Figure 7.4 Illustration of an Internet connection through a NAT (icons by Visual Pharm).

IP addresses. An illustration of this is given in Figure 7.4. This is an important feature, as the number of available IPv4 addresses today is running low. The mapping of a local IP address to a public IP address is most commonly done by using NAT.

It is important to be aware of this type of address translation, as the IP addresses in the log files you examine may be shared by a large number of endpoints.

7.4.3.2 Onion Routing

Sending a request directly from you to the destination endpoint, a web server for instance, may not always be the preferred option. For one thing, authorities may ban requests to the given endpoint, so in this case it becomes preferable to bounce the request through some other endpoint. Furthermore, one may not want to identify their own endpoint to the destination. For those running an illegal operation, suddenly seeing requests from IP addresses belonging to a law enforcement agency may raise some alarms. A technique for sending requests through a set of intermediate endpoints is called *onion routing*. Such routing is illustrated in Figure 7.5, where the black boxes represent the source and destination of the packets. The red circles represent nodes that traffic may be routed through. The solid circles are those that are in fact being used for proxying the data, often referred to as a *circuit*. Finally, solid lines indicate the original packet, whereas stapled lines indicate layers of encryption. In onion-routing networks like Tor (an acronym for "The Onion Router"),[4] there are thousands of nodes that may be chosen as part of the circuit.

Each layer of the onion contains a destination endpoint and an encrypted payload. Once an intermediate endpoint receives a request, it removes the outermost layer and sends the remaining payload to the next endpoint. Once at the final layer, the request is sent to the intended destination.

This type of routing has a number of interesting features. First, the destination endpoint will only see the IP address of the last intermediate endpoint. Second, each

---

4 www.torproject.org.

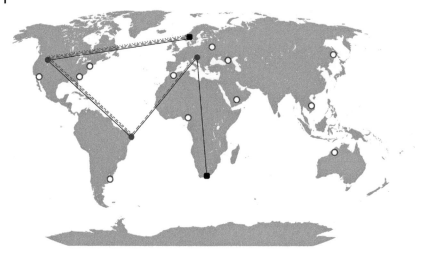

Figure 7.5 Onion routing of a request from Norway to South Africa.

endpoint before that will only know the previous and next endpoints. Finally, due to the encryption used between the source and the intermediate endpoints (though not between the final intermediate endpoint and the destination), it is difficult for a passive listener to determine where the packets are heading. The result is the anonymization of the source and the intended destination of network packets. A common feature of onion routing is services that are only available through the network of the intermediate endpoint. This adds anonymity to the destination endpoint, so the source does not know the actual IP address of the destination.

The anonymity is, however, not absolute. It is trivial to identify from the destination endpoint that it is being visited through an onion router. It is also possible to detect that a certain endpoint is using an onion router.

Example 7.3: Identified by Tor

An example where the user of an onion router actually became *less* anonymous was the student who sent a bomb threat to his school through Tor to avoid taking an exam. His problem was that he connected to Tor through the campus network, and at the time the threat was sent, there was only a single endpoint on that network connected to Tor: his. Had he connected to Tor through the local café, he might not have been caught. See Sandvik (2013) for additional information.

7.4.3.3 Web Shells

A file on a web server that enables the execution of programs on that server is often referred to as a *web shell*. Web shells may be as simple as a single instruction in the popular interpreter PHP:

```
<?php echo passthru($_GET['c']); ?>
```

If the web server at IP address 192.168.0.1 contains this web shell at path/shell.php, an attacker may run a command by executing:

```
curl -X GET http://192.168.0.1/shell.php?c=whoami
```

The command above will return the identity of the user that the web server application is running as on that server. As all interactions with the shell use common web server ports like 80 or 443, it may be difficult to block the commands using a firewall. Adding a web shell to a server is a lot harder than using one. To upload a web shell, the attacker may exploit some vulnerability in software running on the server (e.g., content management software like Drupal or WordPress), or by some means get a hold of credentials that give access. The web shell also needs to be placed at a location where an interpreter like PHP will execute the instructions.

7.5 Tracing Information on the Internet

We divide the gathering of information from the Internet into two distinct activities: *tracing* and *acquisition*. Whereas Internet tracing is the collection of information about endpoints connected to the Internet, acquisition is collection from the endpoints themselves. Tracing often makes use of information publicly available on the Internet, like databases of domain or IP address ownership.

In addition to traces left behind at the origin and the destination of Internet traffic, there is also a range of artifacts on the path between the endpoints that can be valuable to a digital investigation. Such artifacts range from simple things like checking if the endpoint using a certain IP address is online, to geolocation of the IP address based on statistical analysis. It is important to note that all infrastructure artifacts are inherently volatile: things may change rapidly and we inherently influence the crime scene. These changes occur naturally or by intent to hide traces. As an example, owners of a server detecting an ongoing port scan may apply changes accordingly. The remainder of this section is a review of different infrastructure artifacts and how they may be acquired.

7.5.1 DNS and Reverse DNS

You can look up what IP addresses a domain name points to by probing the domain name's DNS server. It is not uncommon for a domain name to use multiple DNS servers and IP addresses. It is important to note that the specific IP addresses you retrieve from such a lookup may depend on where in the world you are asking from. A service that allows one to do DNS lookups through a proxy is called a *looking glass*.

Because a DNS lookup points to the location of an endpoint, it potentially enables law enforcement to remove that endpoint from the Internet. To avoid this, adversaries need to obfuscate the location of the endpoint. While this may be done using anonymization tools like Tor, they can also employ a technique called Fast-Fluxing (Nazario, 2008). With Fast-Flux domains, the TTL of the DNS records is set extremely low, and the domain points to a large number of IP addresses, changing rapidly. These IP addresses usually point to compromised endpoints, in a botnet that perpetrators have access to.

The endpoints are used as proxies for the destination endpoint, making it much harder for law enforcement to follow the traces.

It may also be valuable to determine which domain names are associated with a given IP address. This is called *reverse DNS* and does exactly what its name entails. Given an IP address, it looks through certain databases for DNS records containing that address. Several tools for doing reverse DNS exist, some of the most popular being *nslookup*[5] and *dig.*[6]

7.5.2 Whois and Reverse Whois

In addition to knowing the specific IP addresses a domain name points to, it is useful to know who the registered owner of a domain name is. This information may be looked up using the *whois*-command on UNIX systems, as shown in the example below. While it is quite easy to register a domain name under a false name, the information may provide clues for the investigation.

```
pcbje$ whois hig.no
[...]
NORID Handle...............: HIG240D-NORID
Domain Name................: hig.no
[...]
Type.......................: organization
Name.......................: Høgskolen i Gjøvik
[...]
Post Address...............: Teknologiveien 22
Post Address...............: Postboks 191
Postal Code................: NO-2815
Postal Area................: Gjøvik
Country....................: NO
Email Address..............: hostmaster@hig.no
...
```

Services exist that enable *reverse whois lookups*, where one can search for domains registered to, for example, a name, phone number, or email address. If the domain is registered using a whois protection service, however, this information will not be available.

7.5.3 Ping and Port Scan

When we are dealing with servers connected to the Internet that are not physically available to us, we may want to communicate with the server over the network. The simplest way of doing this is by sending it an Internet Control Message Protocol (ICMP) packet, called a *ping*. A ping can be sent to both an IP address and a domain name, using DNS. In cases where we want to establish whether certain services may be running on a

---

5 $ nslookup 128.39.41.45.
6 $ dig -x 128.39.41.45.

given endpoint, we may use a *port scanner*. Services that must be available on the Internet, such as web and email servers, run on a set of designated ports on the endpoint. If a service is listening on a port, no other service is able to listen on the same port.

For common ports, there are usually a large number of applications that can be used for those services (e.g., web servers and email servers). Therefore, it may not be sufficient to determine that the port is open; we want to identify the exact type and version of the application running on that port. This is done by sending carefully crafted data to the given port and analyzing the response for characteristics unique for various software. This technique is known as *fingerprinting* and is commonly used in vulnerability scanning of networks.

Recently, tools like *masscan*[7] have enabled the scanning of ports across the entire IPv4 address space, providing previously infeasible insight into the deployment of applications and services on the Internet.

7.5.4 Traceroute

To determine the location of an endpoint with ping, port scans and DNS lookups may not be sufficient for an investigation, and you may have to determine exactly how a network packet is transmitted from one endpoint to another. This entails identifying every router receiving and retransmitting the packet. When a network packet is created at an endpoint, it is assigned a number called *time-to-live*. This number determines the maximum number of routers the packet may visit on its way to the destination. Every time a router receives a packet, it decrements the TTL value by one. If the TTL after the decrement is zero, the packet is not retransmitted. Instead, an ICMP packet is sent to the origin of the packet, relating that the packet did not reach the destination in time.

The origin can see at which router the packet timed out. A traceroute uses this information to identify the routers between the origin and destination endpoints. This is done by sending multiple packets with increasing TTL, starting at one. This will generate ICMP timeout messages at every intermittent router. It is important to note that the chosen route of a packet is volatile and may be different over time and at different locations. The chosen route is also dependent on the agreements between the intermittent ISPs, as certain routes may be more expensive than others. The routers will therefore prefer cheaper routes, even if this means a longer and slower path. It is also important to note that routes are asymmetric, and thus the route from origin to destination may be different from the route from destination to origin. Like with DNS lookups, looking-glass services exist to enable traceroutes to an endpoint from different origins around the world.

7.5.5 IP Geolocation

It can be interesting to determine where in the world an IP address is geographically located based on a wide range of sources, and there are several geolocation services available on the Internet. One method for geolocation is by triangulation. If we have access to multiple looking-glass services (i.e., so that we can send packets to a destination

---

7 https://github.com/robertdavidgraham/masscan.

from multiple locations), we can estimate the location of the destination by triangulating the response time. This technique is investigated in Fossen (2005).

It should be noted that IP geolocation is volatile, and the results may and will vary over time. There are two things that may cause a public IP address to move: IP block trading and IP hijacking. As for local IP addresses, these may change due to internal network configurations. As the IPv4 address space is filling up, blocks are becoming a valuable trading asset, and over the last couple of years there has been an increase in IP block trading. The geolocation of the IP address moves along with the ownership. Though we are running out of available IP addresses, some organizations are assigned larger IP blocks than they use, so many IP addresses still go unused. This may tempt others to configure BGP routers to send packets destined for unused IP addresses to their endpoints instead. This is called *IP hijacking*. When an IP address is hijacked, its geographic location will move to the hijacker's network. Because of these benign and malicious changes to IP addresses, the geolocation databases need to be updated regularly to provide sufficient confidence in the results.

7.5.6 Tracing BitTorrent Peers

We have previously described the BitTorrent protocol. In this section, we look at what artifacts can acquire from publicly available BitTorrent swarms. The swarm is the complete set of peers (*seeders* and *leechers*) in the network. The entry point to these swarms is the torrent file containing metadata about the file or files being shared. One of the most significant fields is the *announce*, which points to a URL from which we may retrieve a list of peers. The code below illustrates how a list of IP addresses in a torrent swarm may be acquired using Python. Note that the code is simplified and an actual acquisition tool should support, for example, UDP tracker URLs.

```python
import bencode, sys, hashlib, urllib, socket, struct

with open(sys.argv[1], 'rb') as metafile:
metainfo = bencode.bdecode(metafile.read())

info_hash = hashlib.sha1(bencode.bencode(metainfo['info'])).digest()
params = {
 'peer_id': '1'.zfill(20), 'port': 9999, 'info_hash': info_hash,
 'uploaded': 0, 'downloaded': 0, 'left': 0, 'compact': 1, 'event':
 'started'
}
url = '%s?%s' % (metainfo['announce'], urllib.urlencode(params))
data = bencode.bdecode(urllib.urlopen(url).read())

for i in range(0, len(data['peers']), 6):
 print '%s:%s' % (
  socket.inet_ntoa(data['peers'][i:i + 4]),
  struct.unpack('>H', data['peers'][i + 4:i + 6])[0]
)
```

In the code above, we first parse the announce URL from the torrent file, before making a request to that URL with the parameters encoded in *params*. The response of this request contains the IP addresses in a binary format that we decode in the subsequent lines. Note that we do not necessarily get all peers in a single request, so multiple subsequent requests may be needed to gather the whole swarm. One thing to note is that the anonymization technology Tor does not natively support BitTorrent, making it a little trickier to share files anonymously.

Once we have the list of peers within the swarm, it is possible to connect with each of the peers to determine, for example, how many pieces of the shared file each peer possesses.

7.5.7 Bitcoin Unconfirmed Transaction Tracing

There are multiple ways to receive information from the blockchain. One of them is to participate as a peer on the network and thus receive transaction information like any other peer. Another, possibly simpler approach is to use an *Application Programming Interface* (API) like the one at http://blockchain.info. While this does not give us a guarantee that we receive all data, and it may even curb the amount of data we are sent, it gives us a possible starting point for tracing transactions. Remember that bitcoin transactions are inherently anonymous, and whether or not we are able to extract valuable information from this source depends on a number of factors, especially how often the user generates new addresses (i.e., cryptographic public keys). The code below represents how we can subscribe to new (unconfirmed) transactions on the blockchain using websockets and Python.

```python
import json, websocket

FRAC = 100000000
def format_value(obj):
 return '%s.. (%.2fB)' % (obj['addr'][0:5], float(obj['value']) / FRAC)

def on_message(ws, msg):
 data = json.loads(msg)['x']
 print '\n[%s]' % data['time'],
 for _input_addr in data['inputs']:
 print format_value(_input_addr['prev_out']),
 print '->',
 for _out_addr in data['out']:
 print format_value(_out_addr),

def on_open(ws):
 ws.send('{"op":"unconfirmed_sub"}')

ws = websocket.WebSocketApp('wss://ws.blockchain.info/inv',
 on_message = on_message, on_open = on_open)
ws.run_forever()
```

By running the code, we get an output similar to the one below. Note that, if interested, you should be able to find the listed transactions on the blockchain. See https://blockchain.info/api for more information about the API.

```
$ python trace_bitcoin.py
[1458476339] 1Phbo.. (0.64B) 1Phbo.. (0.26B) -> 18Ws9.. (0.46B) 1Csd4..
(0.4B)
```

```
[1458476339] 1BoXX.. (0.08B) -> 1Luck.. (0.08B)
[1458476339] 31pNj.. (0.04B) -> 3LTi1.. (0.04B)
[1458476340] 1Afpp.. (0.02B) -> 1NHNd.. (0.02B)
[1458476340] 3Eb1q.. (2.29B) -> 3Dq2x.. (0.33B) 3H37f.. (1.96B)
```

If the senders and recipients generate new addresses for each transaction, which is recommended from a privacy perspective, or they let a third party handle this for them, we will not be able to follow a trail of transactions. That is, unless we manage to come up with some spectacular statistical model that may infer the sender and recipient based on a temporal, topological, or some other numeric measure.

We have discussed how we may remotely trace transactions on the blockchain. However, in many cases we may also find bitcoin software on acquired computers. These types of software commonly organize transactions into *wallets*, and we may be able to recover transaction logs, used addresses, and balances.

7.6 Collection Phase – Local Acquisition

The lines between computer and Internet forensics blur when it comes to local acquisition. The artifacts we look for are accessed using the same techniques used for accessing other types of evidence that happen to reside on a computer. So, it makes sense to view this part as a subclass of computer forensics; however, many of these artifacts may be closely related to artifacts acquired elsewhere, e.g., *Dynamic Host Configuration Protocol* (DHCP) logs for dynamic IP address configuration, or the lookup of DNS names. It thus makes sense to give them additional attention here. In this section, we touch upon topics like artifacts generated from the use of the Internet through a web browser, artifacts from email correspondence, and artifacts that may be generated from instant messaging. Finally, we discuss another trend where more and more types of devices are connected to the Internet, what is called the *Internet of Things* (IoT).

Whereas some Internet forensics artifacts are present in disk images and logs, other types of artifacts must be acquired directly from the Internet. With this kind of acquisition, we rely on a remote endpoint, for example a DNS server or web page, to provide us with accurate information. We are not in control of whether relevant information has changed prior to our acquisition, or if it will be modified after. With active acquisition, we run the additional risk of being detected by the suspects (e.g., when communicating with servers under their control). Still, this type of evidence may be sufficiently important to our investigation so as to be necessary. Here, we discuss common sources of Internet artifacts that may be acquired during investigations.

While artifacts discussed here are based on research of browsers on desktop computers, the concepts should be directly transferable to browsers on mobile devices like Android and iPhone. When you access the Internet through a web browser like Chrome or Firefox, the browser normally leaves traces of this activity on your hard drive. However, if you use your browser in *private mode* (also known as *incognito mode*), which most modern browsers support, these traces will not be written to your hard drive. You can also, at any time you want, choose to delete this information from your hard drive. There are three types of traces: history, cache, and cookies.

7.6.1 Browser History

The browser history contains all the URLs you have either typed into the address bar or followed hyperlinks to. The browsers store these URLs as a convenience for the user. This kind of information can be quite useful for determining whether or not a person has accessed certain type of services or information. The browser history also includes information about when the URL was first and last accessed, as well as how many times it has been accessed. Most browsers store browser history in an SQlite database, and are thus easily parseable. However, open source tools exist to make this job easier, such as Plaso[8] (log2timeline) and Autopsy 3.[9] In addition to browser history, browsers also leave other types of artifacts, such as bookmarks, favorite pages, and download history. These artifacts are considered special cases of the browser history artifacts and are thus not discussed separately. These artifacts can be acquired on the same locations and using the same tools as browser history.

7.6.2 Browser Cache

Most of the technology we use on the Internet is motivated by making money. To make money, we need to ensure that we minimize our costs, and transferring data from A to B costs both time and money. Furthermore, much of the information we receive for each HTTP request is unchanged from request to request (e.g., the logo of a website). Therefore, servers and clients agree on caching. Data sent from the server is assigned caching information about how long it will remain valid.

The browser will read this header information and save the object to disk along with its TTL, using the object's URL as a reference key. The next time a request for the given URL is generated, the browser will look in its cache to see if it already contains a valid object. If it does, it will skip the HTTP request and provide the cached object immediately, saving network traffic and reducing response time, pleasing both the user and the server. A cached website logo or style sheet may be of limited value to a digital investigation; however, many objects are cached for somewhat surprising reasons. Much of the technology that is commonly referred to as *Web 2.0* relies on seamless interaction with websites. New information appears on the screen, such as chat messages, without user interaction, and clicking on hyperlinks doesn't necessarily refresh the web page.

These types of features are enabled using scripting technologies like JavaScript. JavaScript also enables much of the third-party services used on many websites, such as visitor analytics, commenting sections, and the Facebook "Like" button. The requests generated by these third-party services often include requests for empty pictures or JavaScript files, where much of the payload of the information is encoded within the URL itself. Because pictures and JavaScript files often are cached to disk, this information is also written to disk. And as the URLs are used as key, this information is fully available, even if both the request and response are encrypted. Figure 7.6 shows an actual example of such information from the popular commenting service Disqus, extracted from a hard drive. We can see that the user has posted something (verb is "post") to a specific forum thread (forum_id is "1244139").

---

8 https://github.com/log2timeline/plaso/wiki.
9 http://www.sleuthkit.org/autopsy/.

```
Remote Address: 23.235.43.134:80
Request URL: http://referrer.disqus.com/juggler/event.js?experiment=default&variant=control
&product=embed&thread=1521270677&forum=pcbje&forum_id=1244139&zone=thread&version=94be1b1e&
page_url=http%3A%2F%2Fpcbje.com%2F2013%2F07%2Fhtml5-activity-chart-inspired-by-github%2F&pa
ge_referrer_domain=pcbje.com&duration=539&object_type=post&object_id=1482882957&verb=post&e
vent=activity&imp=4r0ucni1t7ql5g&prev_imp=&section=default&area=n%2Fa
Request Method: GET
Status Code: ● 200 OK
▶ Request Headers (8)
▶ Query String Parameters (19)
▼ Response Headers     view source
  Connection: keep-alive
  Content-Encoding: gzip
  Content-Type: application/javascript
  Date: Sun, 13 Jul 2014 10:58:08 GMT
  Server: nginx
  Transfer-Encoding: chunked
  Vary: Accept-Encoding
```

Figure 7.6 Information in a cached URL.

Because cache often is stored in custom data formats, it is easiest to access them using tools like Plaso. Plaso is designed to parse information generated by a large number of applications, including web browsers.

7.6.3   Browser Cookies

We briefly mentioned third-party services in Section 7.6.2. Again, as most of the innovation on the Internet is motivated by profit, many third-party services have specialized in brokering advertisement between advertisers and content providers, with an increasing focus on targeted advertising (i.e., providing advertisement suited to the visitor to increase the click rate). To enable this type of targeting, the advertisement brokers need to be able to identify the visitor across multiple content providers. This is enabled by using cookies.

When you download and view a web page, the browser makes a number of requests for objects, like pictures, under the hood. If the provider of the website is affiliated with an advertisement network, the browser will also generate a request to this network. *Cookies* are information that is sent to the server along with an HTTP request; they are specific to a given domain or URL. These cookies are commonly used for remembering states between requests (e.g., user logins or content providers to give visitors a better experience when using their service).

An example of cookie usage is maintaining a shopping cart on an e-commerce site without having to sign up or log in. In the cases of both shopping carts and advertisement, the cookie is usually a unique value identifying the visitor and the browser the visitor is using. Once the customer is identified, scripting on the website can enable analytics, such as where on the screen the cursor is, what the customer is searching for and clicking on, and so forth. If all websites used the same advertisement network, this network could then follow every visit to every site by every visitor. While this may not be the case for any advertisement network as of yet, the Facebook "Like" button enables the same type of identification across websites. Quite a lot of websites use this button.

7.6.4 Email

Jumping from web browsers to emails, we have previously discussed how these may be downloaded from a mail server. The downloaded files are organized by the email applications used on the endpoint (e.g., Microsoft Outlook or OS X Mail). In addition to the contents, these emails contain the email headers, information about the sender, and the disclosed receivers of downloaded emails. The MAC times of the files may further indicate when the emails were downloaded. An example of a case where emails were important as evidence was the Enron investigation starting in 2001. As a result of the investigation, over 600,000 emails sent between 158 employees were made available on the Internet.[10] This dataset has subsequently been an important resource for research on topics such as statistical link analysis, authorship attribution, and approximate matching (Bjelland et al., 2014).

Email correspondence may be an invaluable source of evidence. While email servers are likely to contain much of the same information, mailboxes on a computer provide a closer connection between the email contents and the owner of the computer. Still, while email continues to be an important arena for communication, instant messaging applications and services have also increased in popularity over the last decade.

7.6.5 Messaging and Chats

While email involves a properly defined standard for how messages are pushed between servers and between clients, instant messaging applications are free to implement whatever protocol they see fit. Whereas older instant messaging architectures like Microsoft Network (MSN) were client–server based, modern services like Skype, ICQ, and XMPP are peer-to-peer, where the server functions as a broker for the different peers to find each other. This architecture may make it more difficult to acquire logs of communications between suspects. In addition, multiple layers of encryption may be used. For instance, the network connection between clients may be encrypted using SSL, while messages may be encrypted using technologies such as *pretty good privacy* or *off-the-record* (OTR). In these cases, it may be impossible to recover the messages unless we come across decrypted copies of the messages, or the private keys used for encryption.

At some point, the messages have to be decrypted for the user to read them. Applications may also store chat history as a convenience for the user. These logs may be the decrypted versions of messages, so even if the messages were sent over encrypted channels and used message encryption like OTR, we may be able to recover the plain text if we acquire the endpoint computer.

7.6.6 Internet of Things

IoT is a term for the trend by which a continuously more diverse set of devices are connected to the Internet. For example, Internet-connected fire and burglary alarms, fridges, and power monitors are becoming commonplace gadgets. The difference

---

10 https://www.cs.cmu.edu/~./enron/.

between these devices and conventional Internet-connected devices such as computers is that they are designed to consume significantly less electricity. These devices range from devices that run some sort of server application, like an Internet-connected printer, to tiny, battery-powered devices that only push data on a fixed interval or under some other condition.

Some major challenges with IoT devices are proprietary formats (how data is stored), protocols (how data is transmitted), and interfaces (how data may be acquired). Though some standardization may be put in place at some point, data collection from these sources will likely be a costly and time-consuming process in the time to come.

It seems too soon to conclude how this trend will affect digital forensics, but it is natural to assume that new types of devices will become a ubiquitous part of investigations. Search engines like Shodan[11] make ill-protected devices discoverable from across the globe, and stories like the ones published by the Norwegian newspaper *Dagbladet* in 2014[12] make it seem like large-scale exploitation of IoT devices is inevitable.

7.7 Collection Phase – Network Acquisition

When we are doing investigations of environments where we have access to the local network, valuable artifacts may be found in network logs and captured traffic.

7.7.1 tcpdump and pcap

In high-security environments, it is indeed quite common to store every single packet passing over the network for a certain amount of time. In other scenarios, it might be necessary to capture post-incident network traffic. Both may use the tool *tcpdump*, which listens for packets arriving at a network interface and stores the data in a format called *pcap*. Below is an example command for starting traffic collection on a given interface, and storing the data by minute.

```
$ sudo tcpdump -i en0 -w %Y-%m-%d_%H-%M-%S%z.pcap -G 60
```

By default, an endpoint network interface will only accept network packets destined for itself. Most often, this does not have any practical consequence, as routers make sure that traffic is only sent to the intended recipient anyway. However, under circumstances where the router does not control this (e.g., in wireless networks or with physical interception), we need to tell the network card to accept packets intended for other recipients. This is done by setting the network card in *promiscuous mode*, which tcpdump does by default. Another mode exists, called *monitor*, which operates similarly, but without itself having to connect to the network. Capturing traffic like this may be extremely storage and I/O (input–output) intensive, meaning that on real networks you will only be able to store the data for a short period of time. Once the traffic is captured, it may be analyzed with tools like Wireshark.[13] Below is a Python script to print source and

---

11   www.shodan.io.
12   http://www.dagbladet.no/nullctrl/english.
13   www.wireshark.org.

destination IP addresses from all packets in a pcap file.[14] Another alternative is to write a wrapper around the Wireshark command line tool *tshark*.[15]

```
#!/usr/bin/python
# -*- coding: utf-8 -*-
from datetime import datetime
from pcapfile import savefile
import sys

with open(sys.argv[1]) as cap:
 for packet in savefile.load_savefile(cap, layers=2).packets:
 if packet.packet.type == 2048: # IP packet
 time = datetime.fromtimestamp(packet.timestamp)
 src_ip = packet.packet.payload.src
 dst_ip = packet.packet.payload.dst
 size = packet.packet.payload.len
 print '[%s] %s -> %s (%s bytes)' % (time, src_ip, dst_ip, size)
```

When executed, the output will be something like this:

```
$ python dump_pcap.py 2015-09-05_17-51-48+0200.pcap
[2015-09-05 17:51:48] 192.168.0.1 -> 192.168.0.2 (320 bytes)
[2015-09-05 17:51:49] 192.168.0.2 -> 192.168.0.1 (365 bytes)
[2015-09-05 17:51:51] 192.168.0.2 -> 192.168.0.1 (78 bytes)
[2015-09-05 17:51:51] 192.168.0.1 -> 192.168.0.2 (409 bytes)
```

7.7.1.1 Netflow

Instead of storing the complete network traffic, routers may be configured to log the source and destination of all packets that pass it. Such logs require significantly less storage space, so they can be kept for a longer period of time. Below is an excerpt from a netflow low, showing a request and response between two endpoints.

```
Src IP|Dst IP|Src port|Dst port|Protocol|-|-|-|Start time|End time
192.168.0.1|192.168.0.2|5555|4444|ICMP|1|1|1|1067636618|1067636619
192.168.0.2|192.168.0.1|4444|5555|ICMP|1|1|1|1067636620|1067636621
```

7.7.2 DHCP Logs

For an endpoint to be able to communicate over a network, it needs an IP address. One common way of obtaining this address is through a DHCP server. While this server may run independently, it is common for this service to be integrated into home routers. The server may be configured to keep a log for when an endpoint, identified by a *Media Access Control* (MAC) address, is given a specific IP address.

---

14 Using *pypcapfile*: https://pypi.python.org/pypi/pypcapfile.
15 https://www.wireshark.org/docs/man-pages/tshark.html.

7.8   Collection Phase – Remote Acquisition

The final type of acquisition we discuss in this chapter is remote acquisition. This refers to the acquisition of artifacts that have been generated on endpoints not directly used by those involved, such as web servers, or on endpoints we do not have physical control over, such as websites, social media, and other open sources.

7.8.1   Server

In this discussion, we limit the scope of Internet forensics artifacts on servers to artifacts generated from requests made by web browsers over HTTP, as well as typical artifacts generated by web applications themselves. Other types of artifacts reside closed to computer forensics.

7.8.1.1   Web Server Logs

The artifacts generated on servers from the use of the Internet are usually in the form of logs. These logs are usually in a readable text format that can be parsed and structured by software tools. They are generated by a class of software called *web servers*. Three popular web servers are Nginx, Apache2, and Microsoft IIS. Other, less frequently used web servers also exist; however, these tend to maintain their logs in a manner similar to web application logs, and should thus be somewhat covered by Section 7.8.1.2.

A log entry generated by web servers corresponds to a single HTTP or HTTPS request and usually contains the fields shown in Table 7.3. Each log entry explains, among other things, what resources were requested, who (hyperlink) referred to this resource, how it was requested, and the size and type (OK, Not Found, Forbidden, etc.) of the response.

Log entries are usually grouped together by date (e.g., one log for every hour or every day). Note that closed log files are often automatically compressed to save storage space.

7.8.1.2   Web Application Logs

When the web server receives an incoming request from a client, it determines what running process on the server should handle the request. These processes may be built

Table 7.3   Common web server log fields.

Field	Description	Example
Identity	Identity of the client on its machine	jimmy (though most often "-")
Timestamp	Time when the request was received	10/Sep/2015:16:33:01 +0200
Bytes	Size of the response in bytes	137
Request	A string containing what resource was requested	GET/home.php HTTP/1.1
Auth	The identity of the client on the server	jimmy
Agent	The browser the client says is being used	Mozilla5.0; Windows NT 6.1; [. . .]
Referrer	From where the browser says it came from	http://someothersite.com/page.php
Client IP	The public IP address of the client	128.39.41.45

from a number of different technologies, like PHP, Python, Java, and C#. How some of the common web application technologies maintain their logs is discussed here. Whereas some of these technologies usually run behind a web server, others run a web server of their own. Web application logs often store information about which actions were performed during each request and may provide information about login attempts, user signups, sent and received messages, and so forth.

While each web application is free to maintain (or keep) logs exactly how it chooses, there is a tendency toward a standard logging format. The developers of applications are further free to choose a logging format suited to their needs. As with other log files, web application log files often reside in the operating system's standard log directory (like/ var/log on Linux); however, application developers may choose to store log files where they see fit. Another normal location for application log files is next to where the web application (script or compiled computer code) resides.

7.8.1.3 Virtual Hosts

Web servers such as Apache2 and Nginx allow multiple websites to be served on the same endpoint over the same port. An example of an Apache2 configuration on a Unix system with two virtual hosts is given below. When a HTTP request is sent to an endpoint, the web server looks at the requested domain name, and determines a *document root* based on this value. The different virtual servers may also use different log files, so be sure to look at the virtual server configuration for log file locations.

```
Listen 80
NameVirtualHost *:80

<VirtualHost *:80>
    ServerName www.some-website.com
    DocumentRoot /var/www/example1
</VirtualHost>
<VirtualHost *:80>
    ServerName www.some-other-website.com
    DocumentRoot /var/www/example2
</VirtualHost>
```

7.8.2 Cloud Services

Cloud environments, where a potentially large number of computers cooperate to provide a flexible and scalable computing platform, add additional challenges to an investigation. Cloud forensics may be considered a special case of *remote forensics*, where evidence is obtained from remote endpoints over communication channels like *Secure SHell* (SSH). However, there are some important differences between them. In cloud environments, artifacts from a single virtual machine may be spread across multiple physical machines, so physical disk imaging makes little or no sense. Furthermore, cloud environments often consist of multiple virtual machines. Finally, virtual machines in cloud environments may be spawned, terminated, and moved regularly, so their forensic artifacts should be considered more volatile.

These aspects of cloud forensics add additional requirements on the process, including rapid response, collaboration with service providers such as Amazon and Rackspace, and the automation of tasks to better scale one's efforts. There are also some possibilities that emerge when investigating cloud environments, especially regarding how the environment may be accessed. Virtual machines in cloud environments are often configured with cryptographic keys for access, meaning that there is no username and password in use. The machines, however, are often accessible either through keys stored on the operator's computer or through the service provider's administration panel, accessible through a web browser. It may be possible to access these entry points with known credentials or through collaboration with the service provider. From there, it may be possible to identify and access previously unidentified environments, since all environments will be listed.

7.8.3 Open Sources

The term *open source* is used about information and resources that are publicly available, and this section focuses on information publicly available from remote endpoints. This includes various types of websites on the Internet. Open source artifacts may be deployed in both reactive and proactive investigations. Reactive investigations (let's call them *open source forensics*) are the focus of this section. Proactive use of open source artifacts, demonstrated when the investigation is not a response to a particular incident but rather in preparation for future incidents, is primarily referred to as *open source intelligence*.

We will not attempt an extensive review of how one may use common websites and services in digital investigations. For one thing, such reviews become rapidly outdated, and many resources about their use already exist. Instead, we focus on the types of open source information that may be of interest to an investigation. We categorize them as follows:

- personal information,
- user accounts,
- contact lists,
- publication of content,
- interaction with content,
- public interaction, and
- association with groups and communities.

These types of information may be found all across the Internet, including in social media, forums, news sites, blogs, search engines, and archives. The information may be acquired manually with an investigator using a web browser, or automatically through web scrapers and APIs.

7.8.3.1 Personal Information

Personal information (such as *name, phone number, email address, address, age, sex,* and *employment*) is information that can be tied to an individual. Some of this information is Personally Identifiable Information (PII), such as name, phone number, and email addresses. Personal information that is not PII includes employment and gender. Social media and search engines are great resources for finding such information, and may be valuable in finding easily available clues and context information during investigations.

7.8.3.2 User Accounts

Different user accounts, such as Facebook, Twitter, LinkedIn, email addresses (again), various forums, and Internet communities, may be valuable to identify those user accounts that a person owns. On some services, it may be as easy as searching for the person's name on the service. The results, sometimes including a profile picture, may be compared to known information to validate the results. In other scenarios, it may be trickier to identify the accounts.

It may be possible to determine that a person in fact *has* an account on a service by trying to create an account with the person's email address. If the service tells you that the email address is already registered, you know that the account is there. There are some obvious operational security issues related to this technique, so make sure to check what information the service sends during partial sign-ups. Other services, like the profile picture service Gravatar, use a cryptographic hash of a user's email address to enable a shared profile picture across multiple services. This means that if you know a person's email addresses, you can detect the presence of the person in acquired data by looking at the profile picture references.

7.8.3.3 Contact Lists

Contact lists (such as *friends* on Facebook, *followers* and *following* on Twitter, and *contacts* on LinkedIn) are information about other individuals who in some way are related to a person. These lists are either symmetric or asymmetric. In symmetric contact lists, a relation from person A to person B implies a relation from person B to person A. An example of such relations is friendship on Facebook. In asymmetric contact lists, a relation from A to B does not imply a relation from B to A. Followers on Twitter are an example of asymmetric contact lists. Contact lists can be found on various social media services. The information may provide valuable information about the social context around an individual, and may also provide clues to other individuals who might be of interest to an investigation.

7.8.3.4 Publication of Content

Online content (such as blog posts, personal web pages, tweets, and Facebook posts) published by a person of interest may be valuable to an investigation. Such information includes personal blog posts and other types of self-maintained websites and public posts on sites like Twitter and Facebook. Often this type of information may be found by searching for the person's name in search engines. Other times, the search engines at the given search engine sites (e.g., Facebook) may be used. Furthermore, knowing the user identity of a person allows us to go directly to their personal page.

7.8.3.5 Interaction with Content

In addition to the content the person is publishing, we may be interested in the public interaction that the person has had with other published content (e.g., news articles and other public information like tweets and Facebook posts). Many websites use third-party services like Disqus to let visitors comment on their content. Such services often let us see all comments made by an individual user, so if we find the person of interest's account, we can retrieve the person's comments from all across the Internet. On other services like Facebook, we may have to find the posts that the person may have commented on before finding the person's comments. To narrow down places where one should look for such posts, we can follow links to the person's friends and group memberships and look for comments there.

7.8.3.6 Public Interaction
Another way to further investigate contact lists and interaction with content is to look for any public interaction the person has had with others (such as *forums*, *public posts* on social media profile pages, and Twitter *mentions*). We commonly find this type of information on social media, such as Twitter discussions and posts on Facebook profile pages, as well as Internet forums. Public chat like Internet Relay Chat (IRC) may also fall into this category.

7.8.3.7 Association with Groups and Communities
The final type of open source information we discuss is the type that provides clues to a person's interests and affiliation with communities on the Internet (such as self-written biography, group memberships, and Facebook *likes*). Sometimes this information is provided in the person's biography (e.g., the *About Me* part of a social media account). Other sources of this type of information may be Facebook *likes* and group memberships.

7.9   Other Considerations

Here we discuss some topics that may be relevant to your acquisition and management of artifacts from the Internet. Before starting a discussion on how artifacts may and should be acquired in a forensically sound manner, we describe a technique common for accessing information from applications and services: the APIs.

7.9.1   Application Programming Interfaces (APIs)

While manually browsing and searching for content on various web services is a simple and sometimes valuable technique for acquiring open source information, it is not very efficient. And as the number of sites and services that need to be queried increases, the investigation may become difficult to manage. It therefore makes sense to develop automated tools to do the collection for us. While it certainly is possible to automatically parse the HTML and JavaScript of a website to extract information, many services provide a way for obtaining this information in a structured format. This is called the service's API. These web service APIs accept the same types of requests as the normal service (e.g., GET and POST), but instead of HTML, a JavaScript Object Notation (JSON) or eXtensible Markup Language (XML) document is returned instead. This document is easily parsed by software tools, and may thus help automate the process of acquiring and organizing open source artifacts.

7.9.1.1 Accessing User Accounts
There is a number of ways that an account, such as a Gmail or Facebook account, may become available to an investigator. For one, the computer may be unlocked and logged in to the service when it is acquired. In other cases, login credentials may be found at the

crime scene (e.g., a yellow note sticker next to the computer) or be provided during interrogation. Finally, cookies may be extracted from an acquired disk image and used to re-create a login session on another computer, as illustrated below. Note that cookies are expired after a certain time of inactivity. They are also invalidated when a user signs out.

This is a request without cookies; Facebook wants us to log in:

```
$ curl -X GET https://www.facebook.com/home.php --location \
| sed -n "s/.*<title id=\"pageTitle\">\(.*\)<\/title>.*/\1/p"
Logg inn på Facebook | Facebook
```

This is a request with cookie values extracted from disk image; Facebook considers us logged in:

```
$ curl -X GET https://www.facebook.com/home.php --location \
   --cookie "c_user=<user_id>; xs=<xs_cookie>;" \
      | sed -n "s/.*<title id=\"pageTitle\">\(.*\)<\/title>.*/\1/p"
Facebook
```

Note that accessing Facebook this way may be a violation of their terms of use.

Once logged in to a private account, information about activity and contacts otherwise available may be acquired by the investigators. Note that there may be legal and ethical considerations that must be evaluated before accessing private accounts.

7.9.2 Integrity of Remote Artifacts

The integrity of information traced or acquired from remote endpoints is a question that we need to be aware of every time we collect some new information. In this section, we discuss how we can reduce uncertainty by helping us trace how and when a certain artifact was acquired. As we do not have an original, like a computer or mobile phone on which we can go back and double-check our findings, additional efforts are needed to ensure the integrity after the acquisition. When we are running a command (like traceroute) to trace or acquire information on the Internet, a couple of things should be logged:

- the date and time the command was started,
- the date and time the command finished,
- on which computer (MAC address) it was executed,
- the user executing the command,
- the name of the command executed, and
- the arguments supplied to the command.

All this information should be written to a file (let's call it *input*), and a cryptographic checksum like MD5 or SHA1 should be generated for that file. The results from the command should be written to another file (let's call this one *output*), and another checksum should be generated for that file. Finally, a checksum should be generated for both files. In this way, we know what command and arguments produced a certain result, and we can be certain of this fact as long as the checksums match the *input* and *output* files. The checksums may be written to a file *checksums*, and all three files compressed to a single archive (e.g., Zip). This archive should be given a name containing the date, the command, and the arguments provided to the command. In this way, acquired information is easily organized by time and type. A simple Python program implementing these steps is available online,[16] but note that this technique does not protect against intended tampering with the evidence.

7.10 The Examination and Analysis Phases

We conclude this chapter with a discussion about how Internet forensics artifacts may be examined, analyzed, and presented. We focus the discussion on two commonly used analysis and presentation techniques: networks and timelines. *Networks* are great for showing how various pieces of information or entities are related, and timelines are well suited to see how various events may be related. Much of the artifacts we acquire in Internet forensics may be modeled as networks, also referred to as *link diagrams*. This may be a model of IP addresses having communicated with each other, people communicating with each other in online communities, and DNS relationships such as domain to IP or domain ownership. Other types of artifacts are best organized by the time they occurred (e.g., how an IP address accessed resources on a server). Such visualizations are called *timelines*. Other chapters in this book have introduced network (link) analysis and timelines as analysis techniques. Here we discuss techniques to help make sense of large amounts of artifacts acquired from the Internet.

7.10.1 Finding Interesting Nodes in Large Networks

Once we start acquiring and structuring data from the Internet, we soon find ourselves with a large amount of data that needs to be examined and analyzed. Networks of domain names, IPs, emails, and so on easily contain millions of relations between actors. If you know who your target is, this may be as easy as having a decent search engine available to find data related to this actor. But what do you do when you don't have this luxury? While the answer indeed may be difficult to answer, computational models that rank nodes are a good start. Here we discuss two such computational methods: social network analysis and PageRank.

Social network analysis (SNA) measures how *central* a node or an edge is to a network (Scott, 2012). It can also be used to measure the network as a whole by averaging the centrality of all nodes and edges. There are a number of ways this centrality can be measured. Three such methods are degree, closeness, and betweenness. *Degree* measures centrality as the number of edges originating or terminating at a node. In a network of email correspondence, this is the number of distinct addresses an email address has communicated with. A node with a high degree of centrality is often referred to as a *hub*. The *closeness* centrality of a node is computed based on the total distance to all other nodes in the network. A node with a high closeness centrality has a higher potential for distributing information to the rest of the network. Finally, the *betweenness* centrality of

---

16 https://github.com/pcbje/verify.

a node *B* is computed by measuring the fraction of shortest paths from *A* to *C* that goes through *B*. Nodes *A* and *C* are all pairs of nodes in the network that does not include *B*. A node with a high betweenness centrality may have an important role in transmitting information between parts of the network. From a law enforcement perspective, removing an actor with high betweenness centrality in a criminal network may be an efficient way of disrupting the network.

PageRank was first introduced by the people behind Google (Page et al., 1999). It was originally used to rank search results based on incoming hyperlinks. The assumption the algorithm makes is that high-quality websites tend to be more referenced than lower quality websites (such as spam). Thus, a reference (hyperlink) from a high-quality website is more likely to provide good content than references from low-quality sites.

7.10.2   Divide and Conquer Large Networks

Sometimes the amount of data in a network is too large to make sense of it as a whole. Then we want to break the networks down into manageable parts without losing significant information. Here we discuss two techniques for splitting up a network: *clustering* and *community detection*.

7.10.2.1   Clustering

A large network may consist of multiple completely disjunct graphs, meaning that there is no edge connecting two subgraphs. As both visualization and other computational methods for network analysis tend to be computationally expensive, it makes sense to split the dataset into as many completely disjunct graphs as possible. Splitting a dataset into smaller parts may also help you gain an overview of the available data. The naïve way of doing this splitting is as follows:

```
for each edge
  if edge source and target already are in the same cluster:
  do nothing
  else if edge source is in a cluster and target is not:
  add target to source cluster
  else if edge target is in a cluster and source is not:
  add source to target cluster
  else if edge source and target are in different clusters:
  merge the two clusters
  else if neither edge source and target is in any cluster:
  create a new cluster containing source and target
then write each cluster to file
```

The cluster files may be named according to their metrics, such as the number of nodes, the number of edges, and the number of events, making it easy to detect potentially interesting clusters.

7.10.2.2   Community Detection

In large networks, it makes sense to partition the data into smaller chunks that may be analyzed individually. If the graph is not connected (i.e., we have two or more completely

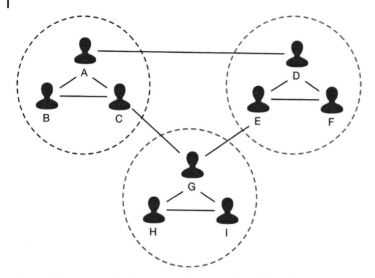

Figure 7.7 Communities in networks (icons by Visual Pharm).

disconnected subgraphs), partitioning is easy, as we have just shown. On large connected graphs, however, we can apply *community detection* (Fortunato, 2010). An illustration of a network containing three easily identifiable communities is given in Figure 7.7. It is important to note that with such techniques, we lose some information in the process as we are removing relations between certain nodes. This potential loss of important information must be accounted for during our analysis. With community detection, we are looking for nodes that are connected with each other to a larger extent than with other nodes. The relationship between the nodes' internal versus external connectivity is called its *clustering coefficient*. Note that community detection is an NP-complete problem, meaning that it does not scale well as the network grows really large (e.g., millions of nodes). In such cases, sampling techniques may be applied to generate approximate communities. If we divide the network into separate communities, we may then be able to investigate each of the communities individually.

7.10.3   Making Sense of Millions of Events

Networks may not be the best way to visualize large datasets. Often it is difficult to identify and understand patterns by looking at a link diagram alone. Here we discuss three techniques that help to identify and understand patterns in datasets. These are based on *when* and *where* events occurred.

7.10.3.1   Aggregated Timelines

Many artifacts we acquire from the Internet share the fact that they are associated with a specific time, a *timestamp*. The timestamps may represent things like the time a domain was registered, or when an email was sent. Based on the timestamps, we can create buckets of an appropriate size (e.g., day or week) and place events into these buckets. The buckets may then be visualized as a time series, where the bucket (i.e., timestamp) is

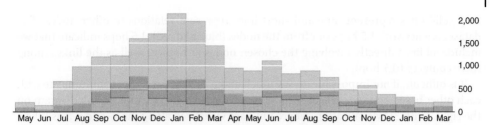

May Jun Jul Aug Sep Oct Nov Dec Jan Feb Mar Apr May Jun Jul Aug Sep Oct Nov Dec Jan Feb Mar

Figure 7.8 An aggregated timeline (data and visualization by D3).[17]

along the *x*-axis, and the number of events is plotted along the *y*-axis. Buckets may also be grouped by some attribute. For example, if we are aware of two interesting email addresses, we may want to visualize the amount of emails they have sent or received. An example of a grouped time series in shown in Figure 7.8.

7.10.3.2 Temporal Networks

Timelines focus on when events occurred, and link analysis focuses on who the events involved. When we combine the two factors (i.e., when we consider the time a link existed between two nodes), we have *temporal networks*. Temporal network theory is currently being applied in physics, biology, and epidemiology (spread of diseases), where the order of events is essential to their significance. A good introduction to temporal networks may be found in Holme (2012). In our analysis, temporal networks may be valuable for both the computational models and visualization.

One question where temporal network theory may be interesting in our investigation is whether our data proves that an actor may have received certain information at a given time. This is relevant in cases like insider trading. Say we have three actors *A*, *B*, and *C*, and links from *A* to *B* and from *B* to *C*. If the link from *B* to *C* occurred *before* the link from *A* to *B*, we cannot say based on these edges that *C* may have received information from *A*.

The visualization of temporal networks may help us identify and understand patterns of links between actors. An example of such a visualization is given in Figure 7.9, where

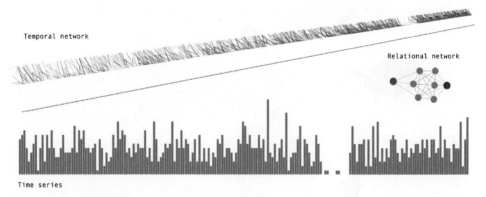

Figure 7.9 Visualization of a 1.5-hop temporal network.

---

17 http://d3js.org.

long solid lines represent time and short lines represent relations to other nodes. The dataset is a network 1.5 hops out from the nodes (blue and red). 1.5 hops indicate that we include all links directly involving the chosen nodes (1 hop), as well as the links among their contacts (0.5 hop).

It is difficult, if not impossible, to say much about how these actors communicate with each other based on the aggregated timeline on the bottom, or from the link diagram on the right. With 3D visualization, where links are visualized along the *x*- and *y*-axis (like a link diagram), and time is along the *z*-axis, it becomes easy to spot how the blue node is repeatedly linked to the same set of other nodes, while the red node is less active.

7.10.3.3 Heat Maps

One other factor it may make sense to visualize is *where* the nodes geographically are at the time of the events. We have previously discussed geolocation of IP addresses, and other artifacts such as Whois may contain geographical information. It may make sense to plot every geolocation on a map, but it is also possible to aggregate data by continent, country, or city. In Figure 7.10, we illustrate aggregation by country. The color of a country represents the number of events geolocated to that country, where gray represents no events, and the scale otherwise goes from yellow (lowest frequency) to red (highest frequency). Such geographically aggregated heat maps may provide quick and valuable insight into where the actors in our investigation are most commonly located (e.g., where the visitors to a web server come from).

Heat maps can also be used to visualize activity over time, either for finding specific dates or weeks someone has been active, or to understand at what hours or on which weekdays two people communicate. An example of the former is shown in Figure 7.11.

The final subject we discuss regarding examination and analysis of Internet artifacts is translation of text. You may encounter situations where the artifacts that are being acquired contain text in a language you do not comprehend. And while human interpreters are a requirement to fully comprehend these texts, machine translation

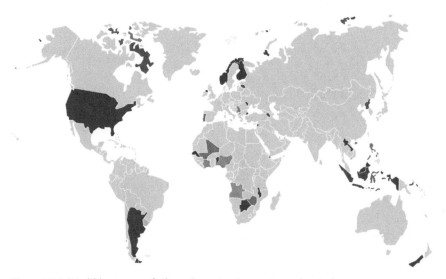

Figure 7.10 World heat map of where the actors in events are located.

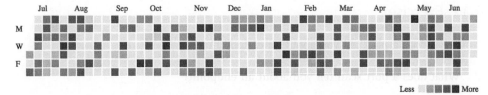

Figure 7.11 A heat map showing the amount of activity over a year's span.

may help you determine the subjects. This may in turn result in more efficient use of interpreters, as we can disregard uninteresting data. Machine translation may also improve the usability of text indexing, as the need for searching in multiple languages is reduced.

We divide machine translation into two classes: *online* and *offline*. Online translation includes commercial tools like Google translate, which provides relatively high-quality translations. In many cases, however, it may be neither possible nor desirable to use a translation service over the Internet. Instead we may deploy our own offline translation service, which may run on closed networks or locally on a single computer. One free and open source tool for doing offline machine translation is *Moses*.[18] You will need to train the translation models yourself, but their site includes easy-to-follow instructions for doing so, as well as datasets for training the system to translate many European languages to English. A description of how Moses works is given in Koehn (2007).

7.11 Summary

This chapter has discussed aspects of computer networking and the Internet that may be relevant during a digital forensic investigation. We have discussed how electronic signals are routed from endpoint to endpoint to websites to determine the identity of an already logged-in user; how various network models enable different kinds of evidence tracing; and how various types of artifacts may be acquired from the Internet infrastructure and open sources. Artifacts found in open sources on the Internet and artifacts generated by Internet activity, such as Internet browser history, were discussed, with examples categorized as local, network, or remote acquisition.

The chapter also touched upon circumstances, or caveats, that may affect the validity and usability of artifacts, like onion routing using Tor or sharing a public IP address with multiple other Internet users behind a NAT. Finally, the chapter presented some ideas for how large amounts of data may be analyzed to support or refute hypotheses during investigations.

As with most information technology, Internet forensics is constantly changing. New types of artifacts emerge as others perish. There is much room for creative and innovative approaches when it comes to reconstructing events based on information available from network and Internet activity. Those who find this subject interesting are encouraged to come up with new and better ways to identify, acquire, and understand the vast amount of information that is out there. Much is yet to be explored and invented.

---

18 www.statmt.org/moses/.

7.12 Exercises

1 What does a ping tell you about an endpoint?

2 What does a port scan tell you about an endpoint?

3 How may a website determine if a user is already logged in?

4 What is a web shell?

5 Why is acquiring artifacts from remote endpoints a challenge in forensic investigations?

6 What types of artifacts may be generated when you visit a website?

7 Why may Network Address Translations (NATs) be a challenge during investigations?

8 Describe some common peer-to-peer networks or applications.

8

Challenges in Digital Forensics

Katrin Franke[1] and André Årnes[2]

[1]*Norwegian University of Science and Technology (NTNU), Gjøvik, Norway*
[2]*Norwegian University of Science and Technology (NTNU), Gjøvik, Norway; and Telenor Group, Oslo, Norway*

One of the key challenges in digital forensics today is the huge amounts of unstructured data, often with inherent uncertainties and errors. Based on the chapters in this textbook, it should be clear that each phase of the digital forensics process can be very time and resource demanding, often exceeding the time and resources available for the investigation. Due to this, there has been substantial interest in leveraging big data, automation, and computational methods as part of the forensic process. For example:

- The *identification phase* can be supported by intelligent detection and identification methods.
- The *collection phase* can be supported by automated remote evidence acquisition tools with built-in evidence integrity assurance.
- The *examination phase* can be supported by automated data recovery and data reduction.
- The *analysis phase* can leverage computational methods and machine learning to identify patterns and data of interest in evidence.
- The *presentation phase* can benefit from a wide range of visualization tools, as well as built-in report generation.

In this chapter, we will give a brief introduction to some open research topics, mainly based on research at the Norwegian Information Security Laboratory (NISLab). The purpose of this chapter is to inspire further studies and research projects within this domain. The reader is also recommended to read the position paper, "Digital Forensics Research: The Next 10 Years," for further inspiration (Garfinkel, 2010).

8.1 Computational Forensics

We will start the discussion with an introduction of computational forensics, as introduced and defined in Franke and Srihari (2007, 2008). It refers to the application of computational methods to forensics. Such methods are becoming a necessity in digital forensics, as the data volume rapidly explodes, the complexity in technology infrastructures increases, the interconnectivity in social networks grows, and finally the digital evidence is often erroneous, uncertain, and partial. In summary, we need to extend our toolkit with more advanced tools and methods, in order to look for tiny pieces of evidence hidden in a chaotic environment – or, if you will, *the needle in the haystack*.

Definition 8.1: Computational Forensics

The hypothesis-driven investigation of a specific forensic problem using computers, with the primary goal of discovery and advancement of forensic knowledge. Computational forensics works toward:

1) In-depth understanding of a forensic discipline
2) Evaluation of a particular scientific method basis
3) Systematic approach to forensic sciences by applying techniques of computer science, applied mathematics, and statistics

It involves modeling and computer simulation (synthesis) and/or computer-based analysis and recognition.

8.1.1 The Objectives of Computational Forensics

The objectives of computational forensics can be examplified as follows.

8.1.1.1 Large-Scale Investigations

Cybercrime investigations and investigations in large multinational corporations share the properties of large volumes of data from a wide range of sources. The ability to efficiently and effectively manage the data during the digital forensics process requires the application of computational methods.

In Flaglien *et al.* (2011), Flaglien researched a method for automatic identification of malware traces across multiple computers, inspired by challenges from large-scale online bank fraud investigations (as exemplified in the SpyEye case in Section 1.3.4). The objective of the research was to efficiently identify patterns in large, complex datasets using link-mining techniques, in a forensically sound fashion.

As part of a PhD project, Shalaginov (Shalaginov & Franke, 2015) researched the use of Neuro-Fuzzy (NF) methods based on large-scale network traffic analysis in digital forensics investigations. The purpose of the research was to identify patterns of benign and malicious activity in network traffic dumps through the use of NF algorithms, handling large-scale datasets with reduced classification model complexity. The research has been continued in several papers.

8.1.1.2 Automation

Digital forensics has to a large degree been dependent on manual processes, supported by checklists, process descriptions, and some built-in automation and scripting in forensic tools. There is, however, a need for more comprehensive automation in order to reduce manual efforts and increase the quality of digital forensics. As we have observed in this textbook, there is extensive potential for automation in all steps of the digital forensics process.

As an example, we studied a method for partial automation of the forensic reconstruction of computer intrusions in Årnes *et al.* (2007). The research utilized a virtual environment to efficiently execute a repeatable forensic reconstruction experience, explained through two scenarios – "The Trojan Did It!" and "A Multistep Attack."

In Fossen and Årnes (2005), Fossen investigated a method for automating the geolocation of IP addresses, using triangulation based on multiple, geographically dispersed measurements. The prototype, referred to as GeoLocate, used the constraint-based geolocation (CBG) method and network Looking Glass services to estimate the location of an IP address in 1 to 2 minutes.

8.1.1.3 Analysis

The analysis of digital evidence can be significantly strengthened through computational methods. Whereas a human analyst can spot anomalies and patterns based on experience, computational methods can establish timelines, perform link analysis, and identify patterns in a predictable manner. Validated computational forensics methods will support human analysts in deducing conclusions based on evidence, in less time and with higher certainties.

As an example, Maartmann-Moe et al. (2009) investigated methods for the identification and extraction of cryptographic keys from volatile memory in computer devices. A new method, *interrogate*, was implemented to allow for a higher success rate for forensic analysis, and the results demonstrated that the chances of locating forensic keys were surprisingly high.

Bjelland *et al.* (2014) studied how approximate *hash-based matching*, also known as *fuzzy hashing*, could be used to identify complex and unstructured data that has a certain amount of byte-level similarity. The research resulted in several analysis and visualization tools and demonstrated that approximate hash-based matching has potential for helping investigators discover information based on data similarity.

As part of a completed PhD thesis project, Nguyen *et al.* (2010) studied the effectiveness of intrusion detection by correlation feature selection (CFS), with the purpose of automatically obtaining a feature set for network traffic without involving expert knowledge. The results successfully demonstrated the ability to remove redundant features while still keeping classification accuracies, leading to improved performance compared to other methods.

8.1.1.4 Forensic Soundness

Any method used for digital forensics must take forensic soundness into consideration. Computational forensics must ensure that evidence integrity and chain of custody are built in, thus reducing the probability of both unintentional mistakes and intentional evidence tampering. In a similar fashion to automated testing for software quality assurance, forensic tool testing should be performed at all levels (from source code validation to unit testing, functional verification, and last but not least software security testing).

It should be further noted that the research area of computational forensics is not limited to digital evidence but also encompasses computational methods for other forensic disciplines. This includes, but is not limited to:

- *Signal and image processing*: Transforming signals and images for better human or machine processing.
- *Computer vision*: The automatic recognition of objects (e.g., face recognition and similarity to other known images) in computer images or video.
- *Computer graphics and data visualization*: The synthesis of two-dimensional images or three-dimensional scenes from multidimensional data for better human understanding.
- *Statistical pattern recognition*: The classification into one or more classes based on abstract measurements, identifying whether a sample belongs to a known class and with what probability.
- *Machine learning*: A mathematical model is learned from examples.
- *Data mining*: Large volumes of data are processed to discover nuggets of information (e.g., the presence of association, number of clusters, and outliers).
- *Robotics*: Human movements are replicated by a machine, for example for the purpose of forensic reconstruction experiments.

8.2   Automation and Standardization

While automation was included as one of the objectives of computational forensics, the problem of automation and standardization deserves additional attention. As we have seen in other domains, automation is required to reduce manual efforts and to increase consistency and quality. Successful automation, however, is dependent on a standardization of, for example, data storage and exchange formats.

In Flaglien *et al.* (2011), we surveyed industry standards and research within digital evidence storage and exchange formats and identified a set of evaluation criteria. The comparative analysis documented a wide range of available formats, in particular for traditional computer forensics. An important observation was that no single industry standard could serve as a generic basis for automation. It is furthermore concluded that a format where data is represented in a standard and structured manner is a prerequisite to improve the efficiency and detection rates where evidence from multiple sources is used.

In recent research at the Netherlands Forensics Institute (NFI), a concept called *digital forensics as a service* (DFaaS) has been experimentally tested (van Baar, van Beek, & van Eijk, 2014). The research documents three years of experience with an approach for processing high data volumes through a standardized process with a high degree of automation. The method has been applied to hundreds of cases.

It should be noted that automation requires that software used as part of the processing of digital evidence must meet certain minimum standards in terms of forensic soundness. A lack of understanding of the weaknesses of individual tools and methods utilized in an automated forensic process could result in large, aggregated uncertainties in the conclusions. The *benchmarking* of forensic tools is thus a critical success factor, achieved through tool testing to identify strengths, weaknesses, and error rates.

8.3 Research Agenda

Digital forensics as a research field is constantly evolving with increasingly complex technologies. Consequently, there is a range of open questions that can be investigated. As an inspiration, we include the research agenda from the Testimon Forensics Group:

- *Large-scale investigations*: Research in the area of large-scale investigations; automatic searching through terabytes of electronic storage within closed systems and the Internet (including the dark net).
- *Internet and cloud forensics*: Research and development for the rapid acquisition, correlation, and analysis of Internet and cloud-related evidence. New tools and methods for evidence acquisition and analysis are constantly needed, with a corresponding need for educating law enforcement and practitioners in the field.
- *Embedded systems and the Internet of Things (IoT)*: Digital forensics involving a mobile device or other embedded systems often involves hardware analysis in addition to software analysis. Hardware is often based on proprietary technology and can be device specific, and forensic acquisition directly from hardware requires customized and well-tested methods. Both the problem of data acquisition and the decoding of binary data represent a continuously developing research area.
- *Cross-media search and data integration*: Technologies for cross-media search and data integration to access diverse sources of information, in particular data enrichment from Internet sources.
- *Encrypted evidence*: Algorithms for the analysis of encrypted evidence and cryptographic credentials.
- *Computational intelligence*: Design of advanced computing technologies to achieve more objective evidence analysis and final decision making by implementing computational intelligence.
- *Attribution and profiling*: Development of methods and tools for digital penetrator attribution and profiling, visualization of serious criminal relationships and associations, and geographical mapping of digital and physical evidence.

8.4 Summary

Digital forensics is a unique field of research, in that new information technology and new ways of exploiting information technology are rapidly introduced. Both researchers and practitioners regularly face new technical challenges, forcing them to develop their inquisitive and creative abilities. Any research within digital forensics should start with this in mind, bringing light to new problems in the field while keeping a keen eye on the principles of chain of custody and evidence integrity.

9

Educational Guide

Stefan Axelsson

Associate Professor, Norwegian University of Science and Technology (NTNU), Gjøvik, Norway

This book has grown out of the need for a textbook for our Introduction to Forensics course that has run for the last several years here at the Norwegian University of Science and Technology (NTNU).

9.1 Teacher's Guide

The course has run in two different versions, both for bachelor's degree students at the end of their studies and as an introductory master's-level course. These students have taken the course as part of engineering programs in information security (some with a specialization in digital forensics) or informatics/systems administration. The course has also been given in an experienced-based master's degree program (run by NTNU and the Norwegian Police University College in cooperation) with students already working in law enforcement with a few years of experience, typically already with a working background in digital forensics. The latter group has consisted of students from different countries, not only Norway, the most notable group (size-wise) being from Germany. The course has been continuously updated based on yearly course evaluations, and the course has generally been well received by the somewhat diverse groups, especially the foreign police students who praised it for being practical in nature without losing track of the overall, bigger picture.

The course follows a traditional format with lectures presenting the material in the book, followed by students choosing a research paper for a group presentation, and then an assignment/project performed in groups of 6–8 students. The idea is that the paper presentation should serve as an introduction to a subfield within digital forensics that the students then can examine in further detail in their project work. In this format, the results of the projects are presented both in class and in the form of a report. Additionally, the students are given lists of possible papers or project topics, but they are free to come up with their own topic if they already have a particular interest. The differences in the treatment of the presentations and projects allow differentiation between the diverse student groups, and this enables the use of the same course book for all topic subgroups. The addition of the project also allows

Digital Forensics, First Edition. Edited by André Årnes.
© 2018 John Wiley & Sons Ltd. Published 2018 by John Wiley & Sons Ltd.

differentiation between the engineering students and the active law enforcement students, as the difference in technological maturity is often substantial between these two groups (and, to be honest, within them as well), especially when it comes to software engineering and programming.

Following the introductory course in digital forensics, students can follow a second-level course in digital forensics that covers certain topics in more depth. Some of these topics are covered in this book or course, and others are not. Memory forensics, for example, is purposely left out of this introductory text. Memory forensics requires a much more detailed and in-depth understanding of, for example, computer internals, hardware and software architecture, and operating systems than we can assume in this course. As such, we only cover that it is possible to learn interesting things from memory dumps, not how and exactly what can be learned. The same is true for other subjects that are covered in other courses on computational forensics (e.g., the use of machine-learning and data-mining techniques to process large amounts of data for evidence of wrongdoing). Thus, this book provides an overview of the subject and gives an introduction to the techniques and challenges of the area, while leaving the deep technical details for other courses or for supplementary research articles (as is done in our introductory course).

Thus, our introductory course covers all the contents of the book, leaving none of the chapters out, in order to give the students a broad overview of the field. Of course, if it is appropriate for the audience, then some chapters may be skipped.

9.2 Student's Guide

For the students of digital forensics, it should be stressed that this book provides a solid foundation on which to build further knowledge in digital forensics in general, as well as in specific fields of digital forensics. Just a few years ago, the field was fairly broad, but already today, a few scant years later, the field has seen further specialization into areas as diverse as the analysis of digital images for signs of "doctoring" (i.e., tampering, or malicious modification), and the de-soldering and analysis of damaged memory chips in a smartphone. Both these tasks are of course highly specialized, and in order to be successful at them, one needs to acquire advanced specialized knowledge and skills that an introductory course cannot provide. So, in order to give a few pointers to the students interested in furthering their knowledge, this section lists a few sources and resources for further learning.

The additional sources can be grouped into a few different areas: journals that publish digital forensics research, organizations that hold conferences on research (including scientific journals) that is pertinent to digital forensics, tools and corpuses of test data, and organizations that provide and/or oversee professional training.

9.2.1 Journals

There are quite a few scientific journals in the field of digital forensics, including a few that are now dead. This alphabetical list presents a few of the longest running journals; they cover most aspects of the field between them, and run the gamut from the theoretical to the applied.

- *Digital Investigation*: One of the flagship journals on general, technological digital forensics. Publishes the conference proceedings of the Digital Forensics Research Workshop (DFRWS) series of conferences as special issues of the journal. Some articles are open access.
- *IEEE Transactions on Information Forensics and Security*: Published by the IEEE Signal Processing Society with support from other IEEE societies. As such, this journal presents many results in, for example, image processing, steganography, biometrics, and other topics, but it is not solely devoted to that task as it also contains more general articles in information security and the like.
- *International Journal of Digital Crime and Forensics*: A general journal in the field but with a slant toward image processing and digital watermarking.
- *Journal of Digital Forensics, Security and Law*: An open access journal (meaning that the articles are freely downloadable from the journal's website) focusing on legal, organizational, and procedural aspects of digital forensics. However, this journal is not solely devoted to such material, as it also has articles of a more technical nature.

9.2.2 Conferences and Organizations

There are a number of professional organizations that primarily promote research in digital forensics and organize scientific conferences in the area. As digital forensics is an area where the distance between research and practice is thankfully small, you will typically see a great deal of applied research with direct application to current problems in digital forensics. One also shouldn't forget that the area relies on academic research results and methods to put the "science" into "forensic science," and hence even as a practitioner one is expected to be able to explain the scientific underpinnings of one's results.

- *DFRWS*: "Bringing together researchers, industry, tool developers, academics, law enforcement, and military to tackle the challenges in digital forensic science." DFRWS started as a workshop on digital forensics in 2001. From that workshop, it grew into an organization that hosts an annual conference at various locations within the United States. Since then, an EU version of the conference has also been held annually. In 2005, the organization formally became a US nonprofit organization. DFRWS is one of the premiere venues for presenting and learning about the most recent advances in digital forensics; it has a decidedly technological slant. All DFRWS conference proceedings are published as open access, and all presented papers can be freely downloaded from the organization's home page.
- *IFIP WG 11.9* – The International Federation for Information Processing (IFIP) is a large organization in information, communications technologies, and sciences. It is recognized by the United Nations and represented by IT societies in 56 countries with a total membership of over half a million professionals, including 3500 scientists, more than 100 working groups, and 13 technical committees. Technical Committee 11 deals with security and privacy protection in information processing systems, and its Working Group 9 deals with forensics, hence the name *WG 11.9*. WG 11.9 has been organizing annual conferences on digital forensics since 2005, and it is rivaled only by DFRWS for its history. The results of each conference are published as an edited book.

- *IAPR* – "The International Association for Pattern Recognition (IAPR) is an international association of non-profit, scientific or professional organizations (being national, multi-national, or international in scope) concerned with pattern recognition, computer vision, and image processing in a broad sense." IAPR holds several conferences that, even though they are not solely devoted to digital forensics (like the two previous bodies), publish many results on digital forensics, such as image recognition and other "big data" approaches that are becoming ever more important.

9.2.3 Professional and Training Organizations

It should be noted that all of these organizations are American and based in the United States, though some hold courses and provide certification internationally (notably, IACIS and SANS).

Before one embarks on a (potentially costly) road to certification, it's imperative to check whether that certification holds any weight in the organization or country with which one is interested in working. Many law enforcement organizations in the United States, for example, have one or several (but not all) of the certifications listed below as requirements for employment (or at least they are considered meritorious), but the value of these certifications varies internationally, as many countries and organizations have their own local requirements and courses. In the corporate arena, certifications can sometimes help to open doors that were otherwise closed. However, since there are so many certifications in different fields, not all of them are accredited, or valued highly; some are even fake. So again, it pays to check with professionals in the industry to learn what is worthwhile. Note also that the popularity of certain certifications waxes and wanes as the field develops and changes. Therefore, many of them require recertification periodically to remain valid.

Even though we don't mention it here, many of the tool providers also offer certification on their respective tools. In the case of industry standard tools, such training should not be overlooked.

- *SANS*: SANS is a large organization that performs training and certification in many areas of computer security, not only forensics but also network security, malware analysis, and related areas that are of interest to the forensic practitioner. SANS provides training for several certifications through Global Information Assurance Certification (GIAC), including: GIAC Certified Forensic Analyst (GCFA), GIAC Certified Forensic Examiner (GCFE), GIAC Network Forensic Analyst (GNFA), and GIAC Advanced Smartphone Forensics (GASF). These require the applicant to sit for specific supervised exams and perform to a set standard.
- *International Association of Computer Investigative Specialists (IACIS)*: IACIS provides training leading to certifications – Certified Forensic Computer Examiner (CFCE) and Certified Advanced Windows Forensic Examiner (CAWFE) – with both peer review and certification testing (including a background check). These certifications are often required by law enforcement organizations in various parts of the world as a prerequisite for presenting digital forensic results in court. IACIS is accredited by the Forensic Specialties Accreditation Board, an organization that accredits professional bodies that certify forensic scientists in all forensic specialties, not only in digital or computer forensics.

- *Information Assurance Certification Review Board (IACRB)*: IACRB provides a number of computer security certifications, including the "certified computer forensic examiner" that is relevant for the digital forensics field. This is a two-part exam with both a proctored written test and a take-home practical part that has to be presented in the form of a report that could be presented to a court.
- *European Network of Forensic Science Institutes (ENFSI)*: ENFSI is an organization that harbors all fields of forensics. They have an active group on digital and computer forensics that runs scientific meetings and other professional activities, including defining and publishing standards of best practice.

9.2.4 Tools

There are several forensics tools with varying quality and capabilities available both commercial and freely. We'll list a few of the freely available ones here, as the commercial ones can be very costly and hence outside the reach of a student (but always check for the possibility of a student license).

The Open Source Digital Forensics Conference (run annually since 2010) is a source of information about open source forensics tools. ForensicsWiki.org is worth a visit; it is a good source of information about tools and corpuses.

- *Disk analysis tools*: No discussion of open source forensics tools would be complete without the Sleuth Kit, a command line tool that is part of Autopsy [a graphical user interface (GUI) that integrates the Sleuth Kit with other tools].
- *Memory analysis tools*: For memory analysis, there are two competing tools, Volatility and Rekall (which started as a fork of Volatility). We would need a whole book to give them justice, and indeed whole books have been written on the subject. For all your memory forensics needs, if these two can't do it, then it probably cannot be done. Rekall is also integrated into GRR, a remote incidence response framework that also leverages Sleuth Kit to make remote live forensics of, for example, large server farms tenable. It is worth a look in itself.
- *Network analysis tools*: When it comes to network analysis tools, Wireshark (formerly Ethereal) stands out. It enables both sniffing and saving of network data, as well as offline analysis of capture files. It provides the analyst with a whole slew of higher level network protocol parsers to extract and recover a variety of data, such as the sound from an IP–telephony conversation and the like. Note that with Wireshark being so popular, there are exploits specifically targeting it, to crash or take over the computer it runs on, so one needs to be aware of such risks before deploying it in an untrusted network.

9.2.5 Corpuses

There are many different corpuses for different uses. We will only mention a few here that are noteworthy.

- *Disk images*: Simson Garfinkel collected "The real data corpus" between 1998 and 2006. It is one of the largest forensic corpuses in existence that contains files of every type, size, and content. It serves as a realistic representation of what might be found on a typical computer or device of the era.

- *Memory images*: The volatility project has several memory images that are openly available.
- *Network traces*: The Wireshark project has a website with many capture files from networks available for download.

9.3 Summary

As the interested reader already has noticed, digital forensics is a rapidly growing field that has already reached a considerable size. Only a short few years ago, the sources of knowledge were few and far between. Today there are many more, and standards and requirements are improving. With the sources given in this chapter, the ambitious reader should be well prepared to go further, be able to gain more in-depth insight into the topics covered in this book, and also be able to find and identify areas that we have not been able to cover. The field does not stand still, however, but keeps moving at a rapid pace. Keeping abreast of current developments takes time and dedication. We wish you the best of luck in your future endeavors.

References

3rd Generation Partnership Program (3GPP). (2015). *3GPP TS 23.040: Digital Cellular Telecommunications System (Phase 2+); Universal Mobile Telecommunications System (UMTS); Technical Realization of the Short Message Service (SMS)*. Technical Specification, ETSI. Sophia Antipolis, France: 3GPP.

Aitken, C., & Taroni, F. (2004). *Statistics and the Evaluation of Evidence for Forensic Scientists*, 2nd ed. Hoboken, NJ: Wiley.

Alendal, G., Kison, C., & modg. (2015, October 1). *Got HW Crypto? On the (In)security of a Self-Encrypting Drive Series*. Retrieved June 29, 2016, from https://eprint.iacr.org/2015/1002.pdf

Altheide, C., & Harlan, C. (2011). *Digital Forensics with Open Source Tools*. Rockland, MA: Syngress, Elsevier.

Alva, A., & Endicott-Popovsky, B. (2012). Digital Evidence Education in Schools of Law. *Journal of Digital Forensics*, **7** (2). Retrieved February 17, 2017, from http://ojs.jdfsl.org/index.php/jdfsl/article/view/120/5

Årnes, A., Haas, P., Vigna, G., & Kemmerer, R. A. (2007). Using a Virtual Security Testbed for Digital Forensic Reconstruction. *Journal in Computer Virology*, 2007 (2/4).

Australian Police to Auction 13m in Confiscated Bitcoin. (2016, May 31). *The Guardian*. Retrieved February 17, 2017, from https://www.theguardian.com/technology/2016/may/31/australian-police-to-auction-13m-in-confiscated-bitcoins

Aviv, A. J., Gibson, K., Mossop, E., Blaze, M., & Smith, J. M. (2010). Smudge Attacks on Smartphone Touch Screens. Paper presented to the 4th USENIX Workshop on Offensive Technologies.

Ballou, S. (2013). *NISTIR 7928: The Biological Evidence Preservation Handbook: Best Practices for Evidence Handlers*. Gaithersburg, MD: National Institute of Standards and Technology.

Bjelland, P. C., Franke, K., & Årnes, A. (2014). Practical Use of Approximate Hash Based Matching in Digital Investigations. *Digital Investigation*, **11**, 18–26.

Bommisety, S., Tamma, R., & Mahalik, H. (2014). *Practical Mobile Forensics*. Birmingham, UK: Packt.

Breeuwsma, M. (2006). Forensic Imaging of Embedded Systems Using JTAG (Boundary-Scan). *Digital Investigation*, **3**, 32–42.

Brenner, S. W., Carrier, B., & Henninger, J. (2004). *The Trojan Horse Defense in Cybercrime Cases*. Santa Clara, CA: Santa Clara High Tech.

Brothers, S. (2008). How Cell Phone "Forensic" Tools Actually Work (Proposed Leveling). Paper presented at Mobile Forensics World.

Digital Forensics, First Edition. Edited by André Årnes.

Carrier, B. (2010). *File System Forensic Analysis*, 9th ed. Reading, MA: Addison-Wesley.

Carrier, B., & Spafford, E. H. (2003). Getting physical with the digital investigation process. *International Journal of Digital Evidence*, **2** (2), 1–20.

Carrier, B. D., & Spafford, E. H. (2004a, August 11–13). An event-based digital forensics investigation process. Paper presented at the Digital Forensics Research Workshop (DFRWS), Baltimore, MD.

Carrier, B. D., & Spafford, E. H. (2004b, November). Defining event reconstruction of a digital crime scene. *Journal of Forensic Sciences*, **49** (6), 1291–1298.

Carrier, B. D., & Spafford, E. H. (2004c). *Defining Searches of Digital Crime Scenes*. Technical Report. West Lafayette, IN: Purdue University, CERIAS.

Carvey, H. (2016). *Windows Registry Forensics: Advanced Digital Forensic Analysis of the Windows Registry*, 2nd ed. Rockland, MA: Syngress.

Casey, E. (2002). Error, Uncertainty and Loss in Digital Forensics. *International Journal of Digital Evidence*, **1** (2).

Chisum, J. W., & Turvey, B. E. (2000). Evidence Dynamics: Locard's Exchange Principle & Crime Reconstruction. *Journal of Behavioral Profiling*, **1** (1).

Chisum, J. W., & Turvey, B. E. (2008). *Crime Reconstruction*. New York: Academic Press.

Ciardhuáin, S. O. (2004, Summer). An Extended Model of Cybercrime Investigation. *International Journal of Digital Evidence*, **3** (1), 1–22.

Council of Europe. (2001). *Explanatory Report to the Cybercrime Convention*. Strasbourg: Council of Europe.

Cybercrime Convention Committee (T-CY). (2014). Guidance Notes. In *Guidance Notes Adopted by the 8th, 9th and 12th Plenary of the T-CY*. Strasbourg: T-CY.

Davidoff, S., & Ham, J. (2012). *Network Forensics, Tracking Hackers through Cyberspace*. Reading, MA: Addison-Wesley.

Digital Forensics Research Workshop. (2001). *A Road Map for Digital Forensic Research*. Retrieved September 1, 2016, from https://dfrws.org/sites/default/files/session-files/a_road_map_for_digital_forensic_research.pdf

DigitalNinja. (2007, April 5). *Fuzzy Clarity: Using Fuzzy Hashing Techniques to Identify Malicious Code*. Shadowserver. Retrieved April 14, 2014, from http://www.shadowserver.org/wiki/uploads/Information/FuzzyHashing.pdf

Dilijonaite, A. (2014). Enterprise Digital Forensics Readiness. M.Sc. thesis, Gjøvik University College, Gjøvik, Norway.

dtSearch. (2015, April 22). *Indexed vs Unindexed Searching*. Retrieved February 17, 2017, from http://www.dtsearch.com/IndexedVsUnindexedSearching.pdf

Ekfeldt, J. (2016). Om Informationstekniskt Bevis. PhD dissertation, Stockholm University, Sweden.

Endicott-Popovsky, B., Frincke, D. A., & Taylor, C. A. (2007). A Theoretical Framework for Organizational Network Forensic Readiness. *Journal of Computers*, **2** (3), 1–11.

Endicott-Popovsky, B., & Horowitz, D. (2012, March). Unintended Consequences: Digital Evidence in Our Legal System. *IEEE Security and Privacy*, **10** (2), 80–83.

European Court of Human Rights Research Division. (2015). *Internet: Case-Law of the European Court of Human Rights*. Strasbourg: European Court of Human Rights.

European Network of Forensic Science Institutes (ENFSI). (2015). *Best Practice Manual for the Forensic Examination of Digital Technology*. ENFSI-BPM-FIT-01. Retrieved February 17, 2017, from http://enfsi.eu/docfile/best-practice-manual-for-the-forensic-examination-of-digital-technology/

European Telecommunications Standards Institute (ETSI). (1996). *Digital Cellular Telecommunications System (Phase 2+): AT Command Set for GSM Mobile Equipment (ME) (GSM 07.07)*, version 5.0.0. Sophia Antipolis, France: ETSI.

Europol. (2014). *The Internet Organised Crime Threat Assessment (IOCTA)* The Hague: Europol.

Europol. (2015). *The Internet Organised Crime Threat Assessment (IOCTA)* The Hague: Europol.

Farmer, D., & Venema, W. (2005). *Forensic Discovery*. Reading, MA: Addison Wesley Professional.

Flaglien, A., Franke, K., & Årnes, A. (2011). Identifying Malware Using Cross-Evidence Correlation. In *Advances in Digital Forensics VII, 7th IFIP WG 11.9 International Conference on Digital Forensics* (pp. 169–182). Berlin: Springer Verlag.

Flaglien, A. O., Mallasvik, A., Mustorp, M., & Årnes, A. (2011). *Storage and Exchange Formats for Digital Evidence*. Amsterdam: Elsevier.

Fortunato, S. (2010). Community Detection in Graphs. *Physics Reports*, **486** (2010), 75–174.

Fossen, E. A., & Årnes, A. (2005). Forensic Geolocation of Internet Addresses Using Network Measurements. Paper presented at Nordsec 2005, 10th Nordic Workshop on Secure IT-Systems.

Franke, K., & Srihari, S. N. (2007). Computational Forensics: Towards Hybrid-Intelligent Crime Investigation. In *Third International Symposium on Information Assurance and Security*. Washington, DC: IEEE Computer Society.

Franke, K., & Srihari, S. N. (2008). Computational Forensics: An Overview. In S. N. Srihari& K. Franke, *Computational Forensics*. Berlin: Springer.

Garfinkel, S. L. (2010). Digital Forensics Research: The Next 10 Years. In *The Proceedings of the Tenth Annual DFRWS Conference*. Amsterdam: Elsevier.

Garfinkel, S. L. (2013). Digital Media Triage with Bulk Data Analysis. *Computers & Security*, **32**, 56–72.

Garijo, J. M. (2014). *Mac OS X Forensics*. London: Royal Holloway, University of London.

Giampaolo, D. (1999). *Practical File System Design with the Be File System*. San Francisco: Morgan Kaufmann.

Graves, M. W. (2014). *Digital Archaeology – The Art and Science of Digital Forensics*. Reading, MA: Addison-Wesley.

Grobler, T., & Louwrens, B. (2007). Digital Forensic Readiness as a Component of Information Security Best Practice. In *New Approaches for Security, Privacy and Trust in Complex Environments, Proceedings of the IFIP TC-11 22nd* (pp. 13–24). Boston: Springer.

Grobler, T., Louwrens, B., & von Solms, S. H. (2010). A Framework to Guide the Implementation of Proactive Digital Forensics in Organisations. In *2010 International Conference on Availability, Reliability and Security* (pp. 687–690). Washington, DC: IEEE Computer Society.

Gruber, T. R. (1993). A Translation Approach to Portable Ontology Specifications. *Knowledge Acquisition*, **5** (2), 199–220.

Gudmundsdottir, H. L. (2015). *Clarifying Broad Hacking Statutes*. Aalborg, Denmark: Aalborg University.

Guo, Y., Slay, J., & Beckett, J. (2009). Validation and Verification of Computer Forensic Software Tools. *Digital Investigation*, 12–22.

Hale-Ligh, M., Case, A., Levy, J., & Walters, A. (2014). *The Art of Memory Forensics*. Hoboken, NJ: John Wiley & Sons.

Hamm, J. (2012). *Carve for Records, Not Files*. Bethesda, MD: SANS. Retrieved April 5, 2014, from https://digital-forensics.sans.org/summit-archives/2012/carve-for-record-not-files.pdf

Hamm, J., & Ballenthin, W. (2012, September 18). *FireEye Threat Research*. Incident Response with NTFS INDX Buffers. Retrieved April 4, 2015, from https://www.fireeye.com/blog/threat-research/2012/09/striking-gold-incident-response-ntfs-indx-buffers-part-1.html

Harrill, D. C., & Mislan, R. P. (2007). A Small Scale Digital Device Forensics Ontology. *Small Scale Digital Device Forensics Journal*, **17**, 341.

Harris, D., O'Boyle, M., & Warbrick, C. (2009). *Law of the European Convention on Human Rights*. Oxford: Oxford University Press.

Hosmer, C. (2002). Proving the Integrity of Digital Evidence with Time. *International Journal of Digital Evidence*, **1** (1).

Hubbart, P. A. (2005). *Making Sense of Search and Seizure Law*. Durham, NC: Carolina Academic Press.

IETF. (1999). *RFC2616 – Hypertext Transfer Protocol – HTTP/1.1*. Fremont, CA: IETF. Retrieved September 18, 2016, from https://www.ietf.org/rfc/rfc2616.txt

International Laboratory Accreditation Cooperation (ILAC). (2002). *ILAC-G19:2002, Guidelines for Forensic Science Laboratories*. ILAC-G19:2002. Silverwater, Australia: ILAC.

International Organization on Computer Evidence (IOCE). (2002). *Guidelines for Best Practice in the Forensic Examination of Digital Technology*. IOCE.

Internet Live Stats. (2016, August 3). *Internet Live Stats*. Retrieved August 3, 2016, from www.internetlivestats.com/internet-users/

ISO. (2008). *ISO 9001:2008 Quality Management Systems – Requirements*. ISO 9001:2008.

ISO/IEC. (2005). *ISO/IEC 17025. 2005. General Requirements for the Competence of Testing and Calibration Laboratories*. ISO/IEC 17025.

ISO/IEC. (2013). *ISO/IEC 27001:2013. 2013. Information Technology – Security Techniques – Information Security Management Systems – Requirements*. ISO/IEC 27001:2013.

ISO/IEC. (2008). *ISO/IEC 27005. 2008. Information Technology – Security Techniques – Information Security Risk Management*. ISO/IEC 27005.

ISO/IEC. (2012). *ISO/IEC 27037. 2012 . Information Technology – Security Techniques – Guidelines for Identification, Collection, Acquisition and Preservation of Digital Evidence*. ISO/IEC 27037.

ISO/IEC. (2015a). *ISO/IEC 27041:2015, Information Technology – Security Techniques – Guidance on Assuring Suitability and Adequacy of Incident Investigative Method*. ISO/IEC 27041:2015.

ISO/IEC. (2015b). *ISO/IEC 27042:2015 Information Technology – Security Techniques – Guidelines for the Analysis and Interpretation of Digital Evidence*. ISO/IEC 27042:2015.

ISO/IEC. (2004). *ISO/IEC Guide 2:2004 Standardization and Related Activities – General Vocabulary*. ISO/IEC Guide 2:2004.

Johnson, L. (2013). *Computer Incident Response and Forensics Team Management*. Rockland, MA: Syngress.

Kent, K., Chevalier, S., Grance, T., & Dang, H. (2006). *Guide to Integrating Forensics into Incident Response*. Special Publication 800-86. Gaithersburg, MD: National Institute of

Standards and Technology, Computer Security Division Information Technology Laboratory.

Kent, K., Chevalier, S., Grance, T., & Dang, H. (2005). *Guide to Integrating Forensic Techniques into Incident Response*. Gaithersburg, MD: National Institute of Standards and Technology. Retrieved August 11, 2015, from http://csrc.nist.gov/publications/nistpubs/800-86/SP800-86.pdf

Kerr, O. S. (2013). *Computer Crime Law*. St. Paul, MN: West Academic.

Kerr, O. S. (2015, May 3). Norms of Computer Trespass. *Columbia Law Review*, **116** (1143).

Klaver, C. (2010). Windows Mobile Advanced Forensics. *Digital Investigation*, **6**, 147–167.

Knijff, R. M. (2010). Embedded Systems Analysis. In E. Casey (Ed.), *Handbook of Digital Forensics and Investigation*. New York: Academic Press.

Knuth, D. (1998). *The Art of Computer Programming, vol. 3: Sorting and Searching*, 2nd ed. Reading, MA: Addison Wesley.

Koehn, P. E. (2007). Moses: Open Source Toolkit for Statistical Machine Translation. In *Proceedings of the 45th Annual Meeting of the ACL on Interactive Poster and Demonstration Sessions*. Stroudsburg, PA: Association for Computational Linguistics.

Kubasiak, R., & Morrissey, S. (2008). *Max OS X, iPod, and iPhone Forensic Analysis DVD Toolkit*. Rockland, MA: Syngress.

Laliberte, S., & Gupta, A. (2004). *The Role of Computer Forensics in Stopping Executive Fraud*. Retrieved February 17, 2017, from http://www.informit.com/articles/article.aspx?p=336258&seqNum=3

Lee, R. (2010, 04 12). *Windows 7 MFT Entry Timestamp Properties*. Bethesda, MD: SANS. Retrieved April 4, 2015, from https://digital-forensics.sans.org/blog/2010/04/12/windows-7-mft-entry-timestamp-properties/

Lock and Code Pty Ltd. (2014). *Computer Forensic Examiner – Quick Reference Guide*. South Melbourne, Australia: Lock and Code, Global Digital Investigation Solutions. Retrieved April 4, 2015, from https://lockandcode.com

Luttgens, J. T., Pepe, M., & Mandia, K. (2014). *Incident Response and Computer Forensics*, 3rd ed. New York: McGraw-Hill.

Maartmann-Moe, C., Thorkildsen, S. E., & Årnes, A. (2009). The Persistence of Memory: Forensic Identification and Extraction of Cryptographic Keys. In *Proceedings of the Ninth Annual DFRWS Conference*. Amsterdam: Elsevier.

Manning, C. (2012, June 1). *How YAFFS Works*. Cambridge: YAFFS. Retrieved September 12, 2015, from http://www.yaffs.net/documents/how-yaffs-works

Mead, S. (2015). *The Impact of RAID on Disk Imaging*. Gaithersburg, MD: National Institute of Standards and Technology. Retrieved September 20, 2015, from http://nvlpubs.nist.gov/nistpubs/ir/2005/ir7276.pdf

Mena, J. (2002). *Investigative Data Mining for Security and Criminal Detection*. Newton, MA: Butterworth Heinemann.

Microsoft. (2013). *A History of Windows*. Retrieved September 27, 2015, from http://windows.microsoft.com/en-us/windows/history#T1=era0

Microsoft. (2015). *Registry*. Microsoft Developers Network. Retrieved April 4, 2015, from https://msdn.microsoft.com/en-us/library/windows/desktop/ms724871(v=vs.85).aspx

Namestnikov, Y. (2009, July 22). *The Economics of Botnets*. Moscow: Securelist, Kaspersky Lab. Retrieved September 30, 2016, from https://securelist.com/large-slider/36257/the-economics-of-botnets/

National Forensic Science Technology Center (NFSTC). (2009). *A Simplified Guide to Digital Evidence.* Retrieved February 17, 2017, from http://www.forensicsciencesimplified.org/digital/DigitalEvidence.pdf

Nelson, B., Phillips, A., & Stewart, C. (2015). *Guide to Computer Forensics and Investigations: Processing Digital Evidence,* 5th ed. Cengage Learning.

NetMarketShare. (2015). *Desktop Operating System Market Share.* Retrieved September 27, 2015, from https://www.netmarketshare.com/operating-system-market-share.aspx?qprid=10&qpcustomd=0

Nguyen, H., Franke, K., & Petrovic, S. (2010). Improving Effectiveness of Intrustion Detection by Correlation Feature Selection. In *2010 International Conference on Availability, Reliability and Security (ARES).* Washington, DC: IEEE Computer Society.

National Institute of Standards and Technology (NIST). (2014, September 18). *Disk Imaging.* Gaithersburg, MD: National Institute of Standards and Technology. Retrieved August 11, 2015, from http://www.cftt.nist.gov/disk_imaging.htm

National Institute of Standards and Technology (NIST). (2006). *Guide to Integrating Forensic Techniques into Incident Response.* NIST SP800-86. Gaithersburg, MD: National Institute of Standards and Technology.

National Institute of Standards and Technology (NIST). (2008). *NIST Special Publication 800-64 Revision 2 – Security Considerations in the System Development Life Cycle.* Gaithersburg, MD: National Institute of Standards and Technology, Information Security.

Page, L., Brin, S., Motwani, R., & Winograd, T. (1999). *The PageRank Citation Ranking: Bringing Order to the Web.* Technical Report. Stanford, CA: InfoLab, Stanford University.

Palmer, G. (2001). A Road Map for Digital Forensic Research. Technical Report DTR-T001-01. In *Digital Forensics Workshop (DFRWS).* Retrieved February 17, 2017, from https://www.dfrws.org/sites/default/files/session-files/a_road_map_for_digital_forensic_research.pdf

Parker, K. P. (2003). *The Boundary-Scan Handbook,* 3rd ed. Alphen aan den Rijn, the Netherlands: Kluwer Academic.

Proctor, P. E. (2014). *How Sony Worked with the FBI to Address a Targeted Attack.* Stamford, CT: Gartner.

Reith, M., Carr, C., & Gunsch, G. (2002). An Examination of Digital Forensics Models. *International Journal of Digital Evidence,* **1** (3).

Richard, G., & Roussev, V. (2005, August 17–19). Scalpel: A Frugal, High-Performance File Carver. In *Proceedings of the 2005 Digital Forensics Research Workshop* (pp. 1–10).

Roussev, V., Quates, C., & Martell, R. (2013, September). Real-Time Digital Forensics and Triage. *Digital Investigations,* **10** (2), 158–167.

Rowlingson, R. (2004, Winter). A Ten Step Process for Forensic Readiness. *International Journal of Digital Evidence,* **2** (3).

Russon, R. (2015). *NTFS.* Retrieved April 15, 2015, from https://flatcap.org/linux-ntfs/ntfs/index.html

Saferstein, R. (2007). *Criminalistics: An Introduction to Forensic Science.* Saddle River, NJ,: Pearson Prentice Hall.

Sammons, J. (2012). *The Basics of Digital Forensics.* Amsterdam: Elsevier.

Sandvik, R. A. (2013, December 18). *Harvard Student Receives F for Tor Failure While Sending "Anonymous" Bomb Threat.* Forbes.com. Retrieved September 18, 2016, from http://www.forbes.com/sites/runasandvik/2013/12/18/harvard-student-receives-f-for-tor-failure-while-sending-anonymous-bomb-threat/#66c5431069f0

SANS. (2012, 09 12). *Best Practices in Digital Evidence Collection.* Bethesda, MD: SANS. Retrieved August 11, 2015, from https://digital-forensics.sans.org/blog/2009/09/12/best-practices-in-digital-evidence-collection/

Schneier, B. (2004). Cryptanalysis of MD5 and SHA: Time for a New Standard. *Computerworld.* Retrieved February 17, 2017, from http://www.computerworld.com/article/2566208/security0/opinion–cryptanalysis-of-md5-and-sha–time-for-a-new-standard.html

Scientific Working Group on Digital Evidence (SWGDE). (2013). *SWGDE Establishing Confidence in Digital Forensics by Error Mitigation Analysis.* Retrieved February 17, 2017, from https://www.swgde.org/documents/Current%20Documents/SWGDE%20Establishing%20Confidence%20in%20Digital%20Forensic%20Results%20by%20Error%20Mitigation%20Analysis

Scott, J. (2012). *Social Network Analysis.* Thousand Oaks, CA: Sage.

Shalaginov, A., & Franke, K. (2015). Automated Generation of Fuzzy Rules from Large-Scale Network Traffic Analysis in Digital Forensics Investigations. In *IEEE 7th International Conference on Soft Computing and Pattern Recognition (SoCPaR).* Piscataway, NJ: IEEE Xplore.

Sikorski, M., & Honig, A. (2012). *Practical Malware Analysis: The Hands-On Guide to Dissecting Malicious Software.* San Francisco: No Starch Press.

SQLite. (2016). *SQLite Home Page.* Retrieved June 26, 2016, from https://www.sqlite.org

Stelfox, P. (2013). *Criminal Investigation: An Introduction to Principles and Practice.* New York: Routledge.

Sunde, I. M. (2010). Automatisert Inndragning [Confiscation by Automation]. PhD dissertation, University of Oslo, Law Faculty, Norway.

Sunde, I. M. (2016). A New Thing under the Sun? Crime in the Digitized Society. In I. A. Kinnunen (Ed.), *NSfK's 58. Research Seminar: New Challenges in Criminology: Can Old Theories Be Used to Explain or Understand New Crimes?* (pp. 60–79). Borgarnes, Iceland: Scandinavian Research Council for Criminology.

Symantec. (2010, 11 02). *Maintaining System Integrity During Forensics.* Mountain View, CA: Symantec. Retrieved August 11, 2015, from http://www.symantec.com/connect/articles/maintaining-system-integrity-during-forensics

Tan, J. (2001). *Forensic Readiness.* Cambridge, MA: @stake. Retrieved from http://citeseerx.ist.psu.edu/viewdoc/download?doi=10.1.1.480.6094&rep=rep1&type=pdf

Tilbury, C. (2011, July 5). *Computer Forensic Artifacts: Windows 7 Shellbags.* Bethesda, MD: SANS. Retrieved April 4, 2015, from https://digital-forensics.sans.org/blog/2011/07/05/shellbags

Tilstone, W. J., Hastrup, M. L., & Hald, C. (2013). *Fischer's Techniques of Crime Scene Investigation.* Boca Raton, FL: CRC Press, Taylor and Francis Group.

Turvey, B. E. (2008). *Criminal Profiling,* 3rd ed. Amsterdam: Elsevier Academic.

UK, Government. (2014). *Codes of Practice and Conduct for Forensic Science Providers and Practitioners in the Criminal Justice System.* London: UK Government. Retrieved February 17, 2017, from https://www.gov.uk/government/publications/forensic-science-providers-codes-of-practice-and-conduct-2014

UN Office on Drugs and Crime (UNODC). (2013). *Comprehensive Study on Cybercrime.* Draft. New York: UNODC.

US Department of Justice (USDOJ. (2014, January 28). *Cyber Criminal Pleads Guilty to Developing and Distributing Notorious Spyeye Malware.* Washington, DC: USDOJ. Retrieved August 4, 2016, from https://www.justice.gov/opa/pr/cyber-criminal-pleads-guilty-developing-and-distributing-notorious-spyeye-malware

US Department of Justice (USDOJ). (2016, April 20). *Two Major International Hackers Who Developed the "SpyEye" Malware Get over 24 Years Combined in Federal Prison.* Washington, DC: USDOJ. Retrieved August 4, 2016, from https://www.justice.gov/usao-ndga/pr/two-major-international-hackers-who-developed-spyeye-malware-get-over-24-years-combined

van Baar, R., van Beek, H., & van Eijk, E. (2014). Digital Forensics as a Service: A Game Changer. In *Proceedings of the First Annual DFRWS Europe* (pp. 54–62). Amsterdam: Elsevier.

Watson, D., & Jones, A. (2013). *Digital Forensics Processing and Procedures: Meeting the requirements of ISO 17020, ISO 17025, ISO 27001 and Best Practice Requirements.* Rockland, MA: Syngress.

Wikipedia. (2015, September 15). *Hard Disk Drive Interfaces.* Retrieved September 20, 2015, from https://en.wikipedia.org/wiki/Hard_disk_drive_interface

Yusoff, Y., Ismail, R., & Hassan, Z. (2011). Common Phases of Computer Forensics Investigation. *International Journal of Computer Science & Information Technology (IJCSIT)*, **3** (3).

Index

Printed and bound by CPI Group (UK) Ltd, Croydon, CR0 4YY

16/04/2025